Copyright © 2021 by Peter Champion -All

No part of this publication may be reproduced, distributed, or transmitted in any form or by any means, including photocopying, recording, or other electronic or mechanical methods, without the prior written permission of the publisher, except in the case of brief quotations embodied in reviews and certain other non-commercial uses permitted by copyright law.

This Book is provided with the sole purpose of providing relevant information on a specific topic for which every reasonable effort has been made to ensure that it is both accurate and reasonable. Nevertheless, by purchasing this Book you consent to the fact that the author, as well as the publisher, are in no way experts on the topics contained herein, regardless of any claims as such that may be made within. It is recommended that you always consult a professional prior to undertaking any of the advice or techniques discussed within.This is a legally binding declaration that is considered both valid and fair by both the Committee of Publishers Association and the American Bar Association and should be considered as legally binding within the United States.

CONTENTS

BREAKFAST RECIPES 8
   1. Glazed Strawberry Toast 8
   2. Ricotta & Chorizo Corn Frittata 8
   3. Peanut Butter & Honey Porridge 8
   4. Quick Paprika Eggs 8
   5. Simple Apple Crisp 8
   6. Cinnamon French Toasts 8
   7. Blackberries Bowls 9
   8. Apple-cinnamon Empanadas 9
   9. Zucchini And Carrot Pudding 9
   10. Fresh Kale & Cottage Omelet 9
   11. Grilled Cheese Sandwich 10
   12. Creamy Mushroom And Spinach Omelet .. 10
   13. Zucchini Omelet 10
   14. Creamy Bacon & Egg Wraps With Spicy Salsa 10
   15. Mushroom Sausage Breakfast Bake 11
   16. Mixed Berry Dutch Baby Pancake 11
   17. Peppered Maple Bacon Knots 11
   18. Banana Oat Muffins 11
   19. Whole Wheat Carrot Bread 12
   20. Spicy Apple Turnovers 12
   21. Quick Mac & Cheese 12
   22. Enchiladas 4 Breakfast 12
   23. Rarebit Air-fried Egg 13
   24. Strawberry Cheesecake Pastries 13
   25. Avocado And Zucchini Mix 13
   26. Chocolate Banana Bread 14
   27. Garlic And Cheese Bread Rolls 14
   28. Fried Cheese Grits 14
   29. Apple Fritter Loaf 14
   30. Mini Brown Rice Quiches 15
   31. Apricot Scones With Almonds 15
   32. Sausage Omelet 15
   33. Tomatta Spinacha Frittata 16
   34. French Toast Delight 16
   35. Tator Tots Casserole 16
   36. Avocado And Tomato Egg Rolls 16
   37. Porridge With Honey & Peanut Butter 17
   38. Easy Egg Bites 17
   39. Nutritious Cinnamon Oat Muffins 17
   40. Healthy Oatmeal Bars 17
   41. Tomato Oatmeal 18
   42. Cheesy Spring Chicken Wraps 18
   43. Spinach Zucchini Egg Muffins 18
   44. Breakfast Potatoes 18
   45. Cabbage And Mushroom Spring Rolls 19
   46. Brioche Breakfast Pudding 19
   47. Peppery Sausage & Parsley Patties 19
   48. Cheesy Bacon And Egg Wraps 20
   49. Almond & Cinnamon Berry Oat Bars 20
   50. Moist Orange Bread Loaf 20
   51. Mushroom & Pepperoncini Omelet 20
   52. Apricot & Almond Scones 21
   53. Basil Dill Egg Muffins 21
   54. Sweet Potato Chickpeas Hash 21
   55. Egg & Bacon Wraps With Salsa 21
   56. Fried Churros With Cinnamon 21
   57. Breakfast Oatmeal Cake 22
   58. Olives, Kale, And Pecorino Baked Eggs 22
   59. Montreal Steak And Seeds Burgers 22
   60. Whole-wheat Blueberry Scones 23
   61. Giant Strawberry Pancake 23
   62. Feta & Spinach Omelet With Mushrooms . 23
   63. Herby Mushrooms With Vermouth 23
   64. Tomato, Basil & Mozzarella Breakfast 23
   65. Cinnamon & Vanilla Toast 24
   66. Raspberries Oatmeal 24
   67. Vanilla Brownies With White Chocolate & Walnuts 24
   68. Delicious Broccoli Quiche 24

LUNCH RECIPES 25
   69. Easy Italian Meatballs 25
   70. Roasted Grape And Goat Cheese Crostinis 25
   71. Air Fried Sausages 25
   72. Lobster Tails 25
   73. Butter Fish With Sake And Miso 26
   74. Lemon Chicken Breasts 26
   75. Turkey And Broccoli Stew 26
   76. Glazed Lamb Chops 26
   77. Turmeric Mushroom(3) 27
   78. Chicken And Celery Stew 27
   79. Parmesan-crusted Pork Loin 27
   80. Herbed Duck Legs 27
   81. Seven-layer Tostadas 27
   82. Beef Steaks With Beans 28
   83. Sweet Potato Chips 28
   84. Spanish Chicken Bake 28
   85. Lemon Pepper Turkey 28
   86. Lime And Mustard Marinated Chicken 29
   87. Turkey Legs 29
   88. Mushroom Meatloaf 29
   89. Green Bean Casserole(2) 29
   90. Persimmon Toast With Sour Cream & Cinnamon 30
   91. Chicken Parmesan 30
   92. Boneless Air Fryer Turkey Breasts 30
   93. Chicken & Rice Casserole 30
   94. Spice-roasted Almonds 31
   95. Chili Chicken Sliders 31
   96. Simple Lamb Bbq With Herbed Salt 31
   97. Onion Omelet 31
   98. Rolled Salmon Sandwich 32
   99. Chicken Legs With Dilled Brussels Sprouts 32
   100. Ricotta Toasts With Salmon 32
   101. Sweet Potato Rosti 32
   102. Fried Chicken Tacos 33
   103. Air Fryer Fish 33
   104. Basic Roasted Tofu 34
   105. Vegetarian Philly Sandwich 34
   106. Tomato And Avocado 34
   107. Sweet & Sour Pork 34
   108. Sweet Potato And Parsnip Spiralized Latkes 35
   109. Moroccan Pork Kebabs 35

110. Chicken Breast With Rosemary 35
111. Pork Stew 35
112. Baked Shrimp Scampi 36
113. Herb-roasted Turkey Breast 36
114. Squash And Zucchini Mini Pizza 36
115. Balsamic Roasted Chicken 36
116. Juicy Turkey Burgers 37
117. Air Fryer Beef Steak 37
118. Portobello Pesto Burgers 37
119. Buttermilk Brined Turkey Breast 37
120. Roasted Fennel, Ditalini, And Shrimp ... 38
121. Coriander Potatoes 38
122. Easy Prosciutto Grilled Cheese 38
123. Chicken Wings With Prawn Paste 38
124. Crispy Breaded Pork Chop 39
125. Zucchini And Cauliflower Stew 39
126. Rosemary Lemon Chicken 39
127. Kalamta Mozarella Pita Melts 39
128. Turkey Meatloaf 40
129. Skinny Black Bean Flautas 40
130. Crisp Chicken Casserole 40
131. Dijon And Swiss Croque Monsieur 40
132. Cheddar & Cream Omelet 41
133. Orange Chicken Rice 41
134. Fried Paprika Tofu 41
135. Saucy Chicken With Leeks 42
136. Roasted Beet Salad With Oranges & Beet Greens 42

DINNER RECIPES 43
137. Lemony Green Beans 43
138. Roasted Lamb 43
139. Grandma's Meatballs With Spicy Sauce .. 43
140. Sage Sausages Balls 43
141. Cheese And Garlic Stuffed Chicken Breasts 43
142. Grilled Tasty Scallops 44
143. Lemongrass Pork Chops 44
144. Venetian Liver 44
145. Curried Eggplant 44
146. One-pan Shrimp And Chorizo Mix Grill ... 45
147. Traditional English Fish And Chips 45
148. Flank Steak Beef 45
149. Cheddar Pork Meatballs 45
150. Pollock With Kalamata Olives And Capers 46
151. Coconut-crusted Haddock With Curried Pumpkin Seeds 46
152. Fish Cakes With Horseradish Sauce 46
153. Rice Flour Coated Shrimp 46
154. Beef Sausage With Grilled Broccoli 47
155. Hot Pork Skewers 47
156. Couscous Stuffed Tomatoes 47
157. Garlic Lamb Shank 47
158. Grilled Halibut With Tomatoes And Hearts Of Palm 48
159. Crispy Scallops 48
160. Herbed Carrots 48
161. Salmon Casserole 48
162. Cinnamon Pork Rinds 49
163. Stuffed Okra 49
164. Zucchini Muffins 49
165. Basil Tomatoes 49
166. Sweet Chicken Breast 50
167. Corned Beef With Carrots 50
168. Smoked Ham With Pears 50
169. Creamy Tuna Cakes 50
170. Pork Belly With Honey 51
171. Cod With Avocado Mayo Sauce 51
172. Paprika Crab Burgers 51
173. Effortless Beef Schnitzel 51
174. Award Winning Breaded Chicken 52
175. Smoked Sausage And Bacon Shashlik ... 52
176. Broccoli Crust Pizza 52
177. Creamy Lemon Turkey 52
178. Homemade Beef Stroganoff 52
179. Roasted Garlic Zucchini Rolls 53
180. Oven-fried Herbed Chicken 53
181. Five Spice Pork 53
182. Broiled Tilapia With Parmesan And Herbs 54
183. Lemon Garlic Shrimps 54
184. Turkey Wontons With Garlic-parmesan Sauce 54
185. Lemon Duck Legs 54
186. Chicken Lasagna With Eggplants 55
187. Buttered Scallops 55
188. Broccoli With Olives 55
189. Sage Beef 55
190. Rich Meatloaf With Mustard And Peppers 56
191. Irish Whisky Steak 56
192. Shrimp Casserole Louisiana Style 56
193. Beef, Mushrooms And Noodles Dish ... 56
194. Sesame Mustard Greens 57
195. Vegetable Cane 57
196. Coconut Crusted Shrimp 57
197. Almond Pork Bites 57
198. Greek-style Monkfish With Vegetables ... 58
199. Almond Asparagus 58
200. Carrot Beef Cake 58
201. Easy Air Fryed Roasted Asparagus 58
202. Easy Marinated London Broil 58
203. Hasselback Potatoes 59
204. Mozzarella & Olive Pizza Bagels 59

MEATLESS RECIPES 60
205. Mushroom Wonton 60
206. Bottle Gourd Flat Cakes 60
207. Roasted Asparagus With Eggs And Tomatoes 60
208. Tasty Polenta Crisps 60
209. Pizza 60
210. Amaranthus French Cuisine Galette 61
211. Mexican Burritos 61
212. Gherkins Flat Cakes 61
213. Dal Mint Spicy Lemon Kebab 62
214. Lemony Wax Beans 62
215. Snake Gourd French Cuisine Galette ... 62
216. Honey Chili Potatoes 62
217. Zucchini Parmesan Crisps 63
218. Cream Cheese Stuffed Bell Peppers ... 63

219. Panko Green Beans 63
220. Vegetable Fried Mix Chips 63
221. Feta & Scallion Triangles 64
222. French Bean Toast 64
223. Mushroom Pops 64
224. Baked Chickpea Stars 64
225. Portobello Steaks 65
226. Barbeque Corn Sandwich 65
227. Cornflakes French Toast 65
228. Simple Polenta Crisps 65
229. Hearty Roasted Veggie Salad 65
230. Asparagus French Cuisine Galette 66
231. Yam French Cuisine Galette 66
232. Eggplant Patties With Mozzarella 66
233. Green Chili Taquitos 66
234. Spicy Sweet Potato Friespotato Fries ... 67
235. Veg Momo's Recipe 67
236. Masala Potato Wedges 67
237. Cauliflower Spicy Lemon Kebab 67
238. Mushroom Homemade Fried Sticks 68
239. Russian-style Eggplant Caviar 68
240. Parmesan Coated Green Beans 68
241. Stuffed Peppers With Beans And Rice .. 68
242. Tortellini With Veggies And Parmesan .. 69
243. Tofu & Pea Cauli Rice 69
244. Black Gram French Cuisine Galette 69
245. Cabbage Steaks With Fennel Seeds 69
246. Gorgonzola Cheese & Pumpkin Salad .. 70
247. Rosemary Butternut Squash Roast 70
248. Rosemary Roasted Squash With Cheese. 70
249. Veggie Mix Fried Chips 70
250. Zucchini Fried Baked Pastry 70
251. Cottage Cheese And Mushroom Mexican Burritos 71
252. Herby Tofu 71
253. Jalapeño & Tomato Gratin 71
254. Easy Cheesy Vegetable Quesadilla 72
255. Caramelized Eggplant With Yogurt Sauce 72
256. Cauliflower Rice With Tofu & Peas 72
257. Baked Turnip And Zucchini 72
258. Cottage Cheese Best Homemade Croquette(2) 73
259. Cheesy Ravioli Lunch 73
260. Cheese And Garlic French Fries 73
261. Cheesy Broccoli Tots 73
262. Stuffed Portobellos With Peppers And Cheese 74
263. Zucchini Parmesan Chips 74
264. Cheese & Vegetable Pizza 74
265. Potato Club Barbeque Sandwich 75
266. Carrot & Chickpea Oat Balls With Cashews 75
267. Tofu, Carrot And Cauliflower Rice 75
268. Spinach Enchiladas With Mozzarella ... 75
269. Grandma´s Ratatouille 76
270. Crispy Fried Okra With Chili 76
271. Asparagus Flat Cakes 76
272. Parmesan Cabbage With Blue Cheese Sauce 76

FISH & SEAFOOD RECIPES 77
273. Party Cod Nuggets 77
274. Thyme Rosemary Shrimp 77
275. Panko-crusted Tilapia 77
276. Old Bay Crab Cakes 77
277. Air Fryer Salmon 77
278. Parmesan Fish Fillets 78
279. Spicy Lemon Cod 78
280. Salmon Fries 78
281. Crispy Cheesy Fish Fingers 78
282. Smoked Paprika Tiger Shrimp 79
283. Fried Cod Nuggets 79
284. Roasted Salmon With Asparagus 79
285. Parmesan-crusted Hake With Garlic Sauce 79
286. Garlic Butter Shrimp Scampi 80
287. Sweet And Savory Breaded Shrimp 80
288. Flavorful Herb Salmon 80
289. Air Fry Prawns 81
290. Baked Tilapia 81
291. Tasty Lemon Pepper Basa 81
292. Herbed Salmon With Asparagus 81
293. Lemon Tilapia 81
294. Cheesy Tuna Patties 82
295. Baked Lemon Swordfish 82
296. Crispy Crab And Fish Cakes 82
297. Spiced Red Snapper 83
298. Lobster Grandma's Easy To Cook Wontons 83
299. Mediterranean Sole 83
300. Parmesan-crusted Halibut Fillets 84
301. Dill Salmon Patties 84
302. Seafood Pizza 84
303. Rosemary Garlic Shrimp 84
304. Baked Halibut Steaks With Parsley 85
305. Sweet & Spicy Lime Salmon 85
306. Rosemary Buttered Prawns 85
307. Sweet Cajun Salmon 85
308. Golden Beer-battered Cod 85
309. Breaded Scallops 86
310. Easy Shrimp And Vegetable Paella 86
311. Firecracker Shrimp 86
312. Prawn Grandma's Easy To Cook Wontons 87
313. Herbed Scallops With Vegetables 87
314. Old Bay Tilapia Fillets 87
315. Prawn French Cuisine Galette 87
316. Basil White Fish 87
317. Cajun And Lemon Pepper Cod 88
318. Old Bay Seasoned Scallops 88
319. Spicy Baked Shrimp 88
320. Lemony Tuna 88
321. Maryland Crab Cakes 88
322. Basil Tomato Salmon 89
323. Prawn Momo's Recipe 89
324. Crispy Fish Sticks 89
325. Panko Crab Sticks With Mayo Sauce ... 89
326. Easy Baked Fish Fillet 90
327. Sticky Hoisin Tuna 90
328. Glazed Tuna And Fruit Kebabs 90

329. Citrus Cilantro Catfish 90
330. Tomato Garlic Shrimp 91
331. Salmon Tandoor 91
332. Crispy Crab Legs 91
333. Fish Cakes With Mango Relish 91
334. Cheesy Tilapia Fillets 91
335. Quick Shrimp Bowl 92
336. Paprika Cod 92
337. Roasted Nicoise Salad 92
338. Paprika Basil Baked Basa 92
339. Tuna Lettuce Wraps 93
340. Caesar Shrimp Salad 93

APPETIZERS AND SIDE DISHES 94
341. Paprika Pickle Chips 94
342. Creamy Fennel(3) 94
343. Homemade Cheddar Biscuits 94
344. Chili Endives 94
345. Delicious Mac And Cheese 94
346. Spicy Pumpkin-ham Fritters 95
347. Zucchini Spaghetti 95
348. Spicy Broccoli With Hot Sauce 95
349. Air Fry Garlic Baby Potatoes 95
350. Pineapple Pork Ribs 95
351. Creamy Corn Casserole 96
352. Herbed Radish Sauté(1) 96
353. Cheese Biscuits 96
354. Easy Broccoli Bread 96
355. Herby Carrot Cookies 96
356. Potato Chips With Lemony Dip 97
357. Classic Cauliflower Hash Browns 97
358. Crunchy Cheese Twists 97
359. Pineapple & Mozzarella Tortillas 97
360. Creamy Fennel(1) 97
361. Garlic Lemon Roasted Chicken 97
362. Creamy Eggplant Cakes 98
363. Healthy Spinach Muffins 98
364. Sausage Mushroom Caps(2) 98
365. Cheddar Broccoli Fritters 98
366. Dijon Zucchini Patties 99
367. Green Beans 99
368. Butternut And Apple Mash 99
369. Crunchy Mozzarella Sticks With Sweet Thai Sauce 99
370. Delicious Chicken Wings With Alfredo Sauce 99
371. Savory Chicken Nuggets With Parmesan Cheese 100
372. Balsamic Keto Vegetables 100
373. Pineapple Spareribs 100
374. Baked Potatoes & Carrots 100
375. Rice And Artichokes 100
376. Whole Chicken With Bbq Sauce 101
377. Poached Fennel 101
378. Rosemary Potato Chips 101
379. Brussels Sprouts With Garlic 101
380. Garlic Asparagus 101
381. Traditional Indian Kofta 102
382. Rosemary & Thyme Roasted Fingerling Potatoes 102
383. Cheddar Cheese Cauliflower Casserole . 102
384. Bbq Chicken Wings 103
385. Healthy Green Beans 103
386. Sweet Coconut Shrimp 103
387. Cabbage Wedges With Parmesan 103
388. Air Fried Green Tomatoes(1) 103
389. Cheese Scones With Chives 104
390. Air Fryer Corn 104
391. Garlic Brussels Sprouts 104
392. Creamy Broccoli Casserole 104
393. Salmon Croquettes 104
394. Savory Parsley Crab Cakes 105
395. Sausage Mushroom Caps(1) 105
396. Simple Baked Potatoes 105
397. Jalapeno Bread 105
398. Cheesy Squash Casserole 106
399. Mixed Nuts With Cinnamon 106
400. Avocado, Tomato, And Grape Salad With Crunchy Potato Croutons 106
401. Bok Choy And Butter Sauce(3) 107
402. Garlic & Olive Oil Spring Vegetables 107
403. Pancetta & Goat Cheese Bombs With Almonds 107
404. Grandma's Apple Cinnamon Chips 107
405. Homemade French Fries 107
406. Bacon Croquettes 107
407. Roasted Brussels Sprouts 108
408. Cheddar & Prosciutto Strips 108

MEAT RECIPES 109
409. Gold Livers 109
410. Chicken Breasts In Onion-mushroom Sauce 109
411. Minty Chicken-fried Pork Chops 109
412. Ranch Chicken Thighs 109
413. Cheesy Pepperoni And Chicken Pizza 110
414. Easy Creamy Chicken 110
415. Pork Wellington 110
416. Chicken Pizza 110
417. Chicken Pasta Broccoli Casserole 111
418. Mustard & Thyme Chicken 111
419. Meatballs(10) 111
420. Sweet & Spicy Chicken 111
421. Caraway Crusted Beef Steaks 112
422. Ham Muffins With Swiss Cheese 112
423. Balsamic Chicken With Mozzarella Cheese 112
424. Pineapple & Ginger Chicken Kabobs 112
425. Mexican Salsa Chicken 113
426. Cayenne Turkey Breasts 113
427. Simple Herbed Hens 113
428. Sweet & Spicy Chicken Wings 113
429. Italian Sausage Jambalaya 114
430. Chicken Oregano Fingers 114
431. Veal Patti With Boiled Peas 114
432. Beef And Spinach Meatloaves 114
433. Parmesan Chicken Fingers With Plum Sauce 115
434. Baked Chicken Fritters 115
435. Rosemary Turkey Scotch Eggs 115
436. Mayo Chicken Breasts With Basil & Cheese 115

437. Barbecue Flavored Pork Ribs 115
438. Baked Beef & Broccoli 116
439. Meatballs(15) 116
440. Spiced Pork Chops 116
441. Air Fried Chicken Wings With Buffalo Sauce 116
442. Korean-style Chicken Wings 117
443. Guacamole Stuffed Chicken 117
444. Easy Baked Chicken Drumsticks 117
445. Tonkatsu 117
446. Spiced Pork Roast 118
447. Tamarind Pork Chops With Green Beans 118
448. Cayenne Chicken Drumsticks 118
449. Cajun Burger Patties 118
450. Parmesan Herb Meatballs 119
451. Perfect Chicken Parmesan 119
452. Turkey Burger Cutlets 119
453. Air Fried Beef And Mushroom Stroganoff 120
454. Chicken Thighs In Waffles 120
455. Juicy & Tender Pork Chops 120
456. Italian Chicken Breasts With Tomatoes 121
457. Juicy Baked Chicken Breast 121
458. Seafood Grandma's Easy To Cook Wontons 121
459. Pork Schnitzel 121
460. Tasty Steak Tips 122
461. Copycat Chicken Sandwich 122
462. Cheesy Bacon Chicken 122
463. Crispy Crusted Pork Chops 123
464. Chicken Momo's Recipe 123
465. Tender Baked Pork Chops 123
466. Chicken Wings With Honey & Cashew Cream 123
467. Ham & Cheese Stuffed Chicken Breasts 124
468. Italian Veggie Chicken 124
469. White Wine Chicken Wings 124
470. Easy Pesto Chicken 124
471. Baked Spinach Cheese Chicken 124
472. Teriyaki Pork Rolls 125
473. Spicy Thai Beef Stir-fry 125
474. Duck Poppers 125
475. Chicken And Eggs 125
476. Beer Corned Beef With Carrots 126

SNACKS AND DESSERTS RECIPES 127
477. Chocolate Donuts 127
478. Strawberry Muffins 127
479. Garlicky-lemon Zucchini 127
480. Toasted Coco Flakes 127
481. Nutella Brownies 127
482. Choco Cookies 128
483. Apple Dumplings 128
484. Three Berry Crumble 128
485. Mozzarella And Tomato Salad 128
486. Sausage And Mushroom Empanadas .. 129
487. Currant Cookies 129
488. Cheese And Ham Stuffed Baby Bella .. 129
489. Lemon Blackberries Cake(2) 129
490. Crispy Cod Fingers 130
491. Rosemary Russet Potato Chips 130
492. Apple-peach Crumble With Honey 130
493. Gooey Chocolate Fudge Cake 130
494. Crispy Eggplant Bites 130
495. Rocky Road Squares 131
496. Moist Baked Donuts 131
497. Keto Mixed Berry Crumble Pots 131
498. Corn And Black Bean Salsa 131
499. Delicious Banana Cake 132
500. Nutella Banana Muffins 132
501. Healthy Carrot Fries 132
502. Pumpkin Bread 133
503. Apricot Crumble With Blackberries 133
504. Chocolate Chip Waffles 133
505. Maple Pecan Pie 133
506. Tasty Gingersnap Cookies 134
507. Sweet Cream Cheese Wontons 134
508. Delicious Jalapeno Poppers 134
509. Yogurt Pumpkin Bread 134
510. Garlic Edamame 135
511. Pan-fried Bananas 135
512. Apple Cake 135
513. Artichoke Cashews Spinach Dip 135
514. Cheese And Leeks Dip 136
515. Tuna Melts With Scallions 136
516. Vegetables Balls 136
517. Vanilla Lemon Cupcakes 136
518. Almond Cookies With Dark Chocolate .. 137
519. Butter Cookies 137
520. Buttermilk Biscuits 137
521. Crab Stuffed Mushrooms 137
522. Peanut Butter Fudge Cake 138
523. Mixed Berry Compote With Coconut Chips 138
524. Chocolate Chip Pan Cookie 138
525. Blueberry Pudding 138
526. Strawberry Tart 139
527. Choco Lava Cakes 139
528. Chocolate Paradise Cake 139
529. Sweet Potato Croquettes 139
530. Crispy Shrimps 139
531. Air Fryer Pepperoni Chips 140
532. Bread Pudding 140
533. Coffee Chocolate Cake 140
534. Sweet Cinnamon Peaches 140
535. Lemon-raspberry Muffins 141
536. Coconut Broccoli Pop-corn 141
537. Crumble With Blackberries & Apricots 141
538. Raspberry-coco Desert 141
539. Mozzarella Pepperoni Pizza Bites 141
540. Caramelized Fruit Kebabs 142
541. Ruderal Swiss Fondue 142
542. Margherita Pizza 142
543. Cinnamon Fried Bananas 142

OTHER FAVORITE RECIPES 144
544. Spinach And Chickpea Casserole 144
545. Fast Cinnamon Toast 144
546. Crispy Cheese Wafer 144
547. Spicy Air Fried Old Bay Shrimp 144
548. Jewish Blintzes 145

549. Crunchy And Beery Onion Rings 145
550. Garlicky Spiralized Zucchini And Squash 145
551. Pastrami Casserole 146
552. Simple Air Fried Okra Chips 146
553. Chocolate And Coconut Macaroons 146
554. Taco Beef And Chile Casserole 146
555. Pão De Queijo 146
556. Corn On The Cob With Mayonnaise 147
557. Goat Cheese And Asparagus Frittata 147
558. Roasted Mushrooms 147
559. Easy Corn And Bell Pepper Casserole 148
560. Simple Cheesy Shrimps 148
561. Chicken Divan 148
562. Cheddar Jalapeño Cornbread 149
563. Ritzy Chicken And Vegetable Casserole 149
564. Shrimp With Sriracha And Worcestershire Sauce 149
565. Asian Dipping Sauce 150
566. Golden Nuggets 150
567. Baked Cherry Tomatoes With Basil 150
568. Classic Churros 150
569. Oven Grits 151
570. Enchilada Sauce 151
571. Citrus Avocado Wedge Fries 151
572. Simple Baked Green Beans 151
573. Chocolate Buttermilk Cake 152
574. Air Fried Crispy Brussels Sprouts 152
575. Dehydrated Bananas With Coconut Sprnikles 152
576. Sumptuous Vegetable Frittata 152
577. Buttery Knots With Parsley 153
578. Creamy Pork Gratin 153
579. Caesar Salad Dressing 153
580. Sweet Cinnamon Chickpeas 153
581. Cauliflower And Pumpkin Casserole 154
582. Potato Chips With Lemony Cream Dip . 154
583. Parmesan Cauliflower Fritters 154
584. Simple Air Fried Edamame 155
585. Crunchy Green Tomatoes Slices 155
586. Sumptuous Beef And Bean Chili Casserole 155
587. Classic Worcestershire Poutine 155
588. Butternut Squash With Hazelnuts 156
589. Salty Tortilla Chips 156
590. Herbed Cheddar Frittata 156
591. Fried Dill Pickles With Buttermilk Dressing 157
592. Golden Salmon And Carrot Croquettes 157
593. Cinnamon Rolls With Cream Glaze 157
594. Banana Cake 158
595. Sausage And Colorful Peppers Casserole 158
596. Southwest Corn And Bell Pepper Roast 158
597. Shrimp Spinach Frittata 159
598. Simple Butter Cake 159
599. Air Fried Blistered Tomatoes 159
600. Lemony And Garlicky Asparagus 160

BREAKFAST RECIPES

1. Glazed Strawberry Toast

Servings: 4 Toasts
Cooking Time: 8 Minutes
Ingredients:
- 4 slices bread, ½-inch thick
- 1 cup sliced strawberries
- 1 teaspoon sugar
- Cooking spray

Directions:
1. On a clean work surface, lay the bread slices and spritz one side of each slice of bread with cooking spray.
2. Place the bread slices in the air fryer basket, sprayed side down. Top with the strawberries and a sprinkle of sugar.
3. Put the air fryer basket on the baking pan and slide into Rack Position 2, select Air Fry, set temperature to 375ºF (190ºC), and set time to 8 minutes.
4. When cooking is complete, the toast should be well browned on each side. Remove from the oven to a plate and serve.

2. Ricotta & Chorizo Corn Frittata

Servings: 2
Cooking Time: 12 Minutes
Ingredients:
- 4 eggs, beaten
- 1 large potato, boiled and cubed
- ½ cup frozen corn
- ½ cup ricotta cheese, crumbled
- 1 tbsp chopped parsley
- ½ chorizo, sliced
- 1 tbsp olive oil
- Salt and black pepper to taste

Directions:
1. Preheat Breville on Bake function to 330 F. Cook the chorizo in a greased skillet over medium heat for 3 minutes; transfer to a baking dish. Mix the eggs, salt, and pepper in a bowl. Stir in the remaining ingredients. Pour the mixture over the chorizo and press Start. Cook for 25 minutes.

3. Peanut Butter & Honey Porridge

Servings: 4
Cooking Time: 5 Minutes
Ingredients:
- 2 cups steel-cut oats
- 1 cup flax seeds
- 1 tbsp peanut butter
- 1 tbsp butter
- 4 cups milk
- 4 tbsp honey

Directions:
1. Preheat Breville on Bake function to 390 F. Combine all of the ingredients in an ovenproof bowl. Place in the Breville oven and press Start. Cook for 7 minutes. Stir and serve.

4. Quick Paprika Eggs

Servings: 4
Cooking Time: 10 Minutes
Ingredients:
- 4 large eggs
- 1 tsp paprika
- Salt and pepper to taste
- ¼ cup cottage cheese, crumbled

Directions:
1. Preheat your fryer to 350 F on Bake function. Crack an egg into a muffin cup. Repeat with the remaining cups. Sprinkle with salt and pepper. Top with cottage cheese. Put the cups in the Air Fryer tray and bake for 8-10 minutes. Remove and sprinkle with paprika to serve.

5. Simple Apple Crisp

Servings: 8
Cooking Time: 35 Minutes
Ingredients:
- 4 medium apples, peel & slice
- 1 tsp cinnamon
- 4 tbsp sugar
- For topping:
- 1/3 cup butter, melted
- 1/2 cup brown sugar
- 3/4 cup all-purpose flour
- 3/4 cup rolled oats

Directions:
1. Fit the oven with the rack in position
2. Add sliced apples, cinnamon, and sugar in a greased 9-inch baking dish and mix well.
3. In a bowl, mix oats, brown sugar, and flour. Add melted butter and mix well.
4. Sprinkle oat mixture over sliced apples.
5. Set to bake at 375 F for 40 minutes. After 5 minutes place the baking dish in the preheated oven.
6. Serve and enjoy.

Nutrition Info: Calories 255 Fat 8.5 g Carbohydrates 44.7 g Sugar 26.5 g Protein 2.6 g Cholesterol 20 mg

6. Cinnamon French Toasts

Servings: 2
Cooking Time: 5 Minutes
Ingredients:
- 2 eggs
- ¼ cup whole milk

- 3 tablespoons sugar
- 2 teaspoons olive oil
- 1/8 teaspoon vanilla extract
- 1/8 teaspoon ground cinnamon
- 4 bread slices

Directions:
1. In a large bowl, mix together all the ingredients except bread slices.
2. Coat the bread slices with egg mixture evenly.
3. Press "Power Button" of Air Fry Oven and turn the dial to select the "Air Fry" mode.
4. Press the Time button and again turn the dial to set the cooking time to 6 minutes.
5. Now push the Temp button and rotate the dial to set the temperature at 390 degrees F.
6. Press "Start/Pause" button to start.
7. When the unit beeps to show that it is preheated, open the lid and lightly, grease the sheet pan.
8. Arrange the bread slices into "Air Fry Basket" and insert in the oven.
9. Flip the bread slices once halfway through.
10. Serve warm.

Nutrition Info: Calories: 238 Cal Total Fat: 10.6 g Saturated Fat: 2.7 g Cholesterol: 167 mg Sodium: 122 mg Total Carbs: 20.8 g Fiber: 0.5 g Sugar: 0.9 g Protein: 7.9 g

7. Blackberries Bowls

Servings: 4
Cooking Time: 30 Minutes
Ingredients:
- 1 ½ cups coconut milk
- ½ cup coconut; shredded
- ½ cup blackberries
- 2 tsp. stevia

Directions:
1. In your air fryer's pan, mix all the ingredients, stir, cover and cook at 360°F for 15 minutes.
2. Divide into bowls and serve

Nutrition Info: Calories: 171; Fat: 4g; Fiber: 2g; Carbs: 3g; Protein: 5g

8. Apple-cinnamon Empanadas

Servings: 2-4
Cooking Time: 30 Minutes
Ingredients:
- 2-3 baking apples, peeled & diced
- 2 tsp.s of cinnamon
- 1/4 cup white sugar
- 1 tablespoon brown sugar
- 1 tablespoon of water
- 1/2 tablespoon cornstarch
- ¼ tsp. of vanilla extract
- 2 tablespoons of margarine or margarine
- 4 pre-made empanada dough shells (Goya)

Directions:
1. In a bowl, add together white sugar, brown sugar, cornstarch and cinnamon; set aside. Put the diced apples in a pot and place on a stovetop.
2. Add the combined dry ingredients to the apples, then add the water, vanilla extract, and margarine; stirring well to mix.
3. Cover pot and cook on high heat. Once it starts boiling, lower heat and simmer, until the apples are soft. Remove from the heat and cool.
4. Lay the empanada shells on a clean counter. Ladle the apple mixture into each of the shells, being careful to prevent spillage over the edges. Fold shells to fully cover apple mixture, seal edges with water, pressing down to secure with a fork.
5. Cover the air fryer basket with tin foil but leave the edges uncovered so that air can circulate through the basket. Place the empanadas shells in the foil lined air fryer basket, set temperature at 350°F and timer for 15 minutes.
6. Halfway through, slide the frying basket out and flip the empanadas using a spatula. Remove when golden, and serve directly from the basket onto plates.

Nutrition Info: Calories 113 Fat 8.2 g Carbohydrates 0.3 g Sugar 0.2 g Protein 5.4 g Cholesterol 18 mg

9. Zucchini And Carrot Pudding

Servings: 4
Cooking Time: 15 Minutes
Ingredients:
- 1 cup carrots, shredded
- 1 cup zucchinis, grated
- 1 cup heavy cream
- 1 cup wild rice
- 2 cups coconut milk
- 1 teaspoon cardamom, ground
- 2 teaspoons sugar
- Cooking spray

Directions:
1. Spray your air fryer with cooking spray, add the carrots, zucchinis and the other ingredients, toss, cover and cook at 365 degrees F for 15 minutes.
2. Divide the pudding into bowls and serve for breakfast.

Nutrition Info: calories 172, fat 7, fiber 4, carbs 14, protein 5

10. Fresh Kale & Cottage Omelet

Servings: 1
Cooking Time: 15 Minutes
Ingredients:
- 3 eggs
- 3 tbsp cottage cheese
- 3 tbsp chopped kale
- ½ tbsp chopped basil

- ½ tbsp chopped parsley
- Salt and black pepper to taste
- 1 tsp olive oil

Directions:
1. Beat the eggs with salt and pepper in a bowl. Stir in the rest of the ingredients. Drizzle a baking pan with olive oil. Pour in the mixture and place it into the oven. Cook for 10-12 minutes on Bake function at 360 F until slightly golden and set. Serve.

11. Grilled Cheese Sandwich

Servings: 1 Person
Cooking Time: 12 Minutes
Ingredients:
- 2 slices of bread
- 2 pieces of bacon
- ½ tsp of olive oil side
- Tomatoes
- Jack cheese
- Peach preserves

Directions:
1. If you have left over bacon from air fried bacon recipe you can get two pieces. However, if you do not have any leftover bacon you can get two pieces and fry them at 200 degree Celsius.
2. Place olive oil on the side of the bread slices. Layer the rest of the ingredients on the non-oiled side following the following steps, peach preserves, tomatoes, jack cheese and cooked bacon.
3. Press down the bread to allow it to cook a little bit and peach side down too to allow the bread and the peel to spread evenly.
4. Place the sandwich in an air fryer and cook it for 12 minutes
5. at 393 degrees Fahrenheit.
6. Serve once you are done.

Nutrition Info: Calories 282 Fats 18g, Carbs 18g, Proteins 12g, Sodium: 830 Mg, Potassium: 250mg

12. Creamy Mushroom And Spinach Omelet

Servings: 2
Cooking Time: 10 Minutes
Ingredients:
- 4 eggs, lightly beaten
- 2 tbsp heavy cream
- 2 cups spinach, chopped
- 1 cup mushrooms, chopped
- 3 oz feta cheese, crumbled
- 1 tbsp fresh parsley, chopped
- Salt and black pepper to taste

Directions:
1. Spray a baking pan with cooking spray. In a bowl, whisk eggs and heavy cream until combined. Stir in spinach, mushrooms, feta, salt, and pepper.
2. Pour into the basket tray and cook in your for 6-10 minutes at 350 F on Bake function until golden and set. Sprinkle with parsley, cut into wedges, and serve.

13. Zucchini Omelet

Servings: 2
Cooking Time: 14 Minutes
Ingredients:
- 1 teaspoon butter
- 1 zucchini, julienned
- 4 eggs
- ¼ teaspoon fresh basil, chopped
- ¼ teaspoon red pepper flakes, crushed
- Salt and ground black pepper, as required

Directions:
1. In a skillet, melt the butter over medium heat and cook the zucchini for about 3-4 minutes.
2. Remove from the heat and set aside to cool slightly.
3. Meanwhile, in a bowl, mix together the eggs, basil, red pepper flakes, salt, and black pepper.
4. Add the cooked zucchini and gently, stir to combine.
5. Place the zucchini mixture into a small baking pan.
6. Press "Power Button" of Air Fry Oven and turn the dial to select the "Air Fry" mode.
7. Press the Time button and again turn the dial to set the cooking time to 10 minutes.
8. Now push the Temp button and rotate the dial to set the temperature at 355 degrees F.
9. Press "Start/Pause" button to start.
10. When the unit beeps to show that it is preheated, open the lid.
11. Arrange pan over the "Wire Rack" and insert in the oven.
12. Cut the omelet into 2 portions and serve hot.

Nutrition Info: Calories 159 Total Fat 10.9 g Saturated Fat 4 g Cholesterol 332 mg Sodium 224 mg Total Carbs 4.1 g Fiber 1.1 g Sugar 2.4 g Protein 12.3 g

14. Creamy Bacon & Egg Wraps With Spicy Salsa

Servings: 3
Cooking Time: 15 Minutes
Ingredients:
- 3 tortillas
- 2 previously scrambled eggs
- 3 slices bacon, cut into strips
- 3 tbsp salsa
- 3 tbsp cream cheese, divided
- 1 cup grated pepper Jack cheese

Directions:

1. Preheat on Air Fry to 390 F. Spread cream cheese onto tortillas. Divide the eggs and bacon between the tortillas. Top with salsa. Sprinkle with cheese. Roll up the tortillas. Place in a greased baking pan and cook for 10 minutes. Serve.

15. Mushroom Sausage Breakfast Bake

Servings: 6
Cooking Time: 30 Minutes
Ingredients:
- 12 eggs
- 2 cups spinach, chopped
- 1 tbsp garlic, minced
- 8 oz mushrooms, sliced
- 1 red bell pepper, diced
- 1 small onion, diced
- 2 tbsp olive oil
- 7 oz sausage links, diced
- Pepper
- Salt

Directions:
1. Fit the oven with the rack in position
2. Spray 9*13-inch baking pan with cooking spray and set aside.
3. Heat oil in a pan over medium-high heat.
4. Add onion and bell pepper and sauté for 2-3 minutes.
5. Add garlic and mushrooms and sauté for 2 minutes.
6. Add sausage and spinach and cook until heated through.
7. Spread pan mixture into the greased baking pan.
8. In a bowl, whisk eggs with pepper and salt.
9. Pour egg mixture over sausage mixture.
10. Set to bake at 350 F for 35 minutes. After 5 minutes place the baking pan in the preheated oven.
11. Serve and enjoy.

Nutrition Info: Calories 293 Fat 23 g Carbohydrates 6 g Sugar 3.2 g Protein 16.9 g Cholesterol 348 mg

16. Mixed Berry Dutch Baby Pancake

Servings: 4
Cooking Time: 14 Minutes
Ingredients:
- 1 tablespoon unsalted butter, at room temperature
- 1 egg
- 2 egg whites
- ½ cup 2% milk
- ½ cup whole-wheat pastry flour
- 1 teaspoon pure vanilla extract
- 1 cup sliced fresh strawberries
- ½ cup fresh raspberries
- ½ cup fresh blueberries

Directions:
1. Grease the baking pan with the butter.
2. Using a hand mixer, beat together the egg, egg whites, milk, pastry flour, and vanilla in a medium mixing bowl until well incorporated.
3. Pour the batter into the pan.
4. Slide the baking pan into Rack Position 1, select Convection Bake, set temperature to 330ºF (166ºC) and set time to 14 minutes.
5. When cooked, the pancake should puff up in the center and the edges should be golden brown
6. Allow the pancake to cool for 5 minutes and serve topped with the berries.

17. Peppered Maple Bacon Knots

Servings: 6
Cooking Time: 7 To 8 Minutes
Ingredients:
- 1 pound (454 g) maple smoked center-cut bacon
- ¼ cup maple syrup
- ¼ cup brown sugar
- Coarsely cracked black peppercorns, to taste

Directions:
1. On a clean work surface, tie each bacon strip in a loose knot.
2. Stir together the maple syrup and brown sugar in a bowl. Generously brush this mixture over the bacon knots.
3. Place the bacon knots in the air fryer basket and sprinkle with the coarsely cracked black peppercorns.
4. Put the air fryer basket on the baking pan and slide into Rack Position 2, select Air Fry, set temperature to 390ºF (199ºC), and set time to 8 minutes.
5. After 5 minutes, remove the pan from the oven and flip the bacon knots. Return to the oven and continue cooking for 2 to 3 minutes more.
6. When cooking is complete, the bacon should be crisp. Remove from the oven to a paper towel-lined plate. Let the bacon knots cool for a few minutes and serve warm.

18. Banana Oat Muffins

Servings: 6
Cooking Time: 25 Minutes
Ingredients:
- 1 egg
- 2 tbsp butter, melted
- 1/2 tsp cinnamon
- 1 tsp vanilla
- 2 tbsp yogurt
- 1 1/2 cup oats
- 1 tsp baking powder
- 2 ripe bananas, mashed

Directions:
1. Fit the oven with the rack in position
2. Line the muffin tray with cupcake liners and set aside.

3. In a bowl, whisk the egg with banana, yogurt, vanilla, cinnamon, baking powder, and butter.
4. Add oats and mix well.
5. Pour mixture into the prepared muffin tray.
6. Set to bake at 350 F for 30 minutes. After 5 minutes place the muffin tray in the preheated oven.
7. Serve and enjoy.
Nutrition Info: Calories 164 Fat 6.1 g Carbohydrates 23.9 g Sugar 5.5 g Protein 4.4 g Cholesterol 38 mg

19. Whole Wheat Carrot Bread

Servings: 10
Cooking Time: 50 Minutes
Ingredients:
- 1 egg
- 3/4 cup whole wheat flour
- 1 cup carrots, shredded
- 3/4 tsp vanilla
- 3/4 cup all-purpose flour
- 1/2 cup brown sugar
- 1 tsp baking powder
- 1/2 tsp nutmeg
- 1 1/2 tsp cinnamon
- 3/4 cup yogurt
- 3 tbsp vegetable oil
- 1 tsp baking soda

Directions:
1. Fit the oven with the rack in position
2. In a large bowl, mix all dry ingredients and set aside.
3. In a separate bowl, whisk the egg with vanilla, sugar, yogurt, and oil.
4. Add carrots and fold well.
5. Add dry ingredient mixture and stir until just combined.
6. Pour mixture into the 9*5-inch greased loaf pan.
7. Set to bake at 350 F for 55 minutes, after 5 minutes, place the loaf pan in the oven.
8. Slice and serve.
Nutrition Info: Calories 159 Fat 5 g Carbohydrates 24.4 g Sugar 9 g Protein 3.7 g Cholesterol 17 mg

20. Spicy Apple Turnovers

Servings: 4
Cooking Time: 20 Minutes
Ingredients:
- 1 cup diced apple
- 1 tablespoon brown sugar
- 1 teaspoon freshly squeezed lemon juice
- 1 teaspoon all-purpose flour, plus more for dusting
- ¼ teaspoon cinnamon
- ⅛ teaspoon allspice
- ½ package frozen puff pastry, thawed
- 1 large egg, beaten
- 2 teaspoons granulated sugar

Directions:
1. Whisk together the apple, brown sugar, lemon juice, flour, cinnamon and allspice in a medium bowl.
2. On a clean work surface, lightly dust with the flour and lay the puff pastry sheet. Using a rolling pin, gently roll the dough to smooth out the folds, seal any tears and form it into a square. Cut the dough into four squares.
3. Spoon a quarter of the apple mixture into the center of each puff pastry square and spread it evenly in a triangle shape over half the pastry, leaving a border of about ½ inch around the edges of the pastry. Fold the pastry diagonally over the filling to form triangles. With a fork, crimp the edges to seal them. Place the turnovers in the baking pan, spacing them evenly.
4. Cut two or three small slits in the top of each turnover. Brush with the egg. Sprinkle evenly with the granulated sugar.
5. Slide the baking pan into Rack Position 1, select Convection Bake, set temperature to 350ºF (180ºC) and set time to 20 minutes.
6. When cooking is complete, remove the pan from the oven. The turnovers should be golden brown and the filling bubbling. Let cool for about 10 minutes before serving.

21. Quick Mac & Cheese

Servings: 2
Cooking Time: 15 Minutes
Ingredients:
- 1 cup macaroni, cooked
- 1 cup cheddar cheese, grated
- ½ cup warm milk
- 1 tbsp Parmesan cheese, grated
- Salt and black pepper to taste

Directions:
1. Preheat Breville on AirFry function to 350 F. Add the macaroni to an ovenproof baking dish. Stir in the cheddar cheese and milk. Season with salt and pepper. Place the dish in the Breville oven and press Start. Cook for 10 minutes. Sprinkle with Parmesan cheese and serve.

22. Enchiladas 4 Breakfast

Servings: 8
Cooking Time: 30 Minutes
Ingredients:
- Nonstick cooking spray
- 1 lb. pork breakfast sausage
- 2 cups hash browns, thawed
- 1/3 cup red bell pepper, chopped
- 1/3 cup poblano pepper, chopped
- 6 green onion, sliced thin
- 2 tsp garlic salt divided
- 10 eggs

- 1 tsp black pepper
- 3 cups pepper jack cheese, grated
- 8 8-inch
- 1 cup salsa Verde
- ½ cup half & half
- ½ tsp cumin
- ½ tsp oregano

Directions:
1. Place the rack in position Lightly spray an 8x11-inch baking dish with cooking spray.
2. In a medium saucepan, over medium heat, cook sausage until no longer pink. Use a slotted spoon to transfer to a paper towel lined plate.
3. Add potatoes, red pepper, poblano, 1 teaspoon garlic salt, and onion (saving 3 tablespoons for garnish) to the pan. Cook until vegetables are fork-tender, about 5-7 minutes. Stir in sausage and stir to combine. Remove from heat.
4. In a medium bowl, whisk eggs, remaining garlic salt, and pepper.
5. Heat a medium skillet over medium heat. Once hot, add eggs and scramble until done. Remove from heat.
6. Place tortillas, one at a time, on work surface. Use 2 cups of cheese for filling. Sprinkle some cheese down the middle. Top with sausage mixture and a little more cheese. Roll up and place seam side down in prepared pan. Repeat with remaining ingredients.
7. In a small bowl, whisk together salsa Verde, half & half, cumin, and oregano. Pour over enchiladas and top with remaining cheese.
8. Set to bake on 375°F for 35 minutes. After 5 minutes, place baking pan on rack and bake 30 minutes or until golden brown and bubbly. Serve garnished with reserved onions.

Nutrition Info: Calories 582, Total Fat 36g, Saturated Fat 15g, Total Carbs 31g, Net Carbs 28g, Protein 31g, Sugar 4g, Fiber 3g, Sodium 1015mg, Potassium 677mg, Phosphorus 512mg

23. Rarebit Air-fried Egg

Servings: 2-4
Cooking Time: 5 Minutes
Ingredients:
- 4 Slices Sourdough
- 4 Eggs
- 1/3 cup ale
- 1 & 1/2 cups cheddar, grated
- 1 tsp. mustard powder
- 1/2 tsp. paprika
- Black Pepper to taste
- 2 tsp. Worcestershire Sauce

Directions:
1. Fry eggs, sunny side up and set to one side. Preheat Air Fryer to 350°F.
2. In a bowl, add together the cheddar, ale, paprika, mustard powder, and Worcestershire sauce.
3. Spread just one side of each slice of sourdough with the cheddar mixture.
4. Place the bread slices into the Air fryer tray. Cook for about 3 minutes until slightly browned.
5. Top the rarebits with fried eggs and spice with pepper to taste.

Nutrition Info: Calories 115 Fat 9.2 g Carbohydrates 0.3 g Sugar 0.3 g Protein 5.4 g Cholesterol 19 mg

24. Strawberry Cheesecake Pastries

Servings: 6
Cooking Time: 20 Minutes
Ingredients:
- 1 sheet puff pastry, thawed
- ¼ cup cream cheese, soft
- 1 tbsp. strawberry jam
- 1 ½ cups strawberries, sliced
- 1 egg
- 1 tbsp. water
- 6 tsp powdered sugar, sifted

Directions:
1. Line the baking pan with parchment paper.
2. Lay the puff pastry on a cutting board and cut into 6 rectangles. Transfer to prepared pan, placing them 1-inch apart.
3. Lightly score the pastry, creating a ½-inch border, do not cut all the way through. Use a fork to prick the center.
4. In a small bowl, combine cream cheese and jam until thoroughly combined. Spoon mixture evenly into centers of the pastry and spread it within the scored area.
5. Top pastries with sliced berries.
6. In a small bowl, whisk together egg and water. Brush edges of pastry with the egg wash.
7. Set to bake at 350°F for 20 minutes. After 5 minutes, place the baking pan in position 1 and bake pastries until golden brown and puffed.
8. Remove from oven and let cool. Dust with powdered sugar before serving.

Nutrition Info: Calories 205, Total Fat 13g, Saturated Fat 4g, Total Carbs 19g, Net Carbs 18g, Protein 3g, Sugar 6g, Fiber 1g, Sodium 107mg, Potassium 97mg, Phosphorus 50mg

25. Avocado And Zucchini Mix

Servings: 4
Cooking Time: 15 Minutes
Ingredients:
- 2 avocados, peeled, pitted and roughly cubed
- 2 zucchinis, roughly cubed
- 1 tablespoon olive oil
- 2 spring onions, chopped
- 8 eggs, whisked
- 1 teaspoon sweet paprika

- A pinch of salt and black pepper
- 1 tablespoon dill, chopped

Directions:
1. Heat up the air fryer with the oil at 350 degrees F, add the zucchinis and the spring onions and cook for 2 minutes.
2. Add the avocados and the other ingredients, cook the mix for 13 minutes more, divide into bowls and serve.

Nutrition Info: calories 232, fat 12, fiber 2, carbs 10, protein 5

26. Chocolate Banana Bread

Servings: 4
Cooking Time: 30 Minutes
Ingredients:
- ¼ cup cocoa powder
- 6 tablespoons plus 2 teaspoons all-purpose flour, divided
- ½ teaspoon kosher salt
- ¼ teaspoon baking soda
- 1½ ripe bananas
- 1 large egg, whisked
- ¼ cup vegetable oil
- ½ cup sugar
- 3 tablespoons buttermilk or plain yogurt (not Greek)
- ½ teaspoon vanilla extract
- 6 tablespoons chopped white chocolate
- 6 tablespoons chopped walnuts

Directions:
1. Mix together the cocoa powder, 6 tablespoons of the flour, salt, and baking soda in a medium bowl.
2. Mash the bananas with a fork in another medium bowl until smooth. Fold in the egg, oil, sugar, buttermilk, and vanilla, and whisk until thoroughly combined. Add the wet mixture to the dry mixture and stir until well incorporated.
3. Combine the white chocolate, walnuts, and the remaining 2 tablespoons of flour in a third bowl and toss to coat. Add this mixture to the batter and stir until well incorporated. Pour the batter into the baking pan and smooth the top with a spatula.
4. Slide the baking pan into Rack Position 1, select Convection Bake, set temperature to 310ºF (154ºC) and set time to 30 minutes.
5. When done, a toothpick inserted into the center of the bread should come out clean.
6. Remove from the oven and allow to cool on a wire rack for 10 minutes before serving.

27. Garlic And Cheese Bread Rolls

Servings: 2
Cooking Time: 5 Minutes
Ingredients:
- 8 tablespoons of grated cheese
- 6 tsp.s of melted margarine
- Garlic bread spice mix
- 2 bread rolls

Directions:
1. Slice the bread rolls from top in a crisscross pattern but not cut through at the bottom.
2. Put all the cheese into the slits and brush the tops of the bread rolls with melted margarine. Sprinkle the garlic mix on the rolls.
3. Heat the air fryer to 350°F. Place the rolls into the basket and cook until cheese is melted for about 5 minutes.

Nutrition Info: Calories 113 Fat 8.2 g Carbohydrates 0.3 g Sugar 0.2 g Protein 5.4 g Cholesterol 18 mg

28. Fried Cheese Grits

Servings: 4
Cooking Time: 11 Minutes
Ingredients:
- $^2/_3$ cup instant grits
- 1 teaspoon salt
- 1 teaspoon freshly ground black pepper
- ¾ cup whole or 2% milk
- 3 ounces (85 g) cream cheese, at room temperature
- 1 large egg, beaten
- 1 tablespoon butter, melted
- 1 cup shredded mild Cheddar cheese
- Cooking spray

Directions:
1. Mix the grits, salt, and black pepper in a large bowl. Add the milk, cream cheese, beaten egg, and melted butter and whisk to combine. Fold in the Cheddar cheese and stir well.
2. Spray the baking pan with cooking spray. Spread the grits mixture into the baking pan.
3. Put the air fryer basket on the baking pan and slide into Rack Position 2, select Air Fry, set temperature to 400ºF (205ºC) and set time to 11 minutes.
4. Stir the mixture halfway through the cooking time.
5. When done, a knife inserted in the center should come out clean.
6. Rest for 5 minutes and serve warm.

29. Apple Fritter Loaf

Servings: 10
Cooking Time: 1 Hour
Ingredients:
- Butter flavored cooking spray
- 1/3 cup brown sugar, packed
- 1 tsp. cinnamon, divided
- 1 ½ cups apples, chopped
- 2/3 cup + 1 tsp. sugar, divided

- ½ cup + ½ tbsp. butter, soft, divided
- 2 eggs
- 2 ¼ tsp. vanilla, divided
- 1 ½ cups flour
- 2 tsp baking powder
- ¼ tsp salt
- ½ cup + 2 tbsp. milk
- 1/2 cup powdered sugar

Directions:
1. Place rack in position 1 of the oven. Spray an 8-inch loaf pan with cooking spray.
2. In a small bowl, combine brown sugar and ½ teaspoon cinnamon.
3. Place apples in a medium bowl and sprinkle with remaining cinnamon and 1 teaspoon sugar, toss to coat.
4. In a large bowl, beat remaining sugar and butter until smooth.
5. Beat in eggs and 2 teaspoons vanilla until combined. Stir in flour, baking powder, and salt until combined.
6. Add ½ cup milk and beat until smooth. Pour half the batter in the prepared pan. Add half the apples then remaining batter. Add the remaining apples over the top, pressing lightly. Sprinkle brown sugar mixture over the apples.
7. Set oven to convection bake at 325°F for 5 minutes. Once timer goes, off place bread on the rack and set timer to 1 hour. Bread is done when it passes the toothpick test.
8. Let cool in pan 10 minutes, then invert onto wire rack to cool.
9. In a small bowl, whisk together powdered sugar and butter until smooth. Whisk in remaining milk and vanilla and drizzle over cooled bread.

Nutrition Info: Calories 418, Total Fat 14g, Saturated Fat 8g, Total Carbs 44g, Net Carbs 43g, Protein 4g, Sugar 28g, Fiber 1g, Sodium 85mg, Potassium 190mg, Phosphorus 128mg

30. Mini Brown Rice Quiches

Servings: 6
Cooking Time: 14 Minutes
Ingredients:
- 4 ounces (113 g) diced green chilies
- 3 cups cooked brown rice
- 1 cup shredded reduced-fat Cheddar cheese, divided
- ½ cup egg whites
- 1/3 cup fat-free milk
- ¼ cup diced pimiento
- ½ teaspoon cumin
- 1 small eggplant, cubed
- 1 bunch fresh cilantro, finely chopped
- Cooking spray

Directions:
1. Spritz a 12-cup muffin pan with cooking spray.
2. In a large bowl, stir together all the ingredients, except for ½ cup of the cheese.
3. Scoop the mixture evenly into the muffin cups and sprinkle the remaining ½ cup of the cheese on top.
4. Put the muffin pan into Rack Position 1, select Convection Bake, set temperature to 400ºF (205ºC) and set time to 14 minutes.
5. When cooking is complete, remove from the oven and check the quiches. They should be set.
6. Carefully transfer the quiches to a platter and serve immediately.

31. Apricot Scones With Almonds

Servings: 4
Cooking Time: 30 Minutes
Ingredients:
- 2 cups flour
- ⅓ cup sugar
- 2 tsp baking powder
- ½ cup sliced almonds
- ¾ cup chopped dried apricots
- ¼ cup cold butter, cut into cubes
- ½ cup milk
- 1 egg
- 1 tsp vanilla extract

Directions:
1. Line a large baking sheet with parchment paper. Mix together flour, sugar, baking powder, almonds, and apricots. Rub the butter into the dry ingredients with hands to form a sandy, crumbly texture. Whisk together egg, milk, and vanilla extract.
2. Pour into the dry ingredients and stir to combine. Sprinkle a working board with flour, lay the dough onto the board and give it a few kneads. Shape into a rectangle and cut into 8 squares. Arrange the squares on the baking sheet and cook for 20-25 minutes at 360 F on Bake function.

32. Sausage Omelet

Servings: 2
Cooking Time: 13 Minutes
Ingredients:
- 4 eggs
- 1 bacon slice, chopped
- 2 sausages, chopped
- 1 yellow onion, chopped

Directions:
1. In a bowl, crack the eggs and beat well.
2. Add the remaining ingredients and gently, stir to combine.
3. Place the mixture into a baking pan.
4. Press "Power Button" of Air Fry Oven and turn the dial to select the "Air Fry" mode.
5. Press the Time button and again turn the dial to set the cooking time to 13 minutes.

6. Now push the Temp button and rotate the dial to set the temperature at 320 degrees F.
7. Press "Start/Pause" button to start.
8. When the unit beeps to show that it is preheated, open the lid.
9. Arrange pan over the "Wire Rack" and insert in the oven.
10. Cut into equal-sized wedges and serve hot.
Nutrition Info: Calories 325 Total Fat 23.1 g Saturated Fat 7.4 g Cholesterol 368 mg Sodium 678 mg Total Carbs 6 g Fiber 1.2 g Sugar 3 g Protein 22.7 g

33. Tomatta Spinacha Frittata

Servings: 4
Cooking Time: 30 Minutes
Ingredients:
- 3 tablespoons olive oil
- 10 large eggs
- 2 teaspoons kosher salt
- 1/2 teaspoon black pepper
- 1 (5-ounce) bag baby spinach
- 1 pint grape tomatoes
- 4 scallions
- 8 ounces feta cheese

Directions:
1. Preheat toaster oven to 350°F.
2. Halve tomatoes and slice scallions into thin pieces.
3. Add oil to a 2-quart oven-safe pan, making sure to brush it on the sides as well as the bottom. Place the dish in toaster oven.
4. Combine the eggs, salt, and pepper in a medium mixing bowl and whisk together for a minute.
5. Add spinach, tomatoes, and scallions to the bowl and mix together until even.
6. Crumble feta cheese into the bowl and mix together gently. Remove the dish from the oven and pour in the egg mixture.
7. Put the dish back into the oven and bake for 25–30 minutes, or until the edges of the frittata are browned.
Nutrition Info: Calories: 448, Sodium: 515 mg, Dietary Fiber: 2.3 g, Total Fat: 35.4 g, Total Carbs: 9.3 g, Protein: 25.9 g.

34. French Toast Delight

Servings: 2
Cooking Time: 10 Minutes
Ingredients:
- 4 bread slices
- 2 tablespoons margarine
- 1/2 tsp. cinnamon
- 2 Eggs
- Pinch salt
- Pinch ground cloves
- Pinch Nutmeg
- Icing sugar and maple syrup, to serve

Directions:
1. Preheat Air fryer to 350°F. Whisk together eggs, cloves, cinnamon, nutmeg, cloves and salt in a bowl. Margarine sides of each bread slice and cut into strips.
2. Soak the margarineed bread strips in the egg mixture one after the other and arrange in the tray. (Cook in two batches, if necessary).
3. Cook 2 minutes and then remove the strips. Lightly coat bread strips with cooking spray on both sides. Place back the tray into the air fryer and cook another 4 minutes, checking to ensure they are cooking evenly.
4. Remove bread from Air fryer once it's golden brown. Sprinkle with icing sugar and drizzle with maple syrup.
Nutrition Info: Calories 118 Fat 9.4 g Carbohydrates 0.2 g Sugar 0.3 g Protein 6 g

35. Tator Tots Casserole

Servings: 8
Cooking Time: 30 Minutes
Ingredients:
- 8 eggs
- 28 oz tator tots
- 8 oz pepper jack cheese, shredded
- 2 green onions, sliced
- 1/4 cup milk
- 1 lb breakfast sausage, cooked
- Pepper
- Salt

Directions:
1. Fit the oven with the rack in position
2. Spray 13*9-inch baking pan with cooking spray and set aside.
3. In a bowl, whisk eggs with milk, pepper, and salt.
4. Layer sausage in a prepared baking pan then pour the egg mixture and sprinkle with half shredded cheese and green onions.
5. Add tator tots on top.
6. Set to bake at 400 F for 35 minutes. After 5 minutes place the baking pan in the preheated oven.
7. Top with remaining cheese and serve.
Nutrition Info: Calories 398 Fat 31.5 g Carbohydrates 2 g Sugar 0.8 g Protein 22.1 g Cholesterol 251 mg

36. Avocado And Tomato Egg Rolls

Servings: 5
Cooking Time: 5 Minutes
Ingredients:
- 10 egg roll wrappers
- 3 avocados, peeled and pitted
- 1 tomato, diced

- Salt and ground black pepper, to taste
- Cooking spray

Directions:
1. Spritz the air fryer basket with cooking spray.
2. Put the tomato and avocados in a food processor. Sprinkle with salt and ground black pepper. Pulse to mix and coarsely mash until smooth.
3. Unfold the wrappers on a clean work surface, then divide the mixture in the center of each wrapper. Roll the wrapper up and press to seal.
4. Transfer the rolls to the pan and spritz with cooking spray.
5. Put the air fryer basket on the baking pan and slide into Rack Position 2, select Air Fry, set temperature to 350ºF (180ºC) and set time to 5 minutes.
6. Flip the rolls halfway through the cooking time.
7. When cooked, the rolls should be golden brown.
8. Serve immediately.

37. Porridge With Honey & Peanut Butter

Servings: 4
Cooking Time: 15 Minutes
Ingredients:
- 2 cups steel-cut oats
- 1 cup flax seeds
- 1 tbsp peanut butter
- 1 tbsp butter
- 4 cups milk
- 4 tbsp honey

Directions:
1. Preheat on Bake function to 390 F. Combine all of the ingredients in an ovenproof bowl. Place in a baking pan and cook for 7 minutes. Stir and serve.

38. Easy Egg Bites

Servings: 6
Cooking Time: 30 Minutes
Ingredients:
- 5 eggs
- 3 bacon slices, cooked & chopped
- 4 tbsp cottage cheese
- 1/2 cup cheddar cheese, shredded
- 1/4 tsp pepper
- 1/4 tsp salt

Directions:
1. Fit the oven with the rack in position
2. Spray 6-cups muffin tin with cooking spray and set aside.
3. Add all ingredients except bacon into the blender and blend for 30 seconds.
4. Pour egg mixture into the prepared muffin tin then divide cooked bacon evenly in all egg cups.
5. Set to bake at 325 F for 35 minutes. After 5 minutes place muffin tin in the preheated oven.
6. Serve and enjoy.

Nutrition Info: Calories 151 Fat 10.9 g Carbohydrates 0.9 g Sugar 0.4 g Protein 11.8 g Cholesterol 158 mg

39. Nutritious Cinnamon Oat Muffins

Servings: 12
Cooking Time: 30 Minutes
Ingredients:
- 2 cups oat flour
- 1/3 cup coconut oil, melted
- 1/2 cup maple syrup
- 1 cup applesauce
- 1 tsp cinnamon
- 2 tsp baking powder
- 1 tsp vanilla
- 1/4 tsp salt

Directions:
1. Fit the oven with the rack in position
2. Line 12-cups muffin tin with cupcake liners and set aside.
3. In a bowl, add applesauce, cinnamon, vanilla, oil, maple syrup, and salt and stir to combine.
4. Add baking powder and oat flour and stir well.
5. Pour batter into the prepared muffin tin.
6. Set to bake at 350 F for 35 minutes, after 5 minutes, place the muffin tin in the oven.
7. Serve and enjoy.

Nutrition Info: Calories 158 Fat 7.1 g Carbohydrates 22.2 g Sugar 9.9 g Protein 2 g Cholesterol 0 mg

40. Healthy Oatmeal Bars

Servings: 18
Cooking Time: 20 Minutes
Ingredients:
- 2 cups oatmeal
- 1/2 tsp allspice
- 1 tsp baking soda
- 1 tbsp maple syrup
- 1 cup butter
- 1 cup of sugar
- 1 cup flour

Directions:
1. Fit the oven with the rack in position
2. Add butter and maple syrup into a bowl and microwave until butter is melted. Stir well.
3. In a mixing bowl, mix oatmeal, sugar, flour, allspice, and baking soda.
4. Add melted butter and maple syrup mixture and mix until well combined.
5. Pour mixture into the parchment-lined 9*12-inch baking dish. Spread well.
6. Set to bake at 350 F for 25 minutes, after 5 minutes, place the baking dish in the oven.
7. Slice and serve.

Nutrition Info: Calories 195 Fat 10.9 g Carbohydrates 23.4 g Sugar 11.9 g Protein 2 g Cholesterol 27 mg

41. Tomato Oatmeal

Servings: 4
Cooking Time: 20 Minutes
Ingredients:
- 1 cup tomatoes, cubed
- 1 cup old fashioned oats
- 2 cups almond milk
- A drizzle of avocado oil
- A pinch of salt and black pepper
- 1 teaspoon cilantro, chopped
- 1 teaspoon basil, chopped
- 2 spring onions, chopped

Directions:
1. In your air fryer, combine the tomatoes with the oats and the other ingredients, toss and cook at 360 degrees F for 20 minutes.
2. Divide the oatmeal into bowls and serve for breakfast.

Nutrition Info: calories 140, fat 2, fiber 3, carbs 8, protein 4

42. Cheesy Spring Chicken Wraps

Servings: 12
Cooking Time: 5 Minutes
Ingredients:
- 2 large-sized chicken breasts, cooked and shredded
- 2 spring onions, chopped
- 10 ounces (284 g) Ricotta cheese
- 1 tablespoon rice vinegar
- 1 tablespoon molasses
- 1 teaspoon grated fresh ginger
- ¼ cup soy sauce
- $^1/_3$ teaspoon sea salt
- ¼ teaspoon ground black pepper, or more to taste
- 48 wonton wrappers
- Cooking spray

Directions:
1. Spritz the air fryer basket with cooking spray.
2. Combine all the ingredients, except for the wrappers in a large bowl. Toss to mix well.
3. Unfold the wrappers on a clean work surface, then divide and spoon the mixture in the middle of the wrappers.
4. Dab a little water on the edges of the wrappers, then fold the edge close to you over the filling. Tuck the edge under the filling and roll up to seal.
5. Arrange the wraps in the pan.
6. Put the air fryer basket on the baking pan and slide into Rack Position 2, select Air Fry, set temperature to 375ºF (190ºC) and set time to 5 minutes.
7. Flip the wraps halfway through the cooking time.
8. When cooking is complete, the wraps should be lightly browned.
9. Serve immediately.

43. Spinach Zucchini Egg Muffins

Servings: 12
Cooking Time: 20 Minutes
Ingredients:
- 8 eggs
- 1 cup baby spinach, chopped
- 1 red bell pepper, diced
- 1/4 cup green onion, chopped
- 12 bacon slices, cooked and crumbled
- 2 small zucchini, sliced
- 1/4 cup almond milk
- 2 tbsp parsley, chopped
- 1 tbsp olive oil
- Pepper
- Salt

Directions:
1. Fit the oven with the rack in position
2. Spray 12-cups muffin tin with cooking spray and set aside.
3. Heat olive oil in a pan over medium heat.
4. Add parsley, spinach, green onion, red bell pepper to the pan and sauté until spinach is wilted.
5. In a bowl, whisk eggs with almond milk, pepper, and salt.
6. Add sautéed vegetables, bacon, and zucchini to the egg mixture and stir well.
7. Pour egg mixture into the greased muffin tin.
8. Set to bake at 350 F for 25 minutes, after 5 minutes, place muffin tin in the oven.
9. Serve and enjoy.

Nutrition Info: Calories 174 Fat 13.3 g Carbohydrates 2.5 g Sugar 1.3 g Protein 11.3 g Cholesterol 130 mg

44. Breakfast Potatoes

Servings: 4
Cooking Time: 35 Minutes
Ingredients:
- 2 lbs potatoes, scrubbed and cut into 1/2-inch cubes
- 1 tsp garlic powder
- 1 tbsp olive oil
- 1/2 tsp sweet paprika
- Pepper
- Salt

Directions:
1. Fit the oven with the rack in position
2. Place potato cubes on the parchment-lined baking pan.

3. Drizzle with oil and season with paprika, garlic powder, pepper, and salt. Toss potatoes well.
4. Set to bake at 425 F for 40 minutes, after 5 minutes, place the baking pan in the oven.
5. Serve and enjoy.
Nutrition Info: Calories 190 Fat 3.8 g Carbohydrates 36.3 g Sugar 2.8 g Protein 4 g Cholesterol 0 mg

45. Cabbage And Mushroom Spring Rolls

Servings: 14 Spring Rolls
Cooking Time: 14 Minutes
Ingredients:
- 2 tablespoons vegetable oil
- 4 cups sliced Napa cabbage
- 5 ounces (142 g) shiitake mushrooms, diced
- 3 carrots, cut into thin matchsticks
- 1 tablespoon minced fresh ginger
- 1 tablespoon minced garlic
- 1 bunch scallions, white and light green parts only, sliced
- 2 tablespoons soy sauce
- 1 (4-ounce / 113-g) package cellophane noodles
- ¼ teaspoon cornstarch
- 1 (12-ounce / 340-g) package frozen spring roll wrappers, thawed
- Cooking spray

Directions:
1. Heat the olive oil in a nonstick skillet over medium-high heat until shimmering.
2. Add the cabbage, mushrooms, and carrots and sauté for 3 minutes or until tender.
3. Add the ginger, garlic, and scallions and sauté for 1 minutes or until fragrant.
4. Mix in the soy sauce and turn off the heat. Discard any liquid remains in the skillet and allow to cool for a few minutes.
5. Bring a pot of water to a boil, then turn off the heat and pour in the noodles. Let sit for 10 minutes or until the noodles are al dente. Transfer 1 cup of the noodles in the skillet and toss with the cooked vegetables. Reserve the remaining noodles for other use.
6. Dissolve the cornstarch in a small dish of water, then place the wrappers on a clean work surface. Dab the edges of the wrappers with cornstarch.
7. Scoop up 3 tablespoons of filling in the center of each wrapper, then fold the corner in front of you over the filling. Tuck the wrapper under the filling, then fold the corners on both sides into the center. Keep rolling to seal the wrapper. Repeat with remaining wrappers.
8. Spritz the air fryer basket with cooking spray. Arrange the wrappers in the pan and spritz with cooking spray.
9. Put the air fryer basket on the baking pan and slide into Rack Position 2, select Air Fry, set temperature to 400ºF (205ºC) and set time to 10 minutes.
10. Flip the wrappers halfway through the cooking time.
11. When cooking is complete, the wrappers will be golden brown.
12. Serve immediately.

46. Brioche Breakfast Pudding

Servings: 8
Cooking Time: 45 Minutes
Ingredients:
- 1 loaf brioche bread, cut in cubes
- ½ tbsp. coconut oil, soft
- 4 cups milk
- 1 can coconut milk
- 6 eggs
- ½ cup sugar
- 2 tsp vanilla
- ¼ tsp salt
- 1 cup coconut, shredded
- ½ cup chocolate chips

Directions:
1. Place rack in position 1 of the oven. Grease an 8x11-inch baking pan with coconut oil.
2. Add the bread cubes to the pan, pressing lightly to settle.
3. In a large bowl, whisk together milk, coconut milk, eggs, sugar, vanilla, and salt until combined.
4. Stir in coconut and chocolate chips. Pour evenly over bread. Cover with plastic wrap and refrigerate 2 hours or overnight.
5. Set oven to bake on 350°F for 50 minutes. After 5 minutes, add the pudding to the oven and bake 40-45 minutes, or until top is beginning to brown and it passes the toothpick test.
6. Remove to wire rack and let cool 5-10 minutes before serving.
Nutrition Info: Calories 476, Total Fat 24g, Saturated Fat 15g, Total Carbs 51g, Net Carbs 48g, Protein 14g, Sugar 30g, Fiber 3g, Sodium 398mg, Potassium 443mg, Phosphorus 288mg

47. Peppery Sausage & Parsley Patties

Servings: 4
Cooking Time: 20 Minutes
Ingredients:
- 1 lb ground Italian sausage
- ¼ cup breadcrumbs
- 1 tsp dried parsley
- 1 tsp red pepper flakes
- ½ tsp salt
- ¼ tsp black pepper
- ¼ tsp garlic powder
- 1 egg, beaten

Directions:
1. Preheat on Bake function to 350 F. Combine all of the ingredients in a large bowl. Line a baking sheet

with parchment paper. Make patties out of the sausage mixture and arrange them on the baking sheet. Cook for 15 minutes, flipping once halfway through cooking. Serve.

48. Cheesy Bacon And Egg Wraps

Servings: 3
Cooking Time: 10 Minutes
Ingredients:
- 3 corn tortillas
- 3 slices bacon, cut into strips
- 2 scrambled eggs
- 3 tablespoons salsa
- 1 cup grated Pepper Jack cheese
- 3 tablespoons cream cheese, divided
- Cooking spray

Directions:
1. Spritz the air fryer basket with cooking spray.
2. Unfold the tortillas on a clean work surface, divide the bacon and eggs in the middle of the tortillas, then spread with salsa and scatter with cheeses. Fold the tortillas over.
3. Arrange the tortillas in the pan.
4. Put the air fryer basket on the baking pan and slide into Rack Position 2, select Air Fry, set temperature to 390ºF (199ºC) and set time to 10 minutes.
5. Flip the tortillas halfway through the cooking time.
6. When cooking is complete, the cheeses will be melted and the tortillas will be lightly browned.
7. Serve immediately.

49. Almond & Cinnamon Berry Oat Bars

Servings: 10
Cooking Time: 40 Minutes
Ingredients:
- 3 cups rolled oats
- ½ cup ground almonds
- ½ cup flour
- 1 tsp baking powder
- 1 tsp ground cinnamon
- 3 eggs, lightly beaten
- ½ cup canola oil
- ⅓ cup milk
- 2 tsp vanilla extract
- 2 cups mixed berries

Directions:
1. Spray the baking pan with cooking spray. In a bowl, add oats, almonds, flour, baking powder and cinnamon into and stir well. In another bowl, whisk eggs, oil, milk, and vanilla.
2. Stir the wet ingredients gently into the oat mixture. Fold in the berries. Pour the mixture in the pan and place in the toaster oven. Cook for 15-20 minutes at 350 F on Bake function until is nice and soft. Let cool and cut into bars to serve.

50. Moist Orange Bread Loaf

Servings: 10
Cooking Time: 50 Minutes
Ingredients:
- 4 eggs
- 4 oz butter, softened
- 1 cup of orange juice
- 1 orange zest, grated
- 1 cup of sugar
- 2 tsp baking powder
- 2 cups all-purpose flour
- 1 tsp vanilla

Directions:
1. Fit the oven with the rack in position
2. In a large bowl, whisk eggs and sugar until creamy.
3. Whisk in vanilla, butter, orange juice, and orange zest.
4. Add flour and baking powder and mix until combined.
5. Pour batter into the greased 9*5-inch loaf pan.
6. Set to bake at 350 F for 55 minutes, after 5 minutes, place the loaf pan in the oven.
7. Slice and serve.

Nutrition Info: Calories 286 Fat 11.3 g Carbohydrates 42.5 g Sugar 22.4 g Protein 5.1 gCholesterol 90 mg

51. Mushroom & Pepperoncini Omelet

Servings: 2
Cooking Time: 20 Minutes
Ingredients:
- 3 large eggs
- ¼ c milk
- Salt and ground black pepper, as required
- ½ cup cheddar cheese, shredded
- ¼ cup cooked mushrooms
- 3 pepperoncini peppers, sliced thinly
- ½ tablespoon scallion, sliced thinly

Directions:
1. In a bowl, add the eggs, milk, salt and black pepper and beat well.
2. Place the mixture into a greased baking pan.
3. Press "Power Button" of Air Fry Oven and turn the dial to select the "Air Bake" mode.
4. Press the Time button and again turn the dial to set the cooking time to 20 minutes.
5. Now push the Temp button and rotate the dial to set the temperature at 350 degrees F.
6. Press "Start/Pause" button to start.
7. When the unit beeps to show that it is preheated, open the lid.

8. Arrange pan over the "Wire Rack" and insert in the oven.
9. Cut into equal-sized wedges and serve hot.
Nutrition Info: Calories 254 Total Fat 17.5 g Saturated Fat 8.7 g Cholesterol 311 mg Sodium 793 mg Total Carbs 7.3 g Fiber 0.1 g Sugar 3.8 g Protein 8.2 g

52. Apricot & Almond Scones

Servings: 4
Cooking Time: 30 Minutes
Ingredients:
- 2 cups flour
- ⅓ cup sugar
- 2 tsp baking powder
- ½ cup sliced almonds
- ¾ cup dried apricots, chopped
- ¼ cup cold butter, cut into cubes
- ½ cup milk
- 1 egg
- 1 tsp vanilla extract

Directions:
1. reheat Breville on AirFry function to 370 F. Line a baking dish with parchment paper. Mix together flour, sugar, baking powder, almonds, and apricots. Rub the butter into the dry ingredients with hands to form a sandy, crumbly texture. Whisk together egg, milk, and vanilla extract.
2. Pour into the dry ingredients and stir to combine. Sprinkle a working board with flour, lay the dough onto the board and give it a few kneads. Shape into a rectangle and cut into 8 squares. Arrange the squares on the baking dish and press Start. Bake for 25 minutes. Serve chilled.

53. Basil Dill Egg Muffins

Servings: 6
Cooking Time: 20 Minutes
Ingredients:
- 6 eggs
- 1 tbsp chives, chopped
- 1 tbsp fresh basil, chopped
- 1 tbsp fresh cilantro, chopped
- 1/4 cup mozzarella cheese, grated
- 1 tbsp fresh dill, chopped
- 1 tbsp fresh parsley, chopped
- Pepper
- Salt

Directions:
1. Fit the oven with the rack in position
2. Spray 6-cups muffin tin with cooking spray and set aside.
3. In a bowl, whisk eggs with pepper and salt.
4. Add remaining ingredients and stir well.
5. Pour egg mixture into the prepared muffin tin.
6. Set to bake at 350 F for 25 minutes. After 5 minutes place muffin tin in the preheated oven.
7. Serve and enjoy.

Nutrition Info: Calories 68 Fat 4.6 g Carbohydrates 0.8 g Sugar 0.4 g Protein 6 g Cholesterol 164 mg

54. Sweet Potato Chickpeas Hash

Servings: 4
Cooking Time: 30 Minutes
Ingredients:
- 14.5 oz can chickpeas, drained
- 1 tsp paprika
- 1 tsp garlic powder
- 1 sweet potato, peeled and cubed
- 1 tbsp olive oil
- 1 bell pepper, chopped
- 1 onion, diced
- 1/2 tsp ground black pepper
- 1 tsp salt

Directions:
1. Fit the oven with the rack in position
2. Spread sweet potato, chickpeas, bell pepper, and onion in a baking pan.
3. Drizzle with oil and season with paprika, garlic powder, pepper, and salt. Stir well.
4. Set to bake at 390 F for 35 minutes, after 5 minutes, place the baking pan in the oven.

Nutrition Info: Calories 203 Fat 4.9 g Carbohydrates 34.9 g Sugar 4.7 g Protein 6.5 g Cholesterol 0 mg

55. Egg & Bacon Wraps With Salsa

Servings: 3
Cooking Time: 15 Minutes
Ingredients:
- 3 tortillas
- 2 previously scrambled eggs
- 3 slices bacon, cut into strips
- 3 tbsp salsa
- 3 tbsp cream cheese
- 1 cup Pepper Jack cheese, grated

Directions:
1. Preheat Breville on AirFry function to 390 F. Spread 1 tbsp of cream cheese onto each tortilla. Divide the eggs and bacon between the tortillas evenly. Top with salsa and sprinkle some grated cheese over. Roll up the tortillas and press Start. Cook for 10 minutes. Serve.

56. Fried Churros With Cinnamon

Ingredients:
- ¼ cup (55g) unsalted butter, melted
- ½ cup (100g) sugar
- ½ teaspoon ground cinnamon
- Special equipment
- Piping bag
- X-inch (1.5cm) closed star pastry tip
- 1 cup (240ml) water
- 1 tablespoon (15g) unsalted butter
- 1 tablespoon sugar

- ½ teaspoon vanilla extract
- ¼ teaspoon kosher salt
- 1 cup (130g) all-purpose flour
- 1 egg
- Scissors

Directions:
1. Combine water, butter, sugar, vanilla, and salt in large saucepan and bring to boil over medium-high heat. Add flour all at once and stir with wooden spoon until well combined, with no streaks of flour remaining. Transfer dough to bowl of Breville stand mixer fitted with paddle attachment.
2. Mix on medium-high speed until cooled slightly, about 1 minute.
3. Reduce speed to low and add egg. Once egg is incorporated, increase speed to high and beat until outside of bowl is cool, about 12–15 minutes. Select AIRFRY/350°F (175°C)/SUPER CONVECTION/20 minutes and press START to preheat oven.
4. Transfer dough to piping bag fitted with X-inch (1.5cm) closed star pastry tip. Pipe 3-inch (7.5cm) lengths of dough onto air fry rack, using scissors to snip dough at tip. Cook in rack position 4 until churros are brown and crisp on the outside, about 20 minutes. Place melted butter in medium bowl. Combine sugar and cinnamon in a second medium bowl.
5. Toss warm churros in melted butter and then in cinnamon sugar. Pipe remaining dough onto air fry rack and repeat steps 5–7. Serve immediately with chocolate sauce or dulce de leche for dipping.

57. Breakfast Oatmeal Cake

Servings: 8
Cooking Time: 25 Minutes
Ingredients:
- 2 eggs
- 1 tbsp coconut oil
- 3 tbsp yogurt
- 1/2 tsp baking powder
- 1 tsp cinnamon
- 1 tsp vanilla
- 3 tbsp honey
- 1/2 tsp baking soda
- 1 apple, peel & chopped
- 1 cup oats

Directions:
1. Fit the oven with the rack in position
2. Line baking dish with parchment paper and set aside.
3. Add 3/4 cup oats and remaining ingredients into the blender and blend until smooth.
4. Add remaining oats and stir well.
5. Pour mixture into the prepared baking dish.
6. Set to bake at 350 F for 30 minutes. After 5 minutes place the baking dish in the preheated oven.
7. Slice and serve.

Nutrition Info: Calories 114 Fat 3.6 g Carbohydrates 18.2 g Sugar 10 g Protein 3.2 g Cholesterol 41 mg

58. Olives, Kale, And Pecorino Baked Eggs

Servings: 2
Cooking Time: 11 Minutes
Ingredients:
- 1 cup roughly chopped kale leaves, stems and center ribs removed
- ¼ cup grated pecorino cheese
- ¼ cup olive oil
- 1 garlic clove, peeled
- 3 tablespoons whole almonds
- Kosher salt and freshly ground black pepper, to taste
- 4 large eggs
- 2 tablespoons heavy cream
- 3 tablespoons chopped pitted mixed olives

Directions:
1. Place the kale, pecorino, olive oil, garlic, almonds, salt, and pepper in a small blender and blitz until well incorporated.
2. One at a time, crack the eggs in the baking pan. Drizzle the kale pesto on top of the egg whites. Top the yolks with the cream and swirl together the yolks and the pesto.
3. Slide the baking pan into Rack Position 1, select Convection Bake, set temperature to 300ºF (150ºC) and set time to 11 minutes.
4. When cooked, the top should begin to brown and the eggs should be set.
5. Allow the eggs to cool for 5 minutes. Scatter the olives on top and serve warm.

59. Montreal Steak And Seeds Burgers

Servings: 4
Cooking Time: 10 Minutes
Ingredients:
- 1 teaspoon cumin seeds
- 1 teaspoon mustard seeds
- 1 teaspoon coriander seeds
- 1 teaspoon dried minced garlic
- 1 teaspoon dried red pepper flakes
- 1 teaspoon kosher salt
- 2 teaspoons ground black pepper
- 1 pound (454 g) 85% lean ground beef
- 2 tablespoons Worcestershire sauce
- 4 hamburger buns
- Mayonnaise, for serving
- Cooking spray

Directions:
1. Spritz the air fryer basket with cooking spray.
2. Put the seeds, garlic, red pepper flakes, salt, and ground black pepper in a food processor. Pulse to coarsely ground the mixture.
3. Put the ground beef in a large bowl. Pour in the seed mixture and drizzle with Worcestershire sauce. Stir to mix well.

4. Divide the mixture into four parts and shape each part into a ball, then bash each ball into a patty. Arrange the patties in the pan.
5. Put the air fryer basket on the baking pan and slide into Rack Position 2, select Air Fry, set temperature to 350ºF (180ºC) and set time to 10 minutes.
6. Flip the patties with tongs halfway through the cooking time.
7. When cooked, the patties will be well browned.
8. Assemble the buns with the patties, then drizzle the mayo over the patties to make the burgers. Serve immediately.

60. Whole-wheat Blueberry Scones

Servings: 14
Cooking Time: 20 Minutes
Ingredients:
- ½ cup low-fat buttermilk
- ¾ cup orange juice
- Zest of 1 orange
- 2¼ cups whole-wheat pastry flour
- ⅓ cup agave nectar
- ¼ cup canola oil
- 1 teaspoon baking soda
- 1 teaspoon cream of tartar
- 1 cup fresh blueberries

Directions:
1. In a small bowl, stir together the buttermilk, orange juice and orange zest.
2. In a large bowl, whisk together the flour, agave nectar, canola oil, baking soda and cream of tartar.
3. Add the buttermilk mixture and blueberries to the bowl with the flour mixture. Mix gently by hand until well combined.
4. Transfer the batter onto a lightly floured baking pan. Pat into a circle about ¾ inch thick and 8 inches across. Use a knife to cut the circle into 14 wedges, cutting almost all the way through.
5. Slide the baking pan into Rack Position 1, select Convection Bake, set temperature to 375ºF (190ºC) and set time to 20 minutes.
6. When cooking is complete, remove the pan and check the scones. They should be lightly browned.
7. Let rest for 5 minutes and cut completely through the wedges before serving.

61. Giant Strawberry Pancake

Servings: 3
Cooking Time: 30 Minutes
Ingredients:
- 3 eggs, beaten
- 2 tbsp butter, melted
- ½ cup flour
- 2 tbsp sugar, powdered
- ½ cup milk
- 1 ½ cups fresh strawberries, sliced

Directions:
1. Preheat on Bake function to 350 F. In a bowl, mix flour, milk, eggs, and vanilla until fully incorporated. Add the mixture a greased with melted butter pan.
2. Place the pan in your toaster oven and cook for 12-16 minutes until the pancake is fluffy and golden brown. Drizzle powdered sugar and toss sliced strawberries on top.

62. Feta & Spinach Omelet With Mushrooms

Servings: 2
Cooking Time: 10 Minutes
Ingredients:
- 4 eggs, lightly beaten
- 2 tbsp heavy cream
- 2 cups spinach, chopped
- 1 cup mushrooms, chopped
- 3 oz feta cheese, crumbled
- A handful of fresh parsley, chopped
- Salt and black pepper to taste

Directions:
1. In a bowl, whisk eggs and stir in spinach, mushrooms, feta, parsley, salt, and pepper. Pour into a greased baking pan and cook in the Breville oven for 12-14 minutes at 350 F on Bake function..

63. Herby Mushrooms With Vermouth

Servings: 4
Cooking Time: 20 Minutes
Ingredients:
- 2 lb portobello mushrooms, sliced
- 2 tbsp vermouth
- ½ tsp garlic powder
- 1 tbsp olive oil
- 2 tsp herbs
- 1 tbsp duck fat, softened

Directions:
1. Mix duck fat, garlic powder, and herbs in a bowl. Pour the mixture over the mushrooms and top with vermouth. Place the mushrooms in a baking dish and press Start. Cook for 15 minutes on Bake function at 350 F. Serve warm.

64. Tomato, Basil & Mozzarella Breakfast

Servings: 1
Cooking Time: 10 Minutes
Ingredients:
- 2 slices of bread
- 4 tomato slices
- 4 mozzarella slices
- 1 tbsp olive oil
- 1 tbsp chopped basil
- Salt and black pepper to taste

Directions:

1. Preheat on Toast function to 350 F. Place the bread slices in the toaster oven and toast for 5 minutes. Arrange two tomato slices on each bread slice. Season with salt and pepper.

65. Cinnamon & Vanilla Toast

Servings: 6
Cooking Time: 10 Minutes
Ingredients:
- 12 bread slices
- ½ cup sugar
- 1 ½ tsp cinnamon
- 1 stick of butter, softened
- 1 tsp vanilla extract

Directions:
1. Preheat Breville on Toast function to 300 F. Combine all ingredients, except the bread, in a bowl. Spread the buttery cinnamon mixture onto the bread slices. Place the bread slices in the oven and press Start. Cook for 8 minutes. Serve.

66. Raspberries Oatmeal

Servings: 4
Cooking Time: 30 Minutes
Ingredients:
- 1 ½ cups coconut; shredded
- ½ cups raspberries
- 2 cups almond milk
- ¼ tsp. nutmeg, ground
- 2 tsp. stevia
- ½ tsp. cinnamon powder
- Cooking spray

Directions:
1. Grease the air fryer's pan with cooking spray, mix all the ingredients inside, cover and cook at 360°F for 15 minutes. Divide into bowls and serve
Nutrition Info: Calories: 172; Fat: 5g; Fiber: 2g; Carbs: 4g; Protein: 6g

67. Vanilla Brownies With White Chocolate & Walnuts

Servings: 4
Cooking Time: 35 Minutes
Ingredients:
- 6 oz dark chocolate, chopped
- 6 oz butter
- ¾ cup white sugar
- 3 eggs, beaten
- 2 tsp vanilla extract
- ¾ cup flour
- ¼ cup cocoa powder
- 1 cup chopped walnuts
- 1 cup white chocolate chips

Directions:
1. Line a baking pan with parchment paper. In a saucepan, melt chocolate and butter over low heat. Do not stop stirring until you obtain a smooth mixture. Let cool slightly and whisk in eggs and vanilla. Sift flour and cocoa and stir to mix well.
2. Sprinkle the walnuts over and add the white chocolate into the batter. Pour the batter into the pan and cook for 20 minutes in the oven at 350 F on Bake function. Serve chilled with raspberry syrup and ice cream.

68. Delicious Broccoli Quiche

Servings: 8
Cooking Time: 45 Minutes
Ingredients:
- 2 eggs
- 2 1/2 cups broccoli, cooked & chopped
- 8 oz cheddar cheese, shredded
- 1/2 cup onion, chopped
- 1 1/2 cups milk
- 1 tsp baking powder
- 1 cup flour
- 1 tsp salt

Directions:
1. Fit the oven with the rack in position
2. In a large bowl, mix flour, baking powder, and salt and set aside.
3. In a separate bowl, whisk eggs. Add onion and stir well.
4. Pour egg mixture into the flour mixture and stir to combine.
5. Stir in broccoli and cheese.
6. Pour egg mixture into the greased 9-inch pie dish.
7. Set to bake at 350 F for 50 minutes. After 5 minutes place the pie dish in the preheated oven.
8. Serve and enjoy.
Nutrition Info: Calories 223 Fat 11.7 g Carbohydrates 17.5 g Sugar 3.1 g Protein 12.4 g Cholesterol 74 mg

LUNCH RECIPES

69. Easy Italian Meatballs

Servings: 4
Cooking Time: 13 Minutes
Ingredients:
- 2-lb. lean ground turkey
- ¼ cup onion, minced
- 2 cloves garlic, minced
- 2 tablespoons parsley, chopped
- 2 eggs
- 1½ cup parmesan cheese, grated
- ½ teaspoon red pepper flakes
- ½ teaspoon Italian seasoning Salt and black pepper to taste

Directions:
1. Toss all the meatball Ingredients: in a bowl and mix well.
2. Make small meatballs out this mixture and place them in the air fryer basket.
3. Press "Power Button" of Air Fry Oven and turn the dial to select the "Air Fry" mode.
4. Press the Time button and again turn the dial to set the cooking time to 13 minutes.
5. Now push the Temp button and rotate the dial to set the temperature at 350 degrees F.
6. Once preheated, place the air fryer basket inside and close its lid.
7. Flip the meatballs when cooked halfway through.
8. Serve warm.

Nutrition Info: Calories 472 Total Fat 25.8 g Saturated Fat .4 g Cholesterol 268 mg Sodium 503 mg Total Carbs 1.7 g Fiber 0.3 g Sugar 0.6 g Protein 59.6 g

70. Roasted Grape And Goat Cheese Crostinis

Servings: 10
Cooking Time: 5 Minutes
Ingredients:
- 1 pound seedless red grapes
- 1 teaspoon chopped rosemary
- 4 tablespoons olive oil
- 1 rustic French baguette
- 1 cup sliced shallots
- 2 tablespoons unsalted butter
- 8 ounces goat cheese
- 1 tablespoon honey

Directions:
1. Start by preheating toaster oven to 400°F.
2. Toss grapes, rosemary, and 1 tablespoon of olive oil in a large bowl.
3. Transfer to a roasting pan and roast for 20 minutes.
4. Remove the pan from the oven and set aside to cool.
5. Slice the baguette into 1/2-inch-thick pieces.
6. Brush each slice with olive oil and place on baking sheet.
7. Bake for 8 minutes, then remove from oven and set aside.
8. In a medium skillet add butter and one tablespoon of olive oil.
9. Add shallots and sauté for about 10 minutes.
10. Mix goat cheese and honey in a medium bowl, then add contents of shallot pan and mix thoroughly.
11. Spread shallot mixture onto baguette, top with grapes, and serve.

Nutrition Info: Calories: 238, Sodium: 139 mg, Dietary Fiber: 0.6 g, Total Fat: 16.3 g, Total Carbs: 16.4 g, Protein: 8.4 g.

71. Air Fried Sausages

Servings: 6
Cooking Time: 13 Minutes
Ingredients:
- 6 sausage
- olive oil spray

Directions:
1. Pour 5 cup of water into Instant Pot Duo Crisp Air Fryer. Place air fryer basket inside the pot, spray inside with nonstick spray and put sausage links inside.
2. Close the Air Fryer lid and steam for about 5 minutes.
3. Remove the lid once done. Spray links with olive oil and close air crisp lid.
4. Set to air crisp at 400°F for 8 min flipping halfway through so both sides get browned.

Nutrition Info: Calories 267, Total Fat 23g, Total Carbs 2g, Protein 13g

72. Lobster Tails

Servings: 2
Cooking Time: 8 Minutes
Ingredients:
- 2 6oz lobster tails
- 1 tsp salt
- 1 tsp chopped chives
- 2 Tbsp unsalted butter melted
- 1 Tbsp minced garlic
- 1 tsp lemon juice

Directions:
1. Combine butter, garlic, salt, chives, and lemon juice to prepare butter mixture.
2. Butterfly lobster tails by cutting through shell followed by removing the meat and resting it on top of the shell.
3. Place them on the tray in the Instant Pot Duo Crisp Air Fryer basket and spread butter over the top of lobster meat. Close the Air Fryer lid, select the Air Fry option and cook on 380°F for 4 minutes.

4. Open the Air Fryer lid and spread more butter on top, cook for extra 2-4 minutes until done.
Nutrition Info: Calories 120, Total Fat 12g, Total Carbs 2g, Protein 1g

73. Butter Fish With Sake And Miso

Servings: 4
Cooking Time: 11 Minutes
Ingredients:
- 4 (7-ounce) pieces of butter fish
- 1/3 cup sake
- 1/3 cup mirin
- 2/3 cup sugar
- 1 cup white miso

Directions:
1. Start by combining sake, mirin, and sugar in a sauce pan and bring to a boil.
2. Allow to boil for 5 minutes, then reduce heat and simmer for another 10 minutes.
3. Remove from heat completely and mix in miso.
4. Marinate the fish in the mixture for as long as possible, up to 3 days if possible.
5. Preheat toaster oven to 450°F and bake fish for 8 minutes.
6. Switch your setting to Broil and broil another 2-3 minutes, until the sauce is caramelized.
Nutrition Info: Calories: 529, Sodium: 2892 mg, Dietary Fiber: 3.7 g, Total Fat: 5.8 g, Total Carbs: 61.9 g, Protein: 53.4 g.

74. Lemon Chicken Breasts

Servings: 4
Cooking Time: 30 Minutes
Ingredients:
- 1/4 cup olive oil
- 3 tablespoons garlic, minced
- 1/3 cup dry white wine
- 1 tablespoon lemon zest, grated
- 2 tablespoons lemon juice
- 1 1/2 teaspoons dried oregano, crushed
- 1 teaspoon thyme leaves, minced
- Salt and black pepper
- 4 skin-on boneless chicken breasts
- 1 lemon, sliced

Directions:
1. Whisk everything in a baking pan to coat the chicken breasts well.
2. Place the lemon slices on top of the chicken breasts.
3. Spread the mustard mixture over the toasted bread slices.
4. Press "Power Button" of Air Fry Oven and turn the dial to select the "Bake" mode.
5. Press the Time button and again turn the dial to set the cooking time to 30 minutes.
6. Now push the Temp button and rotate the dial to set the temperature at 370 degrees F.
7. Once preheated, place the baking pan inside and close its lid.
8. Serve warm.
Nutrition Info: Calories 388 Total Fat 8 g Saturated Fat 1 g Cholesterol 153mg sodium 339 mg Total Carbs 8 g Fiber 1 g Sugar 2 g Protein 13 g

75. Turkey And Broccoli Stew

Servings: 4
Cooking Time: 12 Minutes
Ingredients:
- 1 broccoli head, florets separated
- 1 turkey breast, skinless; boneless and cubed
- 1 cup tomato sauce
- 1 tbsp. parsley; chopped.
- 1 tbsp. olive oil
- Salt and black pepper to taste.

Directions:
1. In a baking dish that fits your air fryer, mix the turkey with the rest of the ingredients except the parsley, toss, introduce the dish in the fryer, bake at 380°F for 25 minutes
2. Divide into bowls, sprinkle the parsley on top and serve.
Nutrition Info: Calories: 250; Fat: 11g; Fiber: 2g; Carbs: 6g; Protein: 12g

76. Glazed Lamb Chops

Servings: 4
Cooking Time: 15 Minutes
Ingredients:
- 1 tablespoon Dijon mustard
- ½ tablespoon fresh lime juice
- 1 teaspoon honey
- ½ teaspoon olive oil
- Salt and ground black pepper, as required
- 4 (4-ounce) lamb loin chops

Directions:
1. In a black pepper large bowl, mix together the mustard, lemon juice, oil, honey, salt, and black pepper.
2. Add the chops and coat with the mixture generously.
3. Place the chops onto the greased "Sheet Pan".
4. Press "Power Button" of Ninja Foodi Digital Air Fry Oven and turn the dial to select the "Air Bake" mode.
5. Press the Time button and again turn the dial to set the cooking time to 15 minutes.
6. Now push the Temp button and rotate the dial to set the temperature at 390 degrees F.
7. Press "Start/Pause" button to start.
8. When the unit beeps to show that it is preheated, open the lid.

9. Insert the "Sheet Pan" in oven.
10. Flip the chops once halfway through.
11. Serve hot.

Nutrition Info: Calories: 224 kcal Total Fat: 9.1 g Saturated Fat: 3.1 g Cholesterol: 102 mg Sodium: 169 mg Total Carbs: 1.7 g Fiber: 0.1 g Sugar: 1.5 g Protein: 32 g

77. Turmeric Mushroom(3)

Servings: 4
Cooking Time: 12 Minutes
Ingredients:
- 1 lb. brown mushrooms
- 4 garlic cloves; minced
- ¼ tsp. cinnamon powder
- 1 tsp. olive oil
- ½ tsp. turmeric powder
- Salt and black pepper to taste.

Directions:
1. In a bowl, combine all the ingredients and toss.
2. Put the mushrooms in your air fryer's basket and cook at 370°F for 15 minutes
3. Divide the mix between plates and serve as a side dish.

Nutrition Info: Calories: 208; Fat: 7g; Fiber: 3g; Carbs: 5g; Protein: 7g

78. Chicken And Celery Stew

Servings: 6
Cooking Time: 12 Minutes
Ingredients:
- 1 lb. chicken breasts, skinless; boneless and cubed
- 4 celery stalks; chopped.
- ½ cup coconut cream
- 2 red bell peppers; chopped.
- 2 tsp. garlic; minced
- 1 tbsp. butter, soft
- Salt and black pepper to taste.

Directions:
1. Grease a baking dish that fits your air fryer with the butter, add all the ingredients in the pan and toss them.
2. Introduce the dish in the fryer, cook at 360°F for 30 minutes, divide into bowls and serve

Nutrition Info: Calories: 246; Fat: 12g; Fiber: 2g; Carbs: 6g; Protein: 12g

79. Parmesan-crusted Pork Loin

Servings: 4
Cooking Time: 20 Minutes
Ingredients:
- 1 pound pork loin
- 1 teaspoon salt
- 1/2 tablespoon garlic powder
- 1/2 tablespoon onion powder
- 2 tablespoons parmesan cheese
- 1 tablespoon olive oil

Directions:
1. Start by preheating toaster oven to 475°F.
2. Place pan in the oven and let it heat while the oven preheats.
3. Mix all ingredients in a shallow dish and roll the pork loin until it is fully coated.
4. Remove pan and sear the pork in the pan on each side.
5. Once seared, bake pork in the pan for 20 minutes.

Nutrition Info: Calories: 334, Sodium: 718 mg, Dietary Fiber: 0 g, Total Fat: 20.8 g, Total Carbs: 1.7 g, Protein: 33.5 g.

80. Herbed Duck Legs

Servings: 2
Cooking Time: 30 Minutes
Ingredients:
- ½ tablespoon fresh thyme, chopped
- ½ tablespoon fresh parsley, chopped
- 2 duck legs
- 1 garlic clove, minced
- 1 teaspoon five spice powder
- Salt and black pepper, as required

Directions:
1. Preheat the Air fryer to 340 degree F and grease an Air fryer basket.
2. Mix the garlic, herbs, five spice powder, salt, and black pepper in a bowl.
3. Rub the duck legs with garlic mixture generously and arrange into the Air fryer basket.
4. Cook for about 25 minutes and set the Air fryer to 390 degree F.
5. Cook for 5 more minutes and dish out to serve hot.

Nutrition Info: Calories: 138, Fat: 4.5g, Carbohydrates: 1g, Sugar: 0g, Protein: 25g, Sodium: 82mg

81. Seven-layer Tostadas

Servings: 6
Cooking Time: 5 Minutes
Ingredients:
- 1 (16-ounce) can refried pinto beans
- 1-1/2 cups guacamole
- 1 cup light sour cream
- 1/2 teaspoon taco seasoning
- 1 cup shredded Mexican cheese blend
- 1 cup chopped tomatoes
- 1/2 cup thinly sliced green onions
- 1/2 cup sliced black olives

- 6-8 whole wheat flour tortillas small enough to fit in your oven
- Olive oil

Directions:
1. Start by placing baking sheet into toaster oven while preheating it to 450°F. Remove pan and drizzle with olive oil.
2. Place tortillas on pan and cook in oven until they are crisp, turn at least once, this should take about 5 minutes or less.
3. In a medium bowl, mash refried beans to break apart any chunks, then microwave for 2 1/2 minutes.
4. Stir taco seasoning into the sour cream. Chop vegetables and halve olives.
5. Top tortillas with ingredients in this order: refried beans, guacamole, sour cream, shredded cheese, tomatoes, onions, and olives.

Nutrition Info: Calories: 657, Sodium: 581 mg, Dietary Fiber: 16.8 g, Total Fat: 31.7 g, Total Carbs: 71.3 g, Protein: 28.9 g.

82. Beef Steaks With Beans

Servings: 4
Cooking Time: 10 Minutes
Ingredients:
- 4 beef steaks, trim the fat and cut into strips
- 1 cup green onions, chopped
- 2 cloves garlic, minced
- 1 red bell pepper, seeded and thinly sliced
- 1 can tomatoes, crushed
- 1 can cannellini beans
- 3/4 cup beef broth
- 1/4 teaspoon dried basil
- 1/2 teaspoon cayenne pepper
- 1/2 teaspoon sea salt
- 1/4 teaspoon ground black pepper, or to taste

Directions:
1. Preparing the ingredients. Add the steaks, green onions and garlic to the instant crisp air fryer basket.
2. Air frying. Close air fryer lid. Cook at 390 degrees f for 10 minutes, working in batches.
3. Stir in the remaining ingredients and cook for an additional 5 minutes.

Nutrition Info: Calories 284 Total fat 7.9 g Saturated fat 1.4 g Cholesterol 36 mg Sodium 704 mg Total carbs 46 g Fiber 3.6 g Sugar 5.5 g Protein 17.9 g

83. Sweet Potato Chips

Servings: 2
Cooking Time: 40 Minutes
Ingredients:
- 2 sweet potatoes
- Salt and pepper to taste
- Olive oil
- Cinnamon

Directions:
1. Start by preheating toaster oven to 400°F.
2. Cut off each end of potato and discard.
3. Cut potatoes into 1/2-inch slices.
4. Brush a pan with olive oil and lay potato slices flat on the pan.
5. Bake for 20 minutes, then flip and bake for another 20.

Nutrition Info: Calories: 139, Sodium: 29 mg, Dietary Fiber: 8.2 g, Total Fat: 0.5 g, Total Carbs: 34.1 g, Protein: 1.9 g.

84. Spanish Chicken Bake

Servings: 4
Cooking Time: 25 Minutes
Ingredients:
- ½ onion, quartered
- ½ red onion, quartered
- ½ lb. potatoes, quartered
- 4 garlic cloves
- 4 tomatoes, quartered
- 1/8 cup chorizo
- ¼ teaspoon paprika powder
- 4 chicken thighs, boneless
- ¼ teaspoon dried oregano
- ½ green bell pepper, julienned
- Salt
- Black pepper

Directions:
1. Toss chicken, veggies, and all the Ingredients: in a baking tray.
2. Press "Power Button" of Air Fry Oven and turn the dial to select the "Bake" mode.
3. Press the Time button and again turn the dial to set the cooking time to 25 minutes.
4. Now push the Temp button and rotate the dial to set the temperature at 425 degrees F.
5. Once preheated, place the baking pan inside and close its lid.
6. Serve warm.

Nutrition Info: Calories 301 Total Fat 8.9 g Saturated Fat 4.5 g Cholesterol 57 mg Sodium 340 mg Total Carbs 24.7 g Fiber 1.2 g Sugar 1.3 g Protein 15.3 g

85. Lemon Pepper Turkey

Servings: 6
Cooking Time: 45 Minutes
Ingredients:
- 3 lbs. turkey breast
- 2 tablespoons oil
- 1 tablespoon Worcestershire sauce
- 1 teaspoon lemon pepper
- 1/2 teaspoon salt

Directions:
1. Whisk everything in a bowl and coat the turkey liberally.

2. Place the turkey in the Air fryer basket.
3. Press "Power Button" of Air Fry Oven and turn the dial to select the "Air Fry" mode.
4. Press the Time button and again turn the dial to set the cooking time to 45 minutes.
5. Now push the Temp button and rotate the dial to set the temperature at 375 degrees F.
6. Once preheated, place the air fryer basket inside and close its lid.
7. Serve warm.
Nutrition Info: Calories 391 Total Fat 2.8 g Saturated Fat 0.6 g Cholesterol 330 mg Sodium 62 mg Total Carbs 36.5 g Fiber 9.2 g Sugar 4.5 g Protein 6.6

86. Lime And Mustard Marinated Chicken

Servings: 4
Cooking Time: 10 Minutes
Ingredients:
- 1/2 teaspoon stone-ground mustard
- 1/2 teaspoon minced fresh oregano
- 1/3 cup freshly squeezed lime juice
- 2 small-sized chicken breasts, skin-on
- 1 teaspoon kosher salt
- 1teaspoon freshly cracked mixed peppercorns

Directions:
1. Preheat your Air Fryer to 345 degrees F.
2. Toss all of the above ingredients in a medium-sized mixing dish; allow it to marinate overnight.
3. Cook in the preheated Air Fryer for 26 minutes.

Nutrition Info: 255 Calories; 15g Fat; 7g Carbs; 33g Protein; 8g Sugars; 3g Fiber

87. Turkey Legs

Servings: 2
Cooking Time: 40 Minutes
Ingredients:
- 2 large turkey legs
- 1 1/2 tsp smoked paprika
- 1 tsp brown sugar
- 1 tsp season salt
- ½ tsp garlic powder
- oil for spraying avocado, canola, etc.

Directions:
1. Mix the smoked paprika, brown sugar, seasoned salt, garlic powder thoroughly.
2. Wash and pat dry the turkey legs.
3. Rub the made seasoning mixture all over the turkey legs making sure to get under the skin also.
4. While preparing for cooking, select the Air Fry option. Press start to begin preheating.
5. Once the preheating temperature is reached, place the turkey legs on the tray in the Instant Pot Duo Crisp Air Fryer basket. Lightly spray them with oil.
6. Air Fry the turkey legs on 400°F for 20 minutes. Then, open the Air Fryer lid and flip the turkey legs and lightly spray with oil. Close the Instant Pot Duo Crisp Air Fryer lid and cook for 20 more minutes.
7. Remove and Enjoy.

Nutrition Info: Calories 958, Total Fat 46g, Total Carbs 3g, Protein 133g

88. Mushroom Meatloaf

Servings: 4
Cooking Time: 25 Minutes
Ingredients:
- 14-ounce lean ground beef
- 1 chorizo sausage, chopped finely
- 1 small onion, chopped
- 1 garlic clove, minced
- 2 tablespoons fresh cilantro, chopped
- 3 tablespoons breadcrumbs
- 1 egg
- Salt and freshly ground black pepper, to taste
- 2 tablespoons fresh mushrooms, sliced thinly
- 3 tablespoons olive oil

Directions:
1. Preparing the ingredients. Preheat the instant crisp air fryer to 390 degrees f.
2. In a large bowl, add all ingredients except mushrooms and mix till well combined.
3. In a baking pan, place the beef mixture.
4. With the back of spatula, smooth the surface.
5. Top with mushroom slices and gently, press into the meatloaf.
6. Drizzle with oil evenly.
7. Air frying. Arrange the pan in the instant crisp air fryer basket, close air fryer lid and cook for about 25 minutes.
8. Cut the meatloaf in desires size wedges and serve.

Nutrition Info: Calories 284 Total fat 7.9 g Saturated fat 1.4 g Cholesterol 36 mg Sodium 704 mg Total carbs 46 g Fiber 3.6 g Sugar 5.5 g Protein 17.9 g

89. Green Bean Casserole(2)

Servings: 4
Cooking Time: 12 Minutes
Ingredients:
- 1 lb. fresh green beans, edges trimmed
- ½ oz. pork rinds, finely ground
- 1 oz. full-fat cream cheese
- ½ cup heavy whipping cream.
- ¼ cup diced yellow onion
- ½ cup chopped white mushrooms
- ½ cup chicken broth
- 4 tbsp. unsalted butter.
- ¼ tsp. xanthan gum

Directions:

1. In a medium skillet over medium heat, melt the butter. Sauté the onion and mushrooms until they become soft and fragrant, about 3–5 minutes.
2. Add the heavy whipping cream, cream cheese and broth to the pan. Whisk until smooth. Bring to a boil and then reduce to a simmer. Sprinkle the xanthan gum into the pan and remove from heat
3. Chop the green beans into 2-inch pieces and place into a 4-cup round baking dish. Pour the sauce mixture over them and stir until coated. Top the dish with ground pork rinds. Place into the air fryer basket
4. Adjust the temperature to 320 Degrees F and set the timer for 15 minutes. Top will be golden and green beans fork tender when fully cooked. Serve warm.
Nutrition Info: Calories: 267; Protein: 6g; Fiber: 2g; Fat: 24g; Carbs: 7g

90. Persimmon Toast With Sour Cream & Cinnamon

Servings: 1
Cooking Time: 5 Minutes
Ingredients:
- 1 slice of wheat bread
- 1/2 persimmon
- Sour cream to taste
- Sugar to taste
- Cinnamon to taste

Directions:
1. Spread a thin layer of sour cream across the bread.
2. Slice the persimmon into 1/4 inch pieces and lay them across the bread.
3. Sprinkle cinnamon and sugar over persimmon.
4. Toast in toaster oven until bread and persimmon begin to brown.
Nutrition Info: Calories: 89, Sodium: 133 mg, Dietary Fiber: 2.0 g, Total Fat: 1.1 g, Total Carbs: 16.5 g, Protein: 3.8 g.

91. Chicken Parmesan

Servings: 4
Cooking Time: 10 Minutes
Ingredients:
- 2 (6-oz.boneless, skinless chicken breasts
- 1 oz. pork rinds, crushed
- ½ cup grated Parmesan cheese, divided.
- 1 cup low-carb, no-sugar-added pasta sauce.
- 1 cup shredded mozzarella cheese, divided.
- 4 tbsp. full-fat mayonnaise, divided.
- ½ tsp. garlic powder.
- ¼ tsp. dried oregano.
- ½ tsp. dried parsley.

Directions:
1. Slice each chicken breast in half lengthwise and lb. out to 3/4-inch thickness. Sprinkle with garlic powder, oregano and parsley
2. Spread 1 tbsp. mayonnaise on top of each piece of chicken, then sprinkle ¼ cup mozzarella on each piece.
3. In a small bowl, mix the crushed pork rinds and Parmesan. Sprinkle the mixture on top of mozzarella
4. Pour sauce into 6-inch round baking pan and place chicken on top. Place pan into the air fryer basket. Adjust the temperature to 320 Degrees F and set the timer for 25 minutes
5. Cheese will be browned and internal temperature of the chicken will be at least 165 Degrees F when fully cooked. Serve warm.
Nutrition Info: Calories: 393; Protein: 32g; Fiber: 1g; Fat: 28g; Carbs: 8g

92. Boneless Air Fryer Turkey Breasts

Servings: 4
Cooking Time: 50 Minutes
Ingredients:
- 3 lb boneless breast
- ¼ cup mayonnaise
- 2 tsp poultry seasoning
- 1 tsp salt
- ½ tsp garlic powder
- ¼ tsp black pepper

Directions:
1. Choose the Air Fry option on the Instant Pot Duo Crisp Air fryer. Set the temperature to 360°F and push start. The preheating will start.
2. Season your boneless turkey breast with mayonnaise, poultry seasoning, salt, garlic powder, and black pepper.
3. Once preheated, Air Fry the turkey breasts on 360°F for 1 hour, turning every 15 minutes or until internal temperature has reached a temperature of 165°F.
Nutrition Info: Calories 558, Total Fat 18g, Total Carbs 1g, Protein 98g

93. Chicken & Rice Casserole

Servings: 6
Cooking Time: 40 Minutes
Ingredients:
- 2 lbs. bone-in chicken thighs
- Salt and black pepper
- 1 teaspoon olive oil
- 5 cloves garlic, chopped
- 2 large onions, chopped
- 2 large red bell peppers, chopped
- 1 tablespoon sweet Hungarian paprika
- 1 teaspoon hot Hungarian paprika
- 2 tablespoons tomato paste
- 2 cups chicken broth

- 3 cups brown rice, thawed
- 2 tablespoons parsley, chopped
- 6 tablespoons sour cream

Directions:
1. Mix broth, tomato paste, and all the spices in a bowl.
2. Add chicken and mix well to coat.
3. Spread the rice in a casserole dish and add chicken along with its marinade.
4. Top the casserole with the rest of the Ingredients:.
5. Press "Power Button" of Air Fry Oven and turn the dial to select the "Bake" mode.
6. Press the Time button and again turn the dial to set the cooking time to 40 minutes.
7. Now push the Temp button and rotate the dial to set the temperature at 350 degrees F.
8. Once preheated, place the baking pan inside and close its lid.
9. Serve warm.

Nutrition Info: Calories 440 Total Fat 7.9 g Saturated Fat 1.8 g Cholesterol 5 mg Sodium 581 mg Total Carbs 21.8 g Sugar 7.1 g Fiber 2.6 g Protein 37.2 g

94. Spice-roasted Almonds

Servings: 32
Cooking Time: 10 Minutes
Ingredients:
- 1 tablespoon chili powder
- 1 tablespoon olive oil
- 1/2 teaspoon salt
- 1/2 teaspoon ground cumin
- 1/2 teaspoon ground coriander
- 1/4 teaspoon ground cinnamon
- 1/4 teaspoon black pepper
- 2 cups whole almonds

Directions:
1. Start by preheating toaster oven to 350°F.
2. Mix olive oil, chili powder, coriander, cinnamon, cumin, salt, and pepper.
3. Add almonds and toss together.
4. Transfer to a baking pan and bake for 10 minutes.

Nutrition Info: Calories: 39, Sodium: 37 mg, Dietary Fiber: 0.8 g, Total Fat: 3.5 g, Total Carbs: 1.4 g, Protein: 1.3 g.

95. Chili Chicken Sliders

Servings: 4
Cooking Time: 10 Minutes
Ingredients:
- 1/3 teaspoon paprika
- 1/3 cup scallions, peeled and chopped
- 3 cloves garlic, peeled and minced
- 1 teaspoon ground black pepper, or to taste
- 1/2 teaspoon fresh basil, minced
- 1 ½ cups chicken, minced
- 1 ½ tablespoons coconut aminos
- 1/2 teaspoon grated fresh ginger
- 1/2 tablespoon chili sauce
- 1 teaspoon salt

Directions:
1. Thoroughly combine all ingredients in a mixing dish. Then, form into 4 patties.
2. Cook in the preheated Air Fryer for 18 minutes at 355 degrees F.
3. Garnish with toppings of choice.

Nutrition Info: 366 Calories; 6g Fat; 4g Carbs; 66g Protein; 3g Sugars; 9g Fiber

96. Simple Lamb Bbq With Herbed Salt

Servings: 8
Cooking Time: 1 Hour 20 Minutes
Ingredients:
- 2 ½ tablespoons herb salt
- 2 tablespoons olive oil
- 4 pounds boneless leg of lamb, cut into 2-inch chunks

Directions:
1. Preheat the air fryer to 390F.
2. Place the grill pan accessory in the air fryer.
3. Season the meat with the herb salt and brush with olive oil.
4. Grill the meat for 20 minutes per batch.
5. Make sure to flip the meat every 10 minutes for even cooking.

Nutrition Info: Calories: 347 kcal Total Fat: 17.8 g Saturated Fat: 0 g Cholesterol: 0 mg Sodium: 0 mg Total Carbs: 0 g Fiber: 0 g Sugar: 0 g Protein: 46.6 g

97. Onion Omelet

Servings: 2
Cooking Time: 15 Minutes
Ingredients:
- 4 eggs
- ¼ teaspoon low-sodium soy sauce
- Ground black pepper, as required
- 1 teaspoon butter
- 1 medium yellow onion, sliced
- ¼ cup Cheddar cheese, grated

Directions:
1. In a skillet, melt the butter over medium heat and cook the onion and cook for about 8-10 minutes.
2. Remove from the heat and set aside to cool slightly.
3. Meanwhile, in a bowl, add the eggs, soy sauce and black pepper and beat well.
4. Add the cooked onion and gently, stir to combine.
5. Place the zucchini mixture into a small baking pan.

6. Press "Power Button" of Air Fry Oven and turn the dial to select the "Air Fry" mode.
7. Press the Time button and again turn the dial to set the cooking time to 5 minutes.
8. Now push the Temp button and rotate the dial to set the temperature at 355 degrees F.
9. Press "Start/Pause" button to start.
10. When the unit beeps to show that it is preheated, open the lid.
11. Arrange pan over the "Wire Rack" and insert in the oven.
12. Cut the omelet into 2 portions and serve hot.
Nutrition Info: Calories: 222 Cal Total Fat: 15.4 g Saturated Fat: 6.9 g Cholesterol: 347 mg Sodium: 264 mg Total Carbs: 6.1 g Fiber: 1.2 g Sugar: 3.1 g Protein: 15.3 g

98. Rolled Salmon Sandwich

Servings: 1
Cooking Time: 5 Minutes
Ingredients:
- 1 piece of flatbread
- 1 salmon filet
- Pinch of salt
- 1 tablespoon green onion, chopped
- 1/4 teaspoon dried sumac
- 1/2 teaspoon thyme
- 1/2 teaspoon sesame seeds
- 1/4 English cucumber
- 1 tablespoon yogurt

Directions:
1. Start by peeling and chopping the cucumber. Cut the salmon at a 45-degree angle into 4 slices and lay them flat on the flatbread.
2. Sprinkle salmon with salt to taste. Sprinkle onions, thyme, sumac, and sesame seeds evenly over the salmon.
3. Broil the salmon for at least 3 minutes, but longer if you want a more well-done fish.
4. While you broil your salmon, mix together the yogurt and cucumber. Remove your flatbread from the toaster oven and put it on a plate, then spoon the yogurt mix over the salmon.
5. Fold the sides of the flatbread in and roll it up for a gourmet lunch that you can take on the go.
Nutrition Info: Calories: 347, Sodium: 397 mg, Dietary Fiber: 1.6 g, Total Fat: 12.4 g, Total Carbs: 20.6 g, Protein: 38.9 g.

99. Chicken Legs With Dilled Brussels Sprouts

Servings: 2
Cooking Time: 10 Minutes
Ingredients:
- 2 chicken legs
- 1/2 teaspoon paprika
- 1/2 teaspoon kosher salt
- 1/2 teaspoon black pepper
- 1/2 pound Brussels sprouts
- 1 teaspoon dill, fresh or dried

Directions:
1. Start by preheating your Air Fryer to 370 degrees F.
2. Now, season your chicken with paprika, salt, and pepper. Transfer the chicken legs to the cooking basket. Cook for 10 minutes.
3. Flip the chicken legs and cook an additional 10 minutes. Reserve.
4. Add the Brussels sprouts to the cooking basket; sprinkle with dill. Cook at 380 degrees F for 15 minutes, shaking the basket halfway through.
5. Serve with the reserved chicken legs.
Nutrition Info: 365 Calories; 21g Fat; 3g Carbs; 36g Protein; 2g Sugars; 3g Fiber

100. Ricotta Toasts With Salmon

Servings: 2
Cooking Time: 4 Minutes
Ingredients:
- 4 bread slices
- 1 garlic clove, minced
- 8 oz. ricotta cheese
- 1 teaspoon lemon zest
- Freshly ground black pepper, to taste
- 4 oz. smoked salmon

Directions:
1. In a food processor, add the garlic, ricotta, lemon zest and black pepper and pulse until smooth.
2. Spread ricotta mixture over each bread slices evenly.
3. Press "Power Button" of Air Fry Oven and turn the dial to select the "Air Fry" mode.
4. Press the Time button and again turn the dial to set the cooking time to 4 minutes.
5. Now push the Temp button and rotate the dial to set the temperature at 355 degrees F.
6. Press "Start/Pause" button to start.
7. When the unit beeps to show that it is preheated, open the lid and lightly, grease the sheet pan.
8. Arrange the bread slices into "Air Fry Basket" and insert in the oven.
9. Top with salmon and serve.
Nutrition Info: Calories: 274 Cal Total Fat: 12 g Saturated Fat: 6.3 g Cholesterol: 48 mg Sodium: 1300 mg Total Carbs: 15.7 g Fiber: 0.5 g Sugar: 1.2 g Protein: 24.8 g

101. Sweet Potato Rosti

Servings: 2
Cooking Time: 15 Minutes
Ingredients:

- ½ lb. sweet potatoes, peeled, grated and squeezed
- 1 tablespoon fresh parsley, chopped finely
- Salt and ground black pepper, as required
- 2 tablespoons sour cream

Directions:
1. In a large bowl, mix together the grated sweet potato, parsley, salt, and black pepper.
2. Press "Power Button" of Air Fry Oven and turn the dial to select the "Air Fry" mode.
3. Press the Time button and again turn the dial to set the cooking time to 15 minutes.
4. Now push the Temp button and rotate the dial to set the temperature at 355 degrees F.
5. Press "Start/Pause" button to start.
6. When the unit beeps to show that it is preheated, open the lid and lightly, grease the sheet pan.
7. Arrange the sweet potato mixture into the "Sheet Pan" and shape it into an even circle.
8. Insert the "Sheet Pan" in the oven.
9. Cut the potato rosti into wedges.
10. Top with the sour cream and serve immediately.

Nutrition Info: Calories: 160 Cal Total Fat: 2.7 g Saturated Fat: 1.6 g Cholesterol: 5 mg Sodium: 95 mg Total Carbs: 32.3 g Fiber: 4.7 g Sugar: 0.6 g Protein: 2.2 g

102. Fried Chicken Tacos

Servings: 4
Cooking Time: 10 Minutes
Ingredients:
- Chicken
- 1 lb. chicken tenders or breast chopped into 2-inch pieces
- 1 tsp garlic powder
- ½ tsp onion powder
- 1 large egg
- 1 ½ tsp salt
- 1 tsp paprika
- 3 Tbsp buttermilk
- ¾ cup All-purpose flour
- 3 Tbsp corn starch
- ½ tsp black pepper
- ½ tsp cayenne pepper
- oil for spraying
- Coleslaw
- ¼ tsp red pepper flakes
- 2 cups coleslaw mix
- 1 Tbsp brown sugar
- ½ tsp salt
- 2 Tbsp apple cider vinegar
- 1 Tbsp water
- Spicy Mayo
- ½ tsp salt
- ¼ cup mayonnaise
- 1 tsp garlic powder
- 2 Tbsp hot sauce
- 1 Tbsp buttermilk
- Tortilla wrappers

Directions:
1. Take a large bowl and mix together coleslaw mix, water, brown sugar, salt, apple cider vinegar, and red pepper flakes. Set aside.
2. Take another small bowl and combine mayonnaise, hot sauce, buttermilk, garlic powder, and salt. Set this mixture aside.
3. Select the Instant Pot Duo Crisp Air Fryer option, adjust the temperature to 360°F and push start. Preheating will start.
4. Create a clear station by placing two large flat pans side by side. Whisk together egg and buttermilk with salt and pepper in one of them. In the second, whisk flour, corn starch, black pepper, garlic powder, onion powder, salt, paprika, and cayenne pepper.
5. Cut the chicken tenders into 1-inch pieces. Season all pieces with a little salt and pepper.
6. Once the Instant Pot Duo Crisp Air Fryer is preheated, remove the tray and lightly spray it with oil. Coat your chicken with egg mixture while shaking off any excess egg, followed by the flour mixture, and place it on the tray and tray in the basket, making sure your chicken pieces don't overlap.
7. Close the Air Fryer lid, and cook on 360°F for 10 minutes
8. while flipping and spraying halfway through cooking.
9. Once the chicken is done, remove and place chicken into warmed tortilla shells. Top with coleslaw and spicy mayonnaise.

Nutrition Info: Calories 375, Total Fat 15g, Total Carbs 31g, Protein 29g

103. Air Fryer Fish

Servings: 4
Cooking Time: 17 Minutes
Ingredients:
- 4-6 Whiting Fish fillets cut in half
- Oil to mist
- Fish Seasoning
- ¾ cup very fine cornmeal
- ¼ cup flour
- 2 tsp old bay
- 1 ½ tsp salt
- 1 tsp paprika
- ½ tsp garlic powder
- ½ tsp black pepper

Directions:
1. Put the Ingredients: for fish seasoning in a Ziplock bag and shake it well. Set aside.
2. Rinse and pat dry the fish fillets with paper towels. Make sure that they still are damp.
3. Place the fish fillets in a ziplock bag and shake until they are completely covered with seasoning.
4. Place the fillets on a baking rack to let any excess flour to fall off.

5. Grease the bottom of the Instant Pot Duo Crisp Air Fryer basket tray and place the fillets on the tray. Close the lid, select the Air Fry option and cook filets on 400°F for 10 minutes.
6. Open the Air Fryer lid and spray the fish with oil on the side facing up before flipping it over, ensure that the fish is fully coated. Flip and cook another side of the fish for 7 minutes. Remove the fish and serve.
Nutrition Info: Calories 193, Total Fat 1g, Total Carbs 27g, Protein 19g

104. Basic Roasted Tofu

Servings: 4
Cooking Time: 45 Minutes
Ingredients:
- 1 or more (16-ounce) containers extra-firm tofu
- 1 tablespoon sesame oil
- 1 tablespoon soy sauce
- 1 tablespoon rice vinegar
- 1 tablespoon water

Directions:
1. Start by drying the tofu: first pat dry with paper towels, then lay on another set of paper towels or a dish towel.
2. Put a plate on top of the tofu then put something heavy on the plate (like a large can of vegetables). Leave it there for at least 20 minutes.
3. While tofu is being pressed, whip up marinade by combining oil, soy sauce, vinegar, and water in a bowl and set aside.
4. Cut the tofu into squares or sticks. Place the tofu in the marinade for at least 30 minutes.
5. Preheat toaster oven to 350°F. Line a pan with parchment paper and add as many pieces of tofu as you can, giving each piece adequate space.
6. Bake 20–45 minutes; tofu is done when the outside edges look golden brown. Time will vary depending on tofu size and shape.
Nutrition Info: Calories: 114, Sodium: 239 mg, Dietary Fiber: 1.1 g, Total Fat: 8.1 g, Total Carbs: 2.2 g, Protein: 9.5 g.

105. Vegetarian Philly Sandwich

Servings: 2
Cooking Time: 20 Minutes
Ingredients:
- 2 tablespoons olive oil
- 8 ounces sliced portabello mushrooms
- 1 vidalia onion, thinly sliced
- 1 green bell pepper, thinly sliced
- 1 red bell pepper, thinly sliced
- Salt and pepper
- 4 slices 2% provolone cheese
- 4 rolls

Directions:
1. Preheat toaster oven to 475°F.
2. Heat the oil in a medium sauce pan over medium heat.
3. Sauté mushrooms about 5 minutes, then add the onions and peppers and sauté another 10 minutes.
4. Slice rolls lengthwise and divide the vegetables into each roll.
5. Add the cheese and toast until the rolls start to brown and the cheese melts.
Nutrition Info: Calories: 645, Sodium: 916 mg, Dietary Fiber: 7.2 g, Total Fat: 33.3 g, Total Carbs: 61.8 g, Protein: 27.1 g.

106. Tomato And Avocado

Servings: 4
Cooking Time: 12 Minutes
Ingredients:
- ½ lb. cherry tomatoes; halved
- 2 avocados, pitted; peeled and cubed
- 1 ¼ cup lettuce; torn
- 1/3 cup coconut cream
- A pinch of salt and black pepper
- Cooking spray

Directions:
1. Grease the air fryer with cooking spray, combine the tomatoes with avocados, salt, pepper and the cream and cook at 350°F for 5 minutes shaking once
2. In a salad bowl, mix the lettuce with the tomatoes and avocado mix, toss and serve.
Nutrition Info: Calories: 226; Fat: 12g; Fiber: 2g; Carbs: 4g; Protein: 8g

107. Sweet & Sour Pork

Servings: 4
Cooking Time: 27 Minutes
Ingredients:
- 2 pounds Pork cut into chunks
- 2 large Eggs
- 1 teaspoon Pure Sesame Oil (optional)
- 1 cup Potato Starch (or cornstarch)
- 1/2 teaspoon Sea Salt
- 1/4 teaspoon Freshly Ground Black Pepper
- 1/16 teaspoon Chinese Five Spice
- 3 Tablespoons Canola Oil
- Oil Mister

Directions:
1. In a mixing bowl, combine salt, potato starch, Chinese Five Spice, and peppers.
2. In another bowl, beat the eggs & add sesame oil.
3. Then dredge the pieces of Pork into the Potato Starch and remove the excess. Then dip each piece into the egg mixture, shake off excess, and then back into the Potato Starch mixture.
4. Place pork pieces into the Instant Pot Duo Crisp Air Fryer Basket after spray the pork with oil.

5. Close the Air Fryer lid and cook at 340°F for approximately 8 to12 minutes (or until pork is cooked), shaking the basket a couple of times for evenly distribution.
Nutrition Info: Calories 521, Total Fat 21g, Total Carbs 23g, Protein 60g

108. Sweet Potato And Parsnip Spiralized Latkes

Servings: 12
Cooking Time: 20 Minutes
Ingredients:
- 1 medium sweet potato
- 1 large parsnip
- 4 cups water
- 1 egg + 1 egg white
- 2 scallions
- 1/2 teaspoon garlic powder
- 1/2 teaspoon sea salt
- 1/2 teaspoon ground pepper

Directions:
1. Start by spiralizing the sweet potato and parsnip and chopping the scallions, reserving only the green parts.
2. Preheat toaster oven to 425°F.
3. Bring 4 cups of water to a boil. Place all of your noodles in a colander and pour the boiling water over the top, draining well.
4. Let the noodles cool, then grab handfuls and place them in a paper towel; squeeze to remove as much liquid as possible.
5. In a large bowl, beat egg and egg white together. Add noodles, scallions, garlic powder, salt, and pepper, mix well.
6. Prepare a baking sheet; scoop out 1/4 cup of mixture at a time and place on sheet.
7. Slightly press down each scoop with your hands, then bake for 20 minutes, flipping halfway through.
Nutrition Info: Calories: 24, Sodium: 91 mg, Dietary Fiber: 1.0 g, Total Fat: 0.4 g, Total Carbs: 4.3 g, Protein: 0.9 g.

109. Moroccan Pork Kebabs

Servings: 4
Cooking Time: 45 Minutes
Ingredients:
- 1/4 cup orange juice
- 1 tablespoon tomato paste
- 1 clove chopped garlic
- 1 tablespoon ground cumin
- 1/8 teaspoon ground cinnamon
- 4 tablespoons olive oil
- 1-1/2 teaspoons salt
- 3/4 teaspoon black pepper
- 1-1/2 pounds boneless pork loin
- 1 small eggplant
- 1 small red onion
- Pita bread (optional)
- 1/2 small cucumber
- 2 tablespoons chopped fresh mint
- Wooden skewers

Directions:
1. Start by placing wooden skewers in water to soak.
2. Cut pork loin and eggplant into 1- to 1-1/2-inch chunks.
3. Preheat toaster oven to 425°F.
4. Cut cucumber and onions into pieces and chop the mint.
5. In a large bowl, combine the orange juice, tomato paste, garlic, cumin, cinnamon, 2 tablespoons of oil, 1 teaspoon of salt, and 1/2 teaspoon of pepper.
6. Add the pork to this mixture and refrigerate for at least 30 minutes, but up to 8 hours.
7. Mix together vegetables, remaining oil, and salt and pepper.
8. Skewer the vegetables and bake for 20 minutes.
9. Add the pork to the skewers and bake for an additional 25 minutes.
10. Remove ingredients from skewers and sprinkle with mint; serve with flatbread if using.
Nutrition Info: Calories: 465, Sodium: 1061 mg, Dietary Fiber: 5.6 g, Total Fat: 20.8 g, Total Carbs: 21.9 g, Protein: 48.2 g.

110. Chicken Breast With Rosemary

Servings: 4
Cooking Time: 60 Minutes
Ingredients:
- 4 bone-in chicken breast halves
- 3 tablespoons softened butter
- 1/2 teaspoon salt
- 1/4 teaspoon pepper
- 1 tablespoon rosemary
- 1 tablespoon extra-virgin olive oil

Directions:
1. Start by preheating toaster oven to 400°F.
2. Mix butter, salt, pepper, and rosemary in a bowl.
3. Coat chicken with the butter mixture and place in a shallow pan.
4. Drizzle oil over chicken and roast for 25 minutes.
5. Flip chicken and roast for another 20 minutes.
6. Flip chicken one more time and roast for a final 15 minutes.
Nutrition Info: Calories: 392, Sodium: 551 mg, Dietary Fiber: 0 g, Total Fat: 18.4 g, Total Carbs: 0.6 g, Protein: 55.4 g.

111. Pork Stew

Servings: 4
Cooking Time: 12 Minutes
Ingredients:

- 2 lb. pork stew meat; cubed
- 1 eggplant; cubed
- ½ cup beef stock
- 2 zucchinis; cubed
- ½ tsp. smoked paprika
- Salt and black pepper to taste.
- A handful cilantro; chopped.

Directions:
1. In a pan that fits your air fryer, mix all the ingredients, toss, introduce in your air fryer and cook at 370°F for 30 minutes
2. Divide into bowls and serve right away.

Nutrition Info: Calories: 245; Fat: 12g; Fiber: 2g; Carbs: 5g; Protein: 14g

112. Baked Shrimp Scampi

Servings: 4
Cooking Time: 10 Minutes
Ingredients:
- 1 lb large shrimp
- 8 tbsp butter
- 1 tbsp minced garlic (use 2 for extra garlic flavor)
- 1/4 cup white wine or cooking sherry
- 1/2 tsp salt
- 1/4 tsp cayenne pepper
- 1/4 tsp paprika
- 1/2 tsp onion powder
- 3/4 cup bread crumbs

Directions:
1. Take a bowl and mix the bread crumbs with dry seasonings.
2. On the stovetop (or in the Instant Pot on saute), melt the butter with the garlic and the white wine.
3. Remove from heat and add the shrimp and the bread crumb mix.
4. Transfer the mix to a casserole dish.
5. Choose the Bake operation and add food to the Instant Pot Duo Crisp Air Fryer. Close the lid and Bake at 350°F for 10 minutes or until they are browned.
6. Serve and enjoy.

Nutrition Info: Calories 422, Total Fat 26g, Total Carbs 18g, Protein 29 g

113. Herb-roasted Turkey Breast

Servings: 8
Cooking Time: 60 Minutes
Ingredients:
- 3 lb turkey breast
- Rub Ingredients:
- 2 tbsp olive oil
- 2 tbsp lemon juice
- 1 tbsp minced Garlic
- 2 tsp ground mustard
- 2 tsp kosher salt
- 1 tsp pepper
- 1 tsp dried rosemary
- 1 tsp dried thyme
- 1 tsp ground sage

Directions:
1. Take a small bowl and thoroughly combine the Rub Ingredients: in it. Rub this on the outside of the turkey breast and under any loose skin.
2. Place the coated turkey breast keeping skin side up on a cooking tray.
3. Place the drip pan at the bottom of the cooking chamber of the Instant Pot Duo Crisp Air Fryer. Select Air Fry option, post this, adjust the temperature to 360°F and the time to one hour, then touch start.
4. When preheated, add the food to the cooking tray in the lowest position. Close the lid for cooking.
5. When the Air Fry program is complete, check to make sure that the thickest portion of the meat reads at least 160°F, remove the turkey and let it rest for 10 minutes before slicing and serving.

Nutrition Info: Calories 214, Total Fat 10g, Total Carbs 2g, Protein 29g

114. Squash And Zucchini Mini Pizza

Servings: 4
Cooking Time: 15 Minutes
Ingredients:
- 1 pizza crust
- 1/2 cup parmesan cheese
- 4 tablespoons oregano
- 1 zucchini
- 1 yellow summer squash
- Olive oil
- Salt and pepper

Directions:
1. Start by preheating toaster oven to 350°F.
2. If you are using homemade crust, roll out 8 mini portions; if crust is store-bought, use a cookie cutter to cut out the portions.
3. Sprinkle parmesan and oregano equally on each piece. Layer the zucchini and squash in a circle – one on top of the other – around the entire circle.
4. Brush with olive oil and sprinkle salt and pepper to taste.
5. Bake for 15 minutes and serve.

Nutrition Info: Calories: 151, Sodium: 327 mg, Dietary Fiber: 3.1 g, Total Fat: 8.6 g, Total Carbs: 10.3 g, Protein: 11.4 g.

115. Balsamic Roasted Chicken

Servings: 4
Cooking Time: 1 Hour
Ingredients:
- 1/2 cup balsamic vinegar
- 1/4 cup Dijon mustard
- 1/3 cup olive oil
- Juice and zest from 1 lemon

- 3 minced garlic cloves
- 1 teaspoon salt
- 1 teaspoon pepper
- 4 bone-in, skin-on chicken thighs
- 4 bone-in, skin-on chicken drumsticks
- 1 tablespoon chopped parsley

Directions:
1. Mix vinegar, lemon juice, mustard, olive oil, garlic, salt, and pepper in a bowl, then pour into a sauce pan.
2. Roll chicken pieces in the pan, then cover and marinate for at least 2 hours, but up to 24 hours.
3. Preheat the toaster oven to 400°F and place the chicken on a fresh baking sheet, reserving the marinade for later.
4. Roast the chicken for 50 minutes.
5. Remove the chicken and cover it with foil to keep it warm. Place the marinade in the toaster oven for about 5 minutes until it simmers down and begins to thicken.
6. Pour marinade over chicken and sprinkle with parsley and lemon zest.

Nutrition Info: Calories: 1537, Sodium: 1383 mg, Dietary Fiber: 0.8 g, Total Fat: 70.5 g, Total Carbs: 2.4 g, Protein: 210.4 g.

116. Juicy Turkey Burgers

Servings: 8
Cooking Time: 25 Minutes
Ingredients:
- 1 lb ground turkey 85% lean / 15% fat
- ¼ cup unsweetened apple sauce
- ½ onion grated
- 1 Tbsp ranch seasoning
- 2 tsp Worcestershire Sauce
- 1 tsp minced garlic
- ¼ cup plain breadcrumbs
- Salt and pepper to taste

Directions:
1. Combine the onion, ground turkey, unsweetened apple sauce, minced garlic, breadcrumbs, ranch seasoning, Worchestire sauce, and salt and pepper. Mix them with your hands until well combined. Form 4 equally sized hamburger patties with them.
2. Place these burgers in the refrigerator for about 30 minutes to have them firm up a bit.
3. While preparing for cooking, select the Air Fry option. Set the temperature of 360°F and the cook time as required. Press start to begin preheating.
4. Once the preheating temperature is reached, place the burgers on the tray in the Air fryer basket, making sure they don't overlap or touch. Cook on for 15 minutes
5. flipping halfway through.

Nutrition Info: Calories 183, Total Fat 3g, Total Carbs 11g, Protein 28g

117. Air Fryer Beef Steak

Servings: 4
Cooking Time: 15 Minutes
Ingredients:
- 1 tbsp. Olive oil
- Pepper and salt
- 2 pounds of ribeye steak

Directions:
1. Preparing the ingredients. Season meat on both sides with pepper and salt.
2. Rub all sides of meat with olive oil.
3. Preheat instant crisp air fryer to 356 degrees and spritz with olive oil.
4. Air frying. Close air fryer lid. Set temperature to 356°f, and set time to 7 minutes. Cook steak 7 minutes. Flip and cook an additional 6 minutes.
5. Let meat sit 2-5 minutes to rest. Slice and serve with salad.

Nutrition Info: Calories: 233; Fat: 19g; Protein:16g; Sugar:0g

118. Portobello Pesto Burgers

Servings: 4
Cooking Time: 26 Minutes
Ingredients:
- 4 portobello mushrooms
- 1/4 cup sundried tomato pesto
- 4 whole-grain hamburger buns
- 1 large ripe tomato
- 1 log fresh goat cheese
- 8 large fresh basil leaves

Directions:
1. Start by preheating toaster oven to 425°F.
2. Place mushrooms on a pan, round sides facing up.
3. Bake for 14 minutes.
4. Pull out tray, flip the mushrooms and spread 1 tablespoon of pesto on each piece.
5. Return to oven and bake for another 10 minutes.
6. Remove the mushrooms and toast the buns for 2 minutes.
7. Remove the buns and build the burger by placing tomatoes, mushroom, 2 slices of cheese, and a sprinkle of basil, then topping with the top bun.

Nutrition Info: Calories: 297, Sodium: 346 mg, Dietary Fiber: 1.8 g, Total Fat: 18.1 g, Total Carbs: 19.7 g, Protein: 14.4 g.

119. Buttermilk Brined Turkey Breast

Servings: 8
Cooking Time: 20 Minutes
Ingredients:
- ¾ cup brine from a can of olives
- 3½ pounds boneless, skinless turkey breast
- 2 fresh thyme sprigs
- 1 fresh rosemary sprig

- ½ cup buttermilk

Directions:
1. Preheat the Air fryer to 350 degree F and grease an Air fryer basket.
2. Mix olive brine and buttermilk in a bowl until well combined.
3. Place the turkey breast, buttermilk mixture and herb sprigs in a resealable plastic bag.
4. Seal the bag and refrigerate for about 12 hours.
5. Remove the turkey breast from bag and arrange the turkey breast into the Air fryer basket.
6. Cook for about 20 minutes, flipping once in between.
7. Dish out the turkey breast onto a cutting board and cut into desired size slices to serve.

Nutrition Info: Calories: 215, Fat: 3.5g, Carbohydrates: 9.4g, Sugar: 7.7g, Protein: 34.4g, Sodium: 2000mg

120. Roasted Fennel, Ditalini, And Shrimp

Servings: 4
Cooking Time: 30 Minutes
Ingredients:
- 1 pound extra large, thawed, tail-on shrimp
- 1 teaspoon fennel seeds
- 1 teaspoon salt
- 1 fennel bulb, halved and sliced crosswise
- 4 garlic cloves, chopped
- 2 tablespoons olive oil
- 1/2 teaspoon freshly ground black pepper
- Grated zest of 1 lemon
- 1/2 pound whole wheat ditalini

Directions:
1. Start by preheating toaster oven to 450°F.
2. Toast the seeds in a medium pan over medium heat for about 5 minutes, then toss with shrimp.
3. Add water and 1/2 teaspoon salt to the pan and bring the mixture to a boil.
4. Reduce heat and simmer for 30 minutes.
5. Combine fennel, garlic, oil, pepper, and remaining salt in a roasting pan.
6. Roast for 20 minutes, then add shrimp mixture and roast for another 5 minutes or until shrimp are cooked.
7. While the fennel is roasting, cook pasta per the directions on the package, drain, and set aside.
8. Remove the shrimp mixture and mix in pasta, roast for another 5 minutes.

Nutrition Info: Calories: 420, Sodium: 890 mg, Dietary Fiber: 4.2 g, Total Fat: 10.2 g, Total Carbs: 49.5 g, Protein: 33.9 g.

121. Coriander Potatoes

Servings: 4
Cooking Time: 25 Minutes
Ingredients:
- 1 pound gold potatoes, peeled and cut into wedges
- Salt and black pepper to the taste
- 1 tablespoon tomato sauce
- 2 tablespoons coriander, chopped
- ½ teaspoon garlic powder
- 1 teaspoon chili powder
- 1 tablespoon olive oil

Directions:
1. In a bowl, combine the potatoes with the tomato sauce and the other Ingredients:, toss, and transfer to the air fryer's basket.
2. Cook at 370 degrees F for 25 minutes, divide between plates and serve as a side dish.

Nutrition Info: Calories 210, fat 5, fiber 7, carbs 12, protein 5

122. Easy Prosciutto Grilled Cheese

Servings: 1
Cooking Time: 5 Minutes
Ingredients:
- 2 slices muenster cheese
- 2 slices white bread
- Four thinly-shaved pieces of prosciutto
- 1 tablespoon sweet and spicy pickles

Directions:
1. Set toaster oven to the Toast setting.
2. Place one slice of cheese on each piece of bread.
3. Put prosciutto on one slice and pickles on the other.
4. Transfer to a baking sheet and toast for 4 minutes or until the cheese is melted.
5. Combine the sides, cut, and serve.

Nutrition Info: Calories: 460, Sodium: 2180 mg, Dietary Fiber: 0 g, Total Fat: 25.2 g, Total Carbs: 11.9 g, Protein: 44.2 g.

123. Chicken Wings With Prawn Paste

Servings: 6
Cooking Time: 8 Minutes
Ingredients:
- Corn flour, as required
- 2 pounds mid-joint chicken wings
- 2 tablespoons prawn paste
- 4 tablespoons olive oil
- 1½ teaspoons sugar
- 2 teaspoons sesame oil
- 1 teaspoon Shaoxing wine
- 2 teaspoons fresh ginger juice

Directions:
1. Preheat the Air fryer to 360 degree F and grease an Air fryer basket.
2. Mix all the ingredients in a bowl except wings and corn flour.
3. Rub the chicken wings generously with marinade and refrigerate overnight.

4. Coat the chicken wings evenly with corn flour and keep aside.
5. Set the Air fryer to 390 degree F and arrange the chicken wings in the Air fryer basket.
6. Cook for about 8 minutes and dish out to serve hot.
Nutrition Info: Calories: 416, Fat: 31.5g, Carbohydrates: 11.2g, Sugar: 1.6g, Protein: 24.4g, Sodium: 661mg

124. Crispy Breaded Pork Chop

Servings: 6
Cooking Time: 12 Minutes
Ingredients:
- olive oil spray
- 6 3/4-inch thick center-cut boneless pork chops, fat trimmed (5 oz each)
- kosher salt
- 1 large egg, beaten
- 1/2 cup panko crumbs, check labels for GF
- 1/3 cup crushed cornflakes crumbs
- 2 tbsp grated parmesan cheese
- 1 1/4 tsp sweet paprika
- 1/2 tsp garlic powder
- 1/2 tsp onion powder
- 1/4 tsp chili powder
- 1/8 tsp black pepper

Directions:
1. Preheat the Instant Pot Duo Crisp Air Fryer for 12 minutes at 400°F.
2. On both sides, season pork chops with half teaspoon kosher salt.
3. Then combine cornflake crumbs, panko, parmesan cheese, 3/4 tsp kosher salt, garlic powder, paprika, onion powder, chili powder, and black pepper in a large bowl.
4. Place the egg beat in another bowl. Dip the pork in the egg & then crumb mixture.
5. When the air fryer is ready, place 3 of the chops into the Instant Pot Duo Crisp Air Fryer Basket and spritz the top with oil.
6. Close the Air Fryer lid and cook for 12 minutes turning halfway, spritzing both sides with oil.
7. Set aside and repeat with the remaining.
Nutrition Info: Calories 281, Total Fat 13g, Total Carbs 8g, Protein 33g

125. Zucchini And Cauliflower Stew

Servings: 4
Cooking Time: 12 Minutes
Ingredients:
- 1 cauliflower head, florets separated
- 1 ½ cups zucchinis; sliced
- 1 handful parsley leaves; chopped.
- ½ cup tomato puree
- 2 green onions; chopped.
- 1 tbsp. balsamic vinegar
- 1 tbsp. olive oil
- Salt and black pepper to taste.

Directions:
1. In a pan that fits your air fryer, mix the zucchinis with the rest of the ingredients except the parsley, toss, introduce the pan in the air fryer and cook at 380°F for 20 minutes
2. Divide into bowls and serve for lunch with parsley sprinkled on top.
Nutrition Info: Calories: 193; Fat: 5g; Fiber: 2g; Carbs: 4g; Protein: 7g

126. Rosemary Lemon Chicken

Servings: 8
Cooking Time: 45 Minutes
Ingredients:
- 4-lb. chicken, cut into pieces
- Salt and black pepper, to taste
- Flour for dredging 3 tablespoons olive oil
- 1 large onion, sliced
- Peel of ½ lemon
- 2 large garlic cloves, minced
- 1 1/2 teaspoons rosemary leaves
- 1 tablespoon honey
- 1/4 cup lemon juice
- 1 cup chicken broth

Directions:
1. Dredges the chicken through the flour then place in the baking pan.
2. Whisk broth with the rest of the Ingredients: in a bowl.
3. Pour this mixture over the dredged chicken in the pan.
4. Press "Power Button" of Air Fry Oven and turn the dial to select the "Bake" mode.
5. Press the Time button and again turn the dial to set the cooking time to 45 minutes.
6. Now push the Temp button and rotate the dial to set the temperature at 400 degrees F.
7. Once preheated, place the baking pan inside and close its lid.
8. Baste the chicken with its sauce every 15 minutes.
9. Serve warm.
Nutrition Info: Calories 405 Total Fat 22.7 g Saturated Fat 6.1 g Cholesterol 4 mg Sodium 227 mg Total Carbs 26.1 g Fiber 1.4 g Sugar 0.9 g Protein 45.2 g

127. Kalamta Mozarella Pita Melts

Servings: 2
Cooking Time: 5 Minutes
Ingredients:
- 2 (6-inch) whole wheat pitas
- 1 teaspoon extra-virgin olive oil

- 1 cup grated part-skim mozzarella cheese
- 1/4 small red onion
- 1/4 cup pitted Kalamata olives
- 2 tablespoons chopped fresh herbs such as parsley, basil, or oregano

Directions:
1. Start by preheating toaster oven to 425°F.
2. Brush the pita on both sides with oil and warm in the oven for one minute.
3. Dice onions and halve olives.
4. Sprinkle mozzarella over each pita and top with onion and olive.
5. Return to the oven for another 5 minutes or until the cheese is melted.
6. Sprinkle herbs over the pita and serve.

Nutrition Info: Calories: 387, Sodium: 828 mg, Dietary Fiber: 7.4 g, Total Fat: 16.2 g, Total Carbs: 42.0 g, Protein: 23.0 g.

128. Turkey Meatloaf

Servings: 4
Cooking Time: 20 Minutes
Ingredients:
- 1 pound ground turkey
- 1 cup kale leaves, trimmed and finely chopped
- 1 cup onion, chopped
- ½ cup fresh breadcrumbs
- 1 cup Monterey Jack cheese, grated
- 2 garlic cloves, minced
- ¼ cup salsa verde
- 1 teaspoon red chili powder
- ½ teaspoon ground cumin
- ½ teaspoon dried oregano, crushed
- Salt and ground black pepper, as required

Directions:
1. Preheat the Air fryer to 400 degree F and grease an Air fryer basket.
2. Mix all the ingredients in a bowl and divide the turkey mixture into 4 equal-sized portions.
3. Shape each into a mini loaf and arrange the loaves into the Air fryer basket.
4. Cook for about 20 minutes and dish out to serve warm.

Nutrition Info: Calories: 435, Fat: 23.1g, Carbohydrates: 18.1g, Sugar: 3.6g, Protein: 42.2g, Sodium: 641mg

129. Skinny Black Bean Flautas

Servings: 10
Cooking Time: 25 Minutes
Ingredients:
- 2 (15-ounce) cans black beans
- 1 cup shredded cheddar
- 1 (4-ounce) can diced green chilies
- 2 teaspoons taco seasoning
- 10 (8-inch) whole wheat flour tortillas
- Olive oil

Directions:
1. Start by preheating toaster oven to 350°F.
2. Drain black beans and mash in a medium bowl with a fork.
3. Mix in cheese, chilies, and taco seasoning until all ingredients are thoroughly combined.
4. Evenly spread the mixture over each tortilla and wrap tightly.
5. Brush each side lightly with olive oil and place on a baking sheet.
6. Bake for 12 minutes, turn, and bake for another 13 minutes.

Nutrition Info: Calories: 367, Sodium: 136 mg, Dietary Fiber: 14.4 g, Total Fat: 2.8 g, Total Carbs: 64.8 g, Protein: 22.6 g.

130. Crisp Chicken Casserole

Servings: 4
Cooking Time: 15 Minutes
Ingredients:
- 3 cup chicken, shredded
- 12 oz bag egg noodles
- 1/2 large onion
- 1/2 cup chopped carrots
- 1/4 cup frozen peas
- 1/4 cup frozen broccoli pieces
- 2 stalks celery chopped
- 5 cup chicken broth
- 1 tsp garlic powder
- salt and pepper to taste
- 1 cup cheddar cheese, shredded
- 1 package French's onions
- 1/4 cup sour cream
- 1 can cream of chicken and mushroom soup

Directions:
1. Place the chicken, vegetables, garlic powder, salt and pepper, and broth and stir. Then place it into the Instant Pot Duo Crisp Air Fryer Basket.
2. Press or lightly stir the egg noodles into the mix until damp/wet.
3. Select the option Air Fryer and cook for 4 minutes.
4. Stir in the sour cream, can of soup, cheese, and 1/3 of the French's onions.
5. Top with the remaining French's onions and close the Air Fryer lid and cook for about 10 more minutes.

Nutrition Info: Calories 301, Total Fat 17g, Total Carbs 17g, Protein 20g

131. Dijon And Swiss Croque Monsieur

Servings: 2
Cooking Time: 13 Minutes
Ingredients:
- 4 slices white bread

- 2 tablespoons unsalted butter
- 1 tablespoon all-purpose flour
- 1/2 cup whole milk
- 3/4 cups shredded Swiss cheese
- 1/4 teaspoon freshly ground black pepper
- 1/8 teaspoon salt
- 1 tablespoon Dijon mustard
- 4 slices ham

Directions:
1. Start by cutting crusts off bread and placing them on a pan lined with parchment paper.
2. Melt 1 tablespoon of butter in a sauce pan, then dab the top sides of each piece of bread with butter.
3. Toast bread inoven for 3-5 minutes until each piece is golden brown.
4. Melt the second tablespoon of butter in the sauce pan and add the flour, mix together until they form a paste.
5. Add the milk and continue to mix until the sauce begins to thicken.
6. Remove from heat and mix in 1 tablespoon of Swiss cheese, salt, and pepper; continue stirring until cheese is melted.
7. Flip the bread over in the pan so the untoasted side is facing up.
8. Set two slices aside and spread Dijon on the other two slices.
9. Add ham and sprinkle 1/4 cup Swiss over each piece.
10. Broil for about 3 minutes.
11. Top the sandwiches off with the other slices of bread, soft-side down.
12. Top with sauce and sprinkle with remaining Swiss. Toast for another 5 minutes or until the cheese is golden brown.
13. Serve immediately.

Nutrition Info: Calories: 452, Sodium: 1273 mg, Dietary Fiber: 1.6 g, Total Fat: 30.5 g, Total Carbs: 19.8 g, Protein: 24.4 g.

132. Cheddar & Cream Omelet

Servings: 2
Cooking Time: 8 Minutes
Ingredients:
- 4 eggs
- ¼ cup cream
- Salt and ground black pepper, as required
- ¼ cup Cheddar cheese, grated

Directions:
1. In a bowl, add the eggs, cream, salt, and black pepper and beat well.
2. Place the egg mixture into a small baking pan.
3. Press "Power Button" of Air Fry Oven and turn the dial to select the "Air Fry" mode.
4. Press the Time button and again turn the dial to set the cooking time to 8 minutes.
5. Now push the Temp button and rotate the dial to set the temperature at 350 degrees F.
6. Press "Start/Pause" button to start.
7. When the unit beeps to show that it is preheated, open the lid.
8. Arrange pan over the "Wire Rack" and insert in the oven.
9. After 4 minutes, sprinkle the omelet with cheese evenly.
10. Cut the omelet into 2 portions and serve hot.
11. Cut into equal-sized wedges and serve hot.

Nutrition Info: Calories: 202 Cal Total Fat: 15.1 g Saturated Fat: 6.8 g Cholesterol: 348 mg Sodium: 298 mg Total Carbs: 1.8 g Fiber: 0 g Sugar: 1.4 g Protein: 14.8 g

133. Orange Chicken Rice

Servings: 4
Cooking Time: 55 Minutes
Ingredients:
- 3 tablespoons olive oil
- 1 medium onion, chopped
- 1 3/4 cups chicken broth
- 1 cup brown basmati rice
- Zest and juice of 2 oranges
- Salt to taste
- 4 (6-oz.) boneless, skinless chicken thighs
- Black pepper, to taste
- 2 tablespoons fresh mint, chopped
- 2 tablespoons pine nuts, toasted

Directions:
1. Spread the rice in a casserole dish and place the chicken on top.
2. Toss the rest of the Ingredients: in a bowl and liberally pour over the chicken.
3. Press "Power Button" of Air Fry Oven and turn the dial to select the "Bake" mode.
4. Press the Time button and again turn the dial to set the cooking time to 55 minutes.
5. Now push the Temp button and rotate the dial to set the temperature at 350 degrees F.
6. Once preheated, place the casserole dish inside and close its lid.
7. Serve warm.

Nutrition Info: Calories 231 Total Fat 20.1 g Saturated Fat 2.4 g Cholesterol 110 mg Sodium 941 mg Total Carbs 30.1 g Fiber 0.9 g Sugar 1.4 g Protein 14.6 g

134. Fried Paprika Tofu

Servings:
Cooking Time: 12 Minutes
Ingredients:
- 1 block extra firm tofu; pressed to remove excess water and cut into cubes
- 1/4 cup cornstarch
- 1 tablespoon smoked paprika
- salt and pepper to taste

Directions:
1. Line the Air Fryer basket with aluminum foil and brush with oil. Preheat the Air Fryer to 370 - degrees Fahrenheit.
2. Mix all ingredients in a bowl. Toss to combine. Place in the Air Fryer basket and cook for 12 minutes.

135. Saucy Chicken With Leeks

Servings: 6
Cooking Time: 10 Minutes
Ingredients:
- 2 leeks, sliced
- 2 large-sized tomatoes, chopped
- 3 cloves garlic, minced
- ½ teaspoon dried oregano
- 6 chicken legs, boneless and skinless
- ½ teaspoon smoked cayenne pepper
- 2 tablespoons olive oil
- A freshly ground nutmeg

Directions:
1. In a mixing dish, thoroughly combine all ingredients, minus the leeks. Place in the refrigerator and let it marinate overnight.
2. Lay the leeks onto the bottom of an Air Fryer cooking basket. Top with the chicken legs.
3. Roast chicken legs at 375 degrees F for 18 minutes, turning halfway through. Serve with hoisin sauce.

Nutrition Info: 390 Calories; 16g Fat; 2g Carbs; 59g Protein; 8g Sugars; 4g Fiber

136. Roasted Beet Salad With Oranges & Beet Greens

Servings: 6
Cooking Time: 1-1/2 Hours
Ingredients:
- 6 medium beets with beet greens attached
- 2 large oranges
- 1 small sweet onion, cut into wedges
- 1/3 cup red wine vinegar
- 1/4 cup extra-virgin olive oil
- 2 garlic cloves, minced
- 1/2 teaspoon grated orange peel

Directions:
1. Start by preheating toaster oven to 400°F.
2. Trim leaves from beets and chop, then set aside.
3. Pierce beets with a fork and place in a roasting pan.
4. Roast beets for 1-1/2 hours.
5. Allow beets to cool, peel, then cut into 8 wedges and put into a bowl.
6. Place beet greens in a sauce pan and cover with just enough water to cover. Heat until water boils, then immediately remove from heat.
7. Drain greens and press to remove liquid from greens, then add to beet bowl.
8. Remove peel and pith from orange and segment, adding each segment to the bowl.
9. Add onion to beet mixture. In a separate bowl mix together vinegar, oil, garlic and orange peel.
10. Combine both bowls and toss, sprinkle with salt and pepper.
11. Let stand for an hour before serving.

Nutrition Info: Calories: 214, Sodium: 183 mg, Dietary Fiber: 6.5 g, Total Fat: 8.9 g, Total Carbs: 32.4 g, Protein: 4.7 g.

DINNER RECIPES

137. Lemony Green Beans

Servings: 3
Cooking Time: 12 Minutes
Ingredients:
- 1 pound green beans, trimmed and halved
- 1 teaspoon butter, melted
- 1 tablespoon fresh lemon juice
- ¼ teaspoon garlic powder

Directions:
1. Preheat the Air fryer to 400F and grease an Air fryer basket.
2. Mix all the ingredients in a bowl and toss to coat well.
3. Arrange the green beans into the Air fryer basket and cook for about 12 minutes.
4. Dish out in a serving plate and serve hot.

Nutrition Info: Calories: 60, Fat: 1.5g, Carbohydrates: 11.1g, Sugar: 2.3g, Protein: 2.8g, Sodium: 70mg

138. Roasted Lamb

Servings: 4
Cooking Time: 1 Hour 30 Minutes
Ingredients:
- 2½ pounds half lamb leg roast, slits carved
- 2 garlic cloves, sliced into smaller slithers
- 1 tablespoon dried rosemary
- 1 tablespoon olive oil
- Cracked Himalayan rock salt and cracked peppercorns, to taste

Directions:
1. Preheat the Air fryer to 400 degree F and grease an Air fryer basket.
2. Insert the garlic slithers in the slits and brush with rosemary, oil, salt, and black pepper.
3. Arrange the lamb in the Air fryer basket and cook for about 15 minutes.
4. Set the Air fryer to 350 degree F on the Roast mode and cook for 1 hour and 15 minutes.
5. Dish out the lamb chops and serve hot.

Nutrition Info: Calories: 246, Fat: 7.4g, Carbohydrates: 9.4g, Sugar: 6.5g, Protein: 37.2g, Sodium: 353mg

139. Grandma's Meatballs With Spicy Sauce

Servings: 4
Cooking Time: 20 Minutes
Ingredients:
- 4 tablespoons pork rinds
- 1/3 cup green onion
- 1 pound beef sausage meat
- 3 garlic cloves, minced
- 1/3 teaspoon ground black pepper
- Sea salt, to taste
- For the sauce:
- 2 tablespoons Worcestershire sauce
- 1/3 yellow onion, minced
- Dash of Tabasco sauce
- 1/3 cup tomato paste
- 1 teaspoon cumin powder
- 1/2 tablespoon balsamic vinegar

Directions:
1. Knead all of the above ingredients until everything is well incorporated.
2. Roll into balls and cook in the preheated Air Fryer at 365 degrees for 13 minutes.
3. In the meantime, in a saucepan, cook the ingredients for the sauce until thoroughly warmed. Serve your meatballs with the tomato sauce and enjoy!

Nutrition Info: 360 Calories; 23g Fat; 6g Carbs; 23g Protein; 4g Sugars; 2g Fiber

140. Sage Sausages Balls

Servings: 4
Cooking Time: 20 Minutes
Ingredients:
- 3 ½ oz sausages, sliced
- Salt and black pepper to taste
- 1 cup onion, chopped
- 3 tbsp breadcrumbs
- ½ tsp garlic puree
- 1 tsp sage

Directions:
1. Preheat your air fryer to 340 f. In a bowl, mix onions, sausage meat, sage, garlic puree, salt and pepper. Add breadcrumbs to a plate. Form balls using the mixture and roll them in breadcrumbs. Add onion balls in your air fryer's cooking basket and cook for 15 minutes. Serve and enjoy!

Nutrition Info: Calories: 162 Cal Total Fat: 12.1 g Saturated Fat: 0 g Cholesterol: 25 mg Sodium: 324 mg Total Carbs: 7.3 g Fiber: 0 g Sugar: 0 g Protein: 6 g

141. Cheese And Garlic Stuffed Chicken Breasts

Servings: 2
Cooking Time: 20 Minutes
Ingredients:
- 1/2 cup Cottage cheese 2 eggs, beaten
- 2 medium-sized chicken breasts, halved
- 2 tablespoons fresh coriander, chopped 1tsp. fine sea salt
- Seasoned breadcrumbs
- 1/3 tsp. freshly ground black pepper, to savor 3 cloves garlic, finely minced

Directions:
1. Firstly, flatten out the chicken breast using a meat tenderizer.
2. In a medium-sized mixing dish, combine the Cottage cheese with the garlic, coriander, salt, and black pepper.
3. Spread 1/3 of the mixture over the first chicken breast. Repeat with the remaining ingredients. Roll the chicken around the filling; make sure to secure with toothpicks.
4. Now, whisk the egg in a shallow bowl. In another shallow bowl, combine the salt, ground black pepper, and seasoned breadcrumbs.
5. Coat the chicken breasts with the whisked egg; now, roll them in the breadcrumbs.
6. Cook in the air fryer cooking basket at 365 °F for 22 minutes. Serve immediately.

Nutrition Info: 424 Calories; 24.5g Fat; 7.5g Carbs; 43.4g Protein; 5.3g Sugars

142. Grilled Tasty Scallops

Servings: 2
Cooking Time: 10 Minutes
Ingredients:
- 1 pound sea scallops, cleaned and patted dry
- Salt and pepper to taste
- 3 dried chilies
- 2 tablespoon dried thyme
- 1 tablespoon dried oregano
- 1 tablespoon ground coriander
- 1 tablespoon ground fennel
- 2 teaspoons chipotle pepper

Directions:
1. Place the instant pot air fryer lid on and preheat the instant pot at 390 degrees F.
2. Place the grill pan accessory in the instant pot.
3. Mix all ingredients in a bowl.
4. Dump the scallops on the grill pan, close the air fryer lid and cook for 10 minutes.

Nutrition Info: Calories:291 ; Carbs: 20.7g; Protein: 48.6g; Fat: 2.5g

143. Lemongrass Pork Chops

Servings: 3
Cooking Time: 2 Hrs 20 Minutes
Ingredients:
- 3 slices pork chops
- 2 garlic cloves, minced
- 1 ½ tbsp sugar
- 4 stalks lemongrass, trimmed and chopped
- 2 shallots, chopped
- 2 tbsp olive oil
- 1 ¼ tsp soy sauce
- 1 ¼ tsp fish sauce
- 1 ½ tsp black pepper

Directions:
1. In a bowl, add the garlic, sugar, lemongrass, shallots, olive oil, soy sauce, fish sauce, and black pepper; mix well. Add the pork chops, coat them with the mixture and allow to marinate for around 2 hours to get nice and savory.
2. Preheat the Air Fryer to 400 F. Cooking in 2 to 3 batches, remove and shake each pork chop from the marinade and place it in the fryer basket. Cook it for 7 minutes. Turn the pork chops with kitchen tongs and cook further for 5 minutes. Remove the chops and serve with a side of sautéed asparagus.

Nutrition Info: 346 Calories; 11g Fat; 4g Carbs; 32g Protein; 1g Sugars; 1g Fiber

144. Venetian Liver

Servings: 6
Cooking Time: 15-30;
Ingredients:
- 500g veal liver
- 2 white onions
- 100g of water
- 2 tbsp vinegar
- Salt and pepper to taste

Directions:
1. Chop the onion and put it inside the pan with the water. Set the air fryer to 1800C and cook for 20 minutes.
2. Add the liver cut into small pieces and vinegar, close the lid, and cook for an additional 10 minutes.
3. Add salt and pepper.

Nutrition Info: Calories 131, Fat 14.19 g, Carbohydrates 16.40 g, Sugars 5.15 g, Protein 25.39 g, Cholesterol 350.41 mg

145. Curried Eggplant

Servings: 2
Cooking Time: 10 Minutes
Ingredients:
- 1 large eggplant, cut into ½-inch thick slices
- 1 garlic clove, minced
- ½ fresh red chili, chopped
- 1 tablespoon vegetable oil
- ¼ teaspoon curry powder
- Salt, to taste

Directions:
1. Preheat the Air fryer to 300 degree F and grease an Air fryer basket.
2. Mix all the ingredients in a bowl and toss to coat well.
3. Arrange the eggplant slices in the Air fryer basket and cook for about 10 minutes, tossing once in between.
4. Dish out onto serving plates and serve hot.

Nutrition Info: Calories: 121, Fat: 7.3g, Carbohydrates: 14.2g, Sugar: 7g, Protein: 2.4g, Sodium: 83mg

146. One-pan Shrimp And Chorizo Mix Grill

Servings: 4
Cooking Time: 15 Minutes
Ingredients:
- 1 ½ pounds large shrimps, peeled and deveined
- Salt and pepper to taste
- 6 links fresh chorizo sausage
- 2 bunches asparagus spears, trimmed
- Lime wedges

Directions:
1. Place the instant pot air fryer lid on and preheat the instant pot at 390 degrees F.
2. Place the grill pan accessory in the instant pot.
3. Season the shrimps with salt and pepper to taste. Set aside.
4. Place the chorizo on the grill pan and the sausage.
5. Place the asparagus on top.
6. Close the air fryer lid and grill for 15 minutes.
7. Serve with lime wedges.

Nutrition Info: Calories:124 ; Carbs: 9.4g; Protein: 8.2g; Fat: 7.1g

147. Traditional English Fish And Chips

Servings: 4
Cooking Time: 17 Minutes
Ingredients:
- 1 3/4 pounds potatoes
- 4 tablespoons olive oil
- 1-1/4 teaspoons kosher salt
- 1-1/4 teaspoons black pepper
- 8 sprigs fresh thyme
- 4 (6-ounce) pieces cod
- 1 lemon
- 1 clove garlic
- 2 tablespoons capers

Directions:
1. Start by preheating toaster oven to 450°F.
2. Cut potatoes into 1-inch chunks.
3. Place potatoes, 2 tablespoons oil, salt, and thyme in a baking tray and toss to combine.
4. Spread in a flat layer and bake for 30 minutes.
5. Wrap mixture in foil to keep warm.
6. Wipe tray with a paper towel and then lay cod in the tray.
7. Slice the lemon and top cod with lemon, salt, pepper, and thyme.
8. Drizzle rest of the oil over the cod and bake for 12 minutes.
9. Place cod and potatoes on separate pans and bake together for an additional 5 minutes.
10. Combine and serve.

Nutrition Info: Calories: 442, Sodium: 1002 mg, Dietary Fiber: 5.4 g, Total Fat: 15.8 g, Total Carbs: 32.7 g, Protein: 42.5 g.

148. Flank Steak Beef

Servings: 4
Cooking Time: 20 Minutes
Ingredients:
- 1 pound flank steaks, sliced
- ¼ cup xanthum gum
- 2 teaspoon vegetable oil
- ½ teaspoon ginger
- ½ cup soy sauce
- 1 tablespoon garlic, minced
- ½ cup water
- ¾ cup swerve, packed

Directions:
1. Preheat the Air fryer to 390 degree F and grease an Air fryer basket.
2. Coat the steaks with xanthum gum on both the sides and transfer into the Air fryer basket.
3. Cook for about 10 minutes and dish out in a platter.
4. Meanwhile, cook rest of the ingredients for the sauce in a saucepan.
5. Bring to a boil and pour over the steak slices to serve.

Nutrition Info: Calories: 372, Fat: 11.8g, Carbohydrates: 1.8g, Sugar: 27.3g, Protein: 34g, Sodium: 871mg

149. Cheddar Pork Meatballs

Servings: 4 To 6
Cooking Time: 25 Minutes
Ingredients:
- 1 lb ground pork
- 1 large onion, chopped
- ½ tsp maple syrup
- 2 tsp mustard
- ½ cup chopped basil leaves
- Salt and black pepper to taste
- 2 tbsp. grated cheddar cheese

Directions:
1. In a mixing bowl, add the ground pork, onion, maple syrup, mustard, basil leaves, salt, pepper, and cheddar cheese; mix well. Use your hands to form bite-size balls. Place in the fryer basket and cook at 400 f for 10 minutes.
2. Slide out the fryer basket and shake it to toss the meatballs. Cook further for 5 minutes. Remove them onto a wire rack and serve with zoodles and marinara sauce.

Nutrition Info: Calories: 300 Cal Total Fat: 24 g Saturated Fat: 9 g Cholesterol: 70 mg Sodium: 860 mg Total Carbs: 3 g Fiber: 0 g Sugar: 0 g Protein: 16 g

150. Pollock With Kalamata Olives And Capers

Servings: 3
Cooking Time: 20 Minutes
Ingredients:
- 2 tablespoons olive oil
- 1 red onion, sliced
- 2 cloves garlic, chopped
- 1 Florina pepper, deveined and minced
- 3 pollock fillets, skinless
- 2 ripe tomatoes, diced
- 12 Kalamata olives, pitted and chopped
- 2 tablespoons capers
- 1 teaspoon oregano
- 1 teaspoon rosemary
- Sea salt, to taste
- 1/2 cup white wine

Directions:
1. Start by preheating your Air Fryer to 360 degrees F. Heat the oil in a baking pan. Once hot, sauté the onion, garlic, and pepper for 2 to 3 minutes or until fragrant.
2. Add the fish fillets to the baking pan. Top with the tomatoes, olives, and capers. Sprinkle with the oregano, rosemary, and salt. Pour in white wine and transfer to the cooking basket.
3. Turn the temperature to 395 degrees F and bake for 10 minutes. Taste for seasoning and serve on individual plates, garnished with some extra Mediterranean herbs if desired. Enjoy!

Nutrition Info: 480 Calories; 37g Fat; 9g Carbs; 49g Protein; 5g Sugars; 2g Fiber

151. Coconut-crusted Haddock With Curried Pumpkin Seeds

Servings: 4
Cooking Time: 10 Minutes
Ingredients:
- 2 teaspoons canola oil
- 2 teaspoons honey
- 1 teaspoon curry powder
- 1/4 teaspoon ground cinnamon
- 1 teaspoon salt
- 1 cup pumpkin seeds
- 1-1/2 pounds haddock or cod filets
- 1/2 cup roughly grated unsweetened coconut
- 3/4 cups panko-style bread crumbs
- 2 tablespoons butter, melted
- 3 tablespoons apricot fruit spread
- 1 tablespoon lime juice

Directions:
1. Start by preheating toaster oven to 350°F.
2. In a medium bowl, mix honey, oil, curry powder, 1/2 teaspoon salt, and cinnamon.
3. Add pumpkin seeds to the bowl and toss to coat, then lay flat on a baking sheet.
4. Toast for 14 minutes, then transfer to a bowl to cool.
5. Increase the oven temperature to 450°F.
6. Brush a baking sheet with oil and lay filets flat.
7. In another medium mixing bowl, mix together bread crumbs, butter, and remaining salt.
8. In a small bowl mash together apricot spread and lime juice.
9. Brush each filet with apricot mixture, then press bread crumb mixture onto each piece.
10. Bake for 10 minutes.
11. Transfer to a plate and top with pumpkin seeds to serve.

Nutrition Info: Calories: 273, Sodium: 491 mg, Dietary Fiber: 6.1 g, Total Fat: 8.4 g, Total Carbs: 47.3 g, Protein: 7.0 g.

152. Fish Cakes With Horseradish Sauce

Servings: 4
Cooking Time: 20 Minutes
Ingredients:
- Halibut Cakes:
- 1 pound halibut
- 2 tablespoons olive oil
- 1/2 teaspoon cayenne pepper
- 1/4 teaspoon black pepper
- Salt, to taste
- 2 tablespoons cilantro, chopped
- 1 shallot, chopped
- 2 garlic cloves, minced
- 1 cup Romano cheese, grated
- 1 egg, whisked
- 1 tablespoon Worcestershire sauce
- Mayo Sauce:
- 1 teaspoon horseradish, grated
- 1/2 cup mayonnaise

Directions:
1. Start by preheating your Air Fryer to 380 degrees F. Spritz the Air Fryer basket with cooking oil.
2. Mix all ingredients for the halibut cakes in a bowl; knead with your hands until everything is well incorporated.
3. Shape the mixture into equally sized patties. Transfer your patties to the Air Fryer basket. Cook the fish patties for 10 minutes, turning them over halfway through.
4. Mix the horseradish and mayonnaise. Serve the halibut cakes with the horseradish mayo.

Nutrition Info: 532 Calories; 32g Fat; 3g Carbs; 28g Protein; 3g Sugars; 6g Fiber

153. Rice Flour Coated Shrimp

Servings: 3
Cooking Time: 20 Minutes
Ingredients:

- 3 tablespoons rice flour
- 1 pound shrimp, peeled and deveined
- 2 tablespoons olive oil
- 1 teaspoon powdered sugar
- Salt and black pepper, as required

Directions:
1. Preheat the Air fryer to 32F and grease an Air fryer basket.
2. Mix rice flour, olive oil, sugar, salt, and black pepper in a bowl.
3. Stir in the shrimp and transfer half of the shrimp to the Air fryer basket.
4. Cook for about 10 minutes, flipping once in between.
5. Dish out the mixture onto serving plates and repeat with the remaining mixture.

Nutrition Info: Calories: 299, Fat: 12g, Carbohydrates: 11.1g, Sugar: 0.8g, Protein: 35g, Sodium: 419mg

154. Beef Sausage With Grilled Broccoli

Servings: 4
Cooking Time: 20 Minutes
Ingredients:
- 1 pound beef Vienna sausage
- 1/2 cup mayonnaise
- 1 teaspoon yellow mustard
- 1 tablespoon fresh lemon juice
- 1 teaspoon garlic powder
- 1/4 teaspoon black pepper
- 1 pound broccoli

Directions:
1. Start by preheating your Air Fryer to 380 degrees F. Spritz the grill pan with cooking oil.
2. Cut the sausages into serving sized pieces. Cook the sausages for 15 minutes, shaking the basket occasionally to get all sides browned. Set aside.
3. In the meantime, whisk the mayonnaise with mustard, lemon juice, garlic powder, and black pepper. Toss the broccoli with the mayo mixture.
4. Turn up temperature to 400 degrees F. Cook broccoli for 6 minutes, turning halfway through the cooking time.
5. Serve the sausage with the grilled broccoli on the side.

Nutrition Info: 477 Calories; 42g Fat; 3g Carbs; 19g Protein; 7g Sugars; 6g Fiber

155. Hot Pork Skewers

Servings: 3 To 4
Cooking Time: 1 Hour 20 Minutes
Ingredients:
- 1 lb pork steak, cut in cubes
- ¼ cup soy sauce
- 2 tsp smoked paprika
- 1 tsp powdered chili
- 1 tsp garlic salt
- 1 tsp red chili flakes
- 1 tbsp white wine vinegar
- 3 tbsp steak sauce
- Skewing:
- 1 green pepper, cut in cubes
- 1 red pepper, cut in cubes
- 1 yellow squash, seeded and cut in cubes
- 1 green squash, seeded and cut in cubes
- Salt and black pepper to taste to season

Directions:
1. In a mixing bowl, add the pork cubes, soy sauce, smoked paprika, powdered chili, garlic salt, red chili flakes, white wine vinegar, and steak sauce. Mix them using a ladle. Refrigerate to marinate them for 1 hour.
2. After one hour, remove the marinated pork from the fridge and preheat the Air Fryer to 370 F.
3. On each skewer, stick the pork cubes and vegetables in the order that you prefer. Have fun doing this. Once the pork cubes and vegetables are finished, arrange the skewers in the fryer basket and grill them for 8 minutes. You can do them in batches. Once ready, remove them onto the serving platter and serve with salad.

Nutrition Info: 456 Calories; 37g Fat; 1g Carbs; 21g Protein; 5g Sugars; 6g Fiber

156. Couscous Stuffed Tomatoes

Servings: 4
Cooking Time: 25 Minutes
Ingredients:
- 4 tomatoes, tops and seeds removed
- 1 parsnip, peeled and finely chopped
- 1 cup mushrooms, chopped
- 1½ cups couscous
- 1 teaspoon olive oil
- 1 garlic clove, minced
- 1 tablespoon mirin sauce

Directions:
1. Preheat the Air fryer to 355 degree F and grease an Air fryer basket.
2. Heat olive oil in a skillet on low heat and add parsnips, mushrooms and garlic.
3. Cook for about 5 minutes and stir in the mirin sauce and couscous.
4. Stuff the couscous mixture into the tomatoes and arrange into the Air fryer basket.
5. Cook for about 20 minutes and dish out to serve warm.

Nutrition Info: Calories: 361, Fat: 2g, Carbohydrates: 75.5g, Sugar: 5.1g, Protein: 10.4g, Sodium: 37mg

157. Garlic Lamb Shank

Servings: 5
Cooking Time: 24 Minutes
Ingredients:

- 17 oz. lamb shanks
- 2 tablespoon garlic, peeled
- 1 teaspoon kosher salt
- 1 tablespoon dried parsley
- 4 oz chive stems, chopped
- ½ cup chicken stock
- 1 teaspoon butter
- 1 teaspoon dried rosemary
- 1 teaspoon nutmeg
- ½ teaspoon ground black pepper

Directions:
1. Chop the garlic roughly.
2. Make the cuts in the lamb shank and fill the cuts with the chopped garlic.
3. Then sprinkle the lamb shank with the kosher salt, dried parsley, dried rosemary, nutmeg, and ground black pepper.
4. Stir the spices on the lamb shank gently.
5. Then put the butter and chicken stock in the air fryer basket tray.
6. Preheat the air fryer to 380 F.
7. Put the chives in the air fryer basket tray.
8. Add the lamb shank and cook the meat for 24 minutes.
9. When the lamb shank is cooked – transfer it to the serving plate and sprinkle with the remaining liquid from the cooked meat.
10. Enjoy!

Nutrition Info: calories 205, fat 8.2, fiber 0.8, carbs 3.8, protein 27.2

158. Grilled Halibut With Tomatoes And Hearts Of Palm

Servings: 4
Cooking Time: 15 Minutes
Ingredients:
- 4 halibut fillets
- Juice from 1 lemon
- Salt and pepper to taste
- 2 tablespoons oil
- ½ cup hearts of palm, rinse and drained
- 1 cup cherry tomatoes

Directions:
1. Place the instant pot air fryer lid on and preheat the instant pot at 390 degrees F.
2. Place the grill pan accessory in the instant pot.
3. Season the halibut fillets with lemon juice, salt, and pepper. Brush with oil.
4. Place the fish on the grill pan.
5. Arrange the hearts of palms and cherry tomatoes on the side and sprinkle with more salt and pepper.
6. Close the air fryer lid and cook for 15 minutes.

Nutrition Info: Calories: 208; Carbs: 7g; Protein: 21 g; Fat: 11g

159. Crispy Scallops

Servings: 4
Cooking Time: 6 Minutes
Ingredients:
- 18 sea scallops, cleaned and patted very dry
- 1/8 cup all-purpose flour
- 1 tablespoon 2% milk
- ½ egg
- ¼ cup cornflakes, crushed
- ½ teaspoon paprika
- Salt and black pepper, as required

Directions:
1. Preheat the Air fryer to 400 degree F and grease an Air fryer basket.
2. Mix flour, paprika, salt, and black pepper in a bowl.
3. Whisk egg with milk in another bowl and place the cornflakes in a third bowl.
4. Coat each scallop with the flour mixture, dip into the egg mixture and finally, dredge in the cornflakes.
5. Arrange scallops in the Air fryer basket and cook for about 6 minutes.
6. Dish out the scallops in a platter and serve hot.

Nutrition Info: Calories: 150, Fat: 1.7g, Carbohydrates: 8g, Sugar: 0.4g, Protein: 24g, Sodium: 278mg

160. Herbed Carrots

Servings: 8
Cooking Time: 14 Minutes
Ingredients:
- 6 large carrots, peeled and sliced lengthwise
- 2 tablespoons olive oil
- ½ tablespoon fresh oregano, chopped
- ½ tablespoon fresh parsley, chopped
- Salt and black pepper, to taste
- 2 tablespoons olive oil, divided
- ½ cup fat-free Italian dressing
- Salt, to taste

Directions:
1. Preheat the Air fryer to 360-degree F and grease an Air fryer basket.
2. Mix the carrot slices and olive oil in a bowl and toss to coat well.
3. Arrange the carrot slices in the Air fryer basket and cook for about 12 minutes.
4. Dish out the carrot slices onto serving plates and sprinkle with herbs, salt and black pepper.
5. Transfer into the Air fryer basket and cook for 2 more minutes.
6. Dish out and serve hot.

Nutrition Info: Calories: 93, Fat: 7.2g, Carbohydrates: 7.3g, Sugar: 3.8g, Protein: 0.7g, Sodium: 252mg

161. Salmon Casserole

Servings: 8

Cooking Time: 12 Minutes
Ingredients:
- 7 oz Cheddar cheese, shredded
- ½ cup cream
- 1-pound salmon fillet
- 1 tablespoon dried dill
- 1 teaspoon dried parsley
- 1 teaspoon salt
- 1 teaspoon ground coriander
- ½ teaspoon ground black pepper
- 2 green pepper, chopped
- 4 oz chive stems, diced
- 7 oz bok choy, chopped
- 1 tablespoon olive oil

Directions:
1. Sprinkle the salmon fillet with the dried dill, dried parsley, ground coriander, and ground black pepper.
2. Massage the salmon fillet gently and leave it for 5 minutes to make the fish soaks the spices.
3. Meanwhile, sprinkle the air fryer casserole tray with the olive oil inside.
4. After this, cut the salmon fillet into the cubes.
5. Separate the salmon cubes into 2 parts.
6. Then place the first part of the salmon cubes in the casserole tray.
7. Sprinkle the fish with the chopped bok choy, diced chives, and chopped green pepper.
8. After this, place the second part of the salmon cubes over the vegetables.
9. Then sprinkle the casserole with the shredded cheese and heavy cream.
10. Preheat the air fryer to 380 F.
11. Cook the salmon casserole for 12 minutes.
12. When the dish is cooked – it will have acrunchy light brown crust.
13. Serve it and enjoy!

Nutrition Info: calories 216, fat 14.4, fiber 1.1, carbs 4.3, protein 18.2

162.Cinnamon Pork Rinds

Servings: 2
Cooking Time: 20 Minutes
Ingredients:
- 2 oz. pork rinds
- ¼ cup powdered erythritol
- 2 tbsp. unsalted butter; melted.
- ½ tsp. ground cinnamon.

Directions:
1. Take a large bowl, toss pork rinds and butter. Sprinkle with cinnamon and erythritol, then toss to evenly coat.
2. Place pork rinds into the air fryer basket. Adjust the temperature to 400 Degrees F and set the timer for 5 minutes. Serve immediately.

Nutrition Info: Calories: 264; Protein: 13g; Fiber: 4g; Fat: 28g; Carbs: 15g

163.Stuffed Okra

Servings: 2
Cooking Time: 12 Minutes
Ingredients:
- 8 ounces large okra
- ¼ cup chickpea flour
- ¼ of onion, chopped
- 2 tablespoons coconut, grated freshly
- 1 teaspoon garam masala powder
- ½ teaspoon ground turmeric
- ½ teaspoon red chili powder
- ½ teaspoon ground cumin
- Salt, to taste

Directions:
1. Preheat the Air fryer to 390F and grease an Air fryer basket.
2. Mix the flour, onion, grated coconut, and spices in a bowl and toss to coat well.
3. Stuff the flour mixture into okra and arrange into the Air fryer basket.
4. Cook for about 12 minutes and dish out in a serving plate.

Nutrition Info: Calories: 166, Fat: 3.7g, Carbohydrates: 26.6g, Sugar: 5.3g, Protein: 7.6g, Sodium: 103mg

164.Zucchini Muffins

Servings: 8
Cooking Time: 20 Minutes
Ingredients:
- 6 eggs
- 4 drops stevia 1/4 cup Swerve
- 1/3 cup coconut oil, melted 1 cup zucchini, grated
- 3/4 cup coconut flour 1/4 tsp ground nutmeg 1 tsp ground cinnamon 1/2 tsp baking soda

Directions:
1. Preheat the air fryer to 325 F.
2. Add all ingredients except zucchini in a bowl and mix well.
3. Add zucchini and stir well.
4. Pour batter into the silicone muffin molds and place into the air fryer basket.
5. Cook muffins for 20 minutes.
6. Serve and enjoy.

Nutrition Info: Calories 136 Fat 12 g Carbohydrates 1 g Sugar 0.6 g Protein 4 g Cholesterol 123 mg

165.Basil Tomatoes

Servings: 2
Cooking Time: 10 Minutes
Ingredients:
- 2 tomatoes, halved
- 1 tablespoon fresh basil, chopped

- Olive oil cooking spray
- Salt and black pepper, as required

Directions:
1. Preheat the Air fryer to 320 degree F and grease an Air fryer basket.
2. Spray the tomato halves evenly with olive oil cooking spray and season with salt, black pepper and basil.
3. Arrange the tomato halves into the Air fryer basket, cut sides up.
4. Cook for about 10 minutes and dish out onto serving plates.

Nutrition Info: Calories: 22, Fat: 4.8g, Carbohydrates: 4.8g, Sugar: 3.2g, Protein: 1.1g, Sodium: 84mg

166. Sweet Chicken Breast

Servings: 4
Cooking Time: 12 Minutes
Ingredients:
- 1-pound chicken breast, boneless, skinless
- 3 tablespoon Stevia extract
- 1 teaspoon ground white pepper
- ½ teaspoon paprika
- 1 teaspoon cayenne pepper
- 1 teaspoon lemongrass
- 1 teaspoon lemon zest
- 1 tablespoon apple cider vinegar
- 1 tablespoon butter

Directions:
1. Sprinkle the chicken breast with the apple cider vinegar.
2. After this, rub the chicken breast with the ground white pepper, paprika, cayenne pepper, lemongrass, and lemon zest.
3. Leave the chicken breast for 5 minutes to marinate.
4. After this, rub the chicken breast with the stevia extract and leave it for 5 minutes more.
5. Preheat the air fryer to 380 F.
6. Rub the prepared chicken breast with the butter and place it in the air fryer basket tray.
7. Cook the chicken breast for 12 minutes.
8. Turn the chicken breast into another side after 6 minutes of cooking.
9. Serve the dish hot!
10. Enjoy!

Nutrition Info: calories 160, fat 5.9, fiber 0.4, carbs 1, protein 24.2

167. Corned Beef With Carrots

Servings: 3
Cooking Time: 35 Minutes
Ingredients:
- 1 tbsp beef spice
- 1 whole onion, chopped
- 4 carrots, chopped
- 12 oz bottle beer
- 1½ cups chicken broth
- 4 pounds corned beef

Directions:
1. Preheat your air fryer to 380 f. Cover beef with beer and set aside for 20 minutes. Place carrots, onion and beef in a pot and heat over high heat. Add in broth and bring to a boil. Drain boiled meat and veggies; set aside.
2. Top with beef spice. Place the meat and veggies in your air fryer's cooking basket and cook for 30 minutes.

Nutrition Info: Calories: 464 Cal Total Fat: 17 g Saturated Fat: 6.8 g Cholesterol: 91.7 mg Sodium: 1904.2 mg Total Carbs: 48.9 g Fiber: 7.2 g Sugar: 5.8 g Protein: 30.6 g

168. Smoked Ham With Pears

Servings: 2
Cooking Time: 30 Minutes
Ingredients:
- 15 oz pears, halved
- 8 pound smoked ham
- 1 ½ cups brown sugar
- ¾ tbsp allspice
- 1 tbsp apple cider vinegar
- 1 tsp black pepper
- 1 tsp vanilla extract

Directions:
1. Preheat your air fryer to 330 f. In a bowl, mix pears, brown sugar, cider vinegar, vanilla extract, pepper, and allspice. Place the mixture in a frying pan and fry for 2-3 minutes. Pour the mixture over ham. Add the ham to the air fryer cooking basket and cook for 15 minutes. Serve ham with hot sauce, to enjoy!

Nutrition Info: Calories: 550 Cal Total Fat: 29 g Saturated Fat: 0 g Cholesterol: 0 mg Sodium: 0 mg Total Carbs: 46 g Fiber: 0 g Sugar: 0 g Protein: 28 g

169. Creamy Tuna Cakes

Servings: 4
Cooking Time: 15 Minutes
Ingredients:
- 2: 6-ouncescans tuna, drained
- 1½ tablespoon almond flour
- 1½ tablespoons mayonnaise
- 1 tablespoon fresh lemon juice
- 1 teaspoon dried dill
- 1 teaspoon garlic powder
- ½ teaspoon onion powder
- Pinch of salt and ground black pepper

Directions:
1. Preheat the Air fryer to 400-degree F and grease an Air fryer basket.
2. Mix the tuna, mayonnaise, almond flour, lemon juice, dill, and spices in a large bowl.

3. Make 4 equal-sized patties from the mixture and arrange in the Air fryer basket.
4. Cook for about 10 minutes and flip the sides.
5. Cook for 5 more minutes and dish out the tuna cakes in serving plates to serve warm.
Nutrition Info: Calories: 200, Fat: 10.1g, Carbohydrates: 2.9g, Sugar: 0.8g, Protein: 23.4g, Sodium: 122mg

170. Pork Belly With Honey

Servings: 8
Cooking Time: 35 Minutes
Ingredients:
- 2 pounds pork belly
- ½ tsp pepper
- 1 tbsp olive oil
- 1 tbsp salt
- 3 tbsp honey

Directions:
1. Preheat your air fryer to 400 f. Season the pork belly with salt and pepper. Grease the basket with oil. Add seasoned meat and cook for 15 minutes. Add honey and cook for 10 minutes more. Serve with green salad.
Nutrition Info: Calories: 274 Cal Total Fat: 18 g Saturated Fat: 0 g Cholesterol: 0 mg Sodium: 0 mg Total Carbs: 8 g Fiber: 0 g Sugar: 0 g Protein: 18 g

171. Cod With Avocado Mayo Sauce

Servings: 2
Cooking Time: 20 Minutes
Ingredients:
- 2 cod fish fillets
- 1 egg
- Sea salt, to taste
- 2 teaspoons olive oil
- 1/2 avocado, peeled, pitted, and mashed
- 1 tablespoon mayonnaise
- 3 tablespoons sour cream
- 1/2 teaspoon yellow mustard
- 1 teaspoon lemon juice
- 1 garlic clove, minced
- 1/4 teaspoon black pepper
- 1/4 teaspoon salt
- 1/4 teaspoon hot pepper sauce

Directions:
1. Start by preheating your Air Fryer to 360 degrees F. Spritz the Air Fryer basket with cooking oil.
2. Pat dry the fish fillets with a kitchen towel. Beat the egg in a shallow bowl. Add in the salt and olive oil.
3. Dip the fish into the egg mixture, making sure to coat thoroughly. Cook in the preheated Air Fryer approximately 12 minutes.
4. Meanwhile, make the avocado sauce by mixing the remaining ingredients in a bowl. Place in your refrigerator until ready to serve.
5. Serve the fish fillets with chilled avocado sauce on the side.
Nutrition Info: 344 Calories; 27g Fat; 8g Carbs; 21g Protein; 8g Sugars; 7g Fiber

172. Paprika Crab Burgers

Servings: 3
Cooking Time: 20 Minutes
Ingredients:
- 2 eggs, beaten
- 1 shallot, chopped
- 2 garlic cloves, crushed
- 1 tablespoon olive oil
- 1 teaspoon yellow mustard
- 1 teaspoon fresh cilantro, chopped
- 10 ounces crab meat
- 1 teaspoon smoked paprika
- 1/2 teaspoon ground black pepper
- Sea salt, to taste
- 3/4 cup parmesan cheese

Directions:
1. In a mixing bowl, thoroughly combine the eggs, shallot, garlic, olive oil, mustard, cilantro, crab meat, paprika, black pepper, and salt. Mix until well combined.
2. Shape the mixture into 6 patties. Roll the crab patties over grated parmesan cheese, coating well on all sides. Place in your refrigerator for 2 hours.
3. Spritz the crab patties with cooking oil on both sides. Cook in the preheated Air Fryer at 360 degrees F for 14 minutes. Serve on dinner rolls if desired.
Nutrition Info: 279 Calories; 14g Fat; 7g Carbs; 23g Protein; 5g Sugars; 6g Fiber

173. Effortless Beef Schnitzel

Servings: 2
Cooking Time: 25 Minutes
Ingredients:
- 2 tbsp vegetable oil
- 2 oz breadcrumbs
- 1 whole egg, whisked
- 1 thin beef schnitzel, cut into strips
- 1 whole lemon

Directions:
1. Preheat your fryer to 356 F. In a bowl, add breadcrumbs and oil and stir well to get a loose mixture. Dip schnitzel in egg, then dip in breadcrumbs coat well. Place the prepared schnitzel your Air Fryer's cooking basket and cook for 12 minutes. Serve with a drizzle of lemon juice.
Nutrition Info: 346 Calories; 11g Fat; 4g Carbs; 32g Protein; 1g Sugars; 1g Fiber

174. Award Winning Breaded Chicken

Servings: 4
Cooking Time: 20 Minutes
Ingredients:
- 1 1/2 tsp.s olive oil
- 1 tsp. red pepper flakes, crushed 1/3 tsp. chicken bouillon granules 1/3 tsp. shallot powder
- 1 1/2 tablespoons tamari soy sauce 1/3 tsp. cumin powder
- 1½ tablespoons mayo 1 tsp. kosher salt
- For the chicken:
- 2 beaten eggs Breadcrumbs
- 1½ chicken breasts, boneless and skinless 1 ½ tablespoons plain flour

Directions:
1. Margarine fly the chicken breasts, and then, marinate them for at least 55 minutes. Coat the chicken with plain flour; then, coat with the beaten eggs; finally, roll them in the breadcrumbs.
2. Lightly grease the cooking basket. Air-fry the breaded chicken at 345 °F for 12 minutes, flipping them halfway.

Nutrition Info: 262 Calories; 14.9g Fat; 2.7g Carbs; 27.5g Protein; 0.3g Sugars

175. Smoked Sausage And Bacon Shashlik

Servings: 4
Cooking Time: 20 Minutes
Ingredients:
- 1 pound smoked Polish beef sausage, sliced
- 1 tablespoon mustard
- 1 tablespoon olive oil
- 2 tablespoons Worcestershire sauce
- 2 bell peppers, sliced
- Salt and ground black pepper, to taste

Directions:
1. Toss the sausage with the mustard, olive, and Worcestershire sauce. Thread sausage and peppers onto skewers.
2. Sprinkle with salt and black pepper.
3. Cook in the preheated Air Fryer at 360 degrees Ffor 11 minutes. Brush the skewers with the reserved marinade.

Nutrition Info: 422 Calories; 36g Fat; 9g Carbs; 18g Protein; 6g Sugars; 7g Fiber

176. Broccoli Crust Pizza

Servings: 4
Cooking Time: 20 Minutes
Ingredients:
- 3 cups riced broccoli, steamed and drained well
- ½ cup shredded mozzarella cheese
- ½ cup grated vegetarian Parmesan cheese.
- 1 large egg.
- 3 tbsp. low-carb Alfredo sauce

Directions:
1. Take a large bowl, mix broccoli, egg and Parmesan.
2. Cut a piece of parchment to fit your air fryer basket. Press out the pizza mixture to fit on the parchment, working in two batches if necessary. Place into the air fryer basket. Adjust the temperature to 370 Degrees F and set the timer for 5 minutes.
3. When the timer beeps, the crust should be firm enough to flip. If not, add 2 additional minutes. Flip crust.
4. Top with Alfredo sauce and mozzarella. Return to the air fryer basket and cook an additional 7 minutes or until cheese is golden and bubbling. Serve warm.

Nutrition Info: Calories: 136; Protein: 9g; Fiber: 3g; Fat: 6g; Carbs:7g

177. Creamy Lemon Turkey

Servings: 4
Cooking Time: 20 Minutes
Ingredients:
- 1/3 cup sour cream
- 2 cloves garlic, finely minced 1/3 tsp. lemon zest
- 2 small-sized turkey breasts, skinless and cubed 1/3 cup thickened cream
- 2 tablespoons lemon juice
- 1 tsp. fresh marjoram, chopped
- Salt and freshly cracked mixed peppercorns, to taste 1/2 cup scallion, chopped
- 1/2 can tomatoes, diced
- 1½ tablespoons canola oil

Directions:
1. Firstly, pat dry the turkey breast. Mix the remaining items; marinate the turkey for 2 hours.
2. Set the air fryer to cook at 355 °F. Brush the turkey with a nonstick spray; cook for 23 minutes, turning once. Serve with naan and enjoy!

Nutrition Info: 260 Calories; 15.3g Fat; 8.9g Carbs; 28.6g Protein; 1.9g Sugars

178. Homemade Beef Stroganoff

Servings: 3
Cooking Time: 20 Minutes
Ingredients:
- 1 pound thin steak
- 4 tbsp butter
- 1 whole onion, chopped
- 1 cup sour cream
- 8 oz mushrooms, sliced
- 4 cups beef broth
- 16 oz egg noodles, cooked

Directions:
1. Preheat your Air Fryer to 400 F. Using a microwave proof bowl, melt butter in a microwave

oven. In a mixing bowl, mix the melted butter, sliced mushrooms, cream, onion, and beef broth.
2. Pour the mixture over steak and set aside for 10 minutes. Place the marinated beef in your fryer's cooking basket, and cook for 10 minutes. Serve with cooked egg noodles and enjoy!
Nutrition Info: 456 Calories; 37g Fat; 1g Carbs; 21g Protein; 5g Sugars; 6g Fiber

179. Roasted Garlic Zucchini Rolls

Servings: 4
Cooking Time: 20 Minutes
Ingredients:
- 2 medium zucchinis
- ½ cup full-fat ricotta cheese
- ¼ white onion; peeled. And diced
- 2 cups spinach; chopped
- ¼ cup heavy cream
- ½ cup sliced baby portobello mushrooms
- ¾ cup shredded mozzarella cheese, divided.
- 2 tbsp. unsalted butter.
- 2 tbsp. vegetable broth.
- ½ tsp. finely minced roasted garlic
- ¼ tsp. dried oregano.
- ⅛ tsp. xanthan gum
- ¼ tsp. salt
- ½ tsp. garlic powder.

Directions:
1. Using a mandoline or sharp knife, slice zucchini into long strips lengthwise. Place strips between paper towels to absorb moisture. Set aside
2. In a medium saucepan over medium heat, melt butter. Add onion and sauté until fragrant. Add garlic and sauté 30 seconds.
3. Pour in heavy cream, broth and xanthan gum. Turn off heat and whisk mixture until it begins to thicken, about 3 minutes.
4. Take a medium bowl, add ricotta, salt, garlic powder and oregano and mix well. Fold in spinach, mushrooms and ½ cup mozzarella
5. Pour half of the sauce into a 6-inch round baking pan. To assemble the rolls, place two strips of zucchini on a work surface. Spoon 2 tbsp. of ricotta mixture onto the slices and roll up. Place seam side down on top of sauce. Repeat with remaining ingredients
6. Pour remaining sauce over the rolls and sprinkle with remaining mozzarella. Cover with foil and place into the air fryer basket. Adjust the temperature to 350 Degrees F and set the timer for 20 minutes. In the last 5 minutes, remove the foil to brown the cheese. Serve immediately.
Nutrition Info: Calories: 245; Protein: 15g; Fiber: 8g; Fat: 19g; Carbs: 1g

180. Oven-fried Herbed Chicken

Servings: 2
Cooking Time: 15 Minutes
Ingredients:
- 1/2 cup buttermilk
- 2 cloves garlic, minced
- 1-1/2 teaspoons salt
- 1 tablespoon oil
- 1/2 pound boneless, skinless chicken breasts
- 1 cup rolled oats
- 1/2 teaspoon red pepper flakes
- 1/2 cup grated parmesan cheese
- 1/4 cup fresh basil leaves or rosemary needles
- Olive oil spray

Directions:
1. Mix together buttermilk, oil, 1/2 teaspoon salt, and garlic in a shallow bowl.
2. Roll chicken in buttermilk and refrigerate in bowl overnight.
3. Preheat your toaster oven to 425°F.
4. Mix together the oats, red pepper, salt, parmesan, and basil, and mix roughly to break up oats.
5. Place the mixture on a plate.
6. Remove the chicken from the buttermilk mixture and let any excess drip off.
7. Roll the chicken in the oat mixture and transfer to a baking sheet lightly coated with olive oil spray.
8. Spray the chicken with oil spray and bake for 15 minutes.
Nutrition Info: Calories: 651, Sodium: 713 mg, Dietary Fiber: 4.4 g, Total Fat: 31.2 g, Total Carbs: 34.1 g, Protein: 59.5 g.

181. Five Spice Pork

Servings: 4
Cooking Time: 20 Minutes
Ingredients:
- 1-pound pork belly
- 2 tablespoons swerve
- 2 tablespoons dark soy sauce
- 1 tablespoon Shaoxing: cooking wine
- 2 teaspoons garlic, minced
- 2 teaspoons ginger, minced
- 1 tablespoon hoisin sauce
- 1 teaspoon Chinese Five Spice

Directions:
1. Preheat the Air fryer to 390 degree F and grease an Air fryer basket.
2. Mix all the ingredients in a bowl and place in the Ziplock bag.
3. Seal the bag, shake it well and refrigerate to marinate for about 1 hour.
4. Remove the pork from the bag and arrange it in the Air fryer basket.
5. Cook for about 15 minutes and dish out in a bowl to serve warm.

Nutrition Info: Calories: 604, Fat: 30.6g, Carbohydrates: 1.4g, Sugar: 20.3g, Protein: 19.8g, Sodium: 834mg

182. Broiled Tilapia With Parmesan And Herbs

Servings: 4
Cooking Time: 8 Minutes
Ingredients:
- 4 (6- to 8-ounce) farm-raised tilapia filets
- 1/2 cup freshly grated parmesan cheese
- 2 tablespoons low-fat mayonnaise
- 2 tablespoons light sour cream
- 2 tablespoons melted unsalted butter
- 2 tablespoons lemon juice
- 1/2 teaspoon dried basil
- 1/2 teaspoon dried tarragon
- 1/8 teaspoon onion powder
- Salt and pepper to taste

Directions:
1. Mix together 1/4 cup parmesan and all other ingredients, except tilapia.
2. Place mixture in a plastic zipper bag, add fish and toss.
3. Pour fish mixture into a shallow pan and set aside to marinate for 20 minutes.
4. Place the fish in a broiler pan, top with a few spoonful of marinade, and sprinkle the rest of the parmesan over the fish.
5. Broil until lightly browned, around 8 minutes.

Nutrition Info: Calories: 369, Sodium: 459 mg, Dietary Fiber: 0 g, Total Fat: 17.7 g, Total Carbs: 2.0 g, Protein: 51.6 g.

183. Lemon Garlic Shrimps

Servings: 2
Cooking Time: 8 Minutes
Ingredients:
- ¾ pound medium shrimp, peeled and deveined
- 1½ tablespoons fresh lemon juice
- 1 tablespoon olive oil
- 1 teaspoon lemon pepper
- ¼ teaspoon paprika
- ¼ teaspoon garlic powder

Directions:
1. Preheat the Air fryer to 400 degree F and grease an Air fryer basket.
2. Mix lemon juice, olive oil, lemon pepper, paprika and garlic powder in a large bowl.
3. Stir in the shrimp and toss until well combined.
4. Arrange shrimp into the Air fryer basket in a single layer and cook for about 8 minutes.
5. Dish out the shrimp in serving plates and serve warm.

Nutrition Info: Calories: 260, Fat: 12.4g, Carbohydrates: 0.3g, Sugar: 0.1g, Protein: 35.6g, Sodium: 619mg

184. Turkey Wontons With Garlic-parmesan Sauce

Servings: 8
Cooking Time: 20 Minutes
Ingredients:
- 8 ounces cooked turkey breasts, shredded 16 wonton wrappers
- 1½ tablespoons margarine, melted
- 1/3 cup cream cheese, room temperature 8 ounces Asiago cheese, shredded
- 3 tablespoons Parmesan cheese, grated
- 1 tsp. garlic powder
- Fine sea salt and freshly ground black pepper, to taste

Directions:
1. In a small-sized bowl, mix the margarine, Parmesan, garlic powder, salt, and black pepper; give it a good stir.
2. Lightly grease a mini muffin pan; lay 1 wonton wrapper in each mini muffin cup. Fill each cup with the cream cheese and turkey mixture.
3. Air-fry for 8 minutes at 335 °F. Immediately top with Asiago cheese and serve warm.

Nutrition Info: 362 Calories; 13.5g Fat; 40.4g Carbs; 18.5g Protein; 1.2g Sugars

185. Lemon Duck Legs

Servings: 6
Cooking Time: 25 Minutes
Ingredients:
- 1 lemon
- 2-pound duck legs
- 1 teaspoon ground coriander
- 1 teaspoon ground nutmeg
- 1 teaspoon kosher salt
- ½ teaspoon dried rosemary
- 1 tablespoon olive oil
- 1 teaspoon stevia extract
- ¼ teaspoon sage

Directions:
1. Squeeze the juice from the lemon and grate the zest.
2. Combine the lemon juice and lemon zest together in the big mixing bowl.
3. Add the ground coriander, ground nutmeg, kosher salt, dried rosemary, and sage.
4. Sprinkle the liquid with the olive oil and stevia extract.
5. Whisk it carefully and put the duck legs there.
6. Stir the duck legs and leave them for 15 minutes to marinate.
7. Meanwhile, preheat the air fryer to 380 F.

8. Put the marinated duck legs in the air fryer and cook them for 25 minutes.
9. Turn the duck legs into another side after 15 minutes of cooking.
10. When the duck legs are cooked – let them cool little.
11. Serve and enjoy!
Nutrition Info: calories 296, fat 11.5, fiber 0.5, carbs 1.6, protein 44.2

186. Chicken Lasagna With Eggplants

Servings: 10
Cooking Time: 17 Minutes
Ingredients:
- 6 oz Cheddar cheese, shredded
- 7 oz Parmesan cheese, shredded
- 2 eggplants
- 1-pound ground chicken
- 1 teaspoon paprika
- 1 teaspoon salt
- ½ teaspoon cayenne pepper
- ½ cup heavy cream
- 2 teaspoon butter
- 4 oz chive stems, diced

Directions:
1. Take the air fryer basket tray and spread it with the butter.
2. Then peel the eggplants and slice them.
3. Separate the sliced eggplants into 3 parts.
4. Combine the ground chicken with the paprika, salt, cayenne pepper, and diced chives.
5. Mix the mixture up.
6. Separate the ground chicken mixture into 2 parts.
7. Make the layer of the first part of the sliced eggplant in the air fryer basket tray.
8. Then make the layer of the ground chicken mixture.
9. After this, sprinkle the ground chicken layer with the half of the shredded Cheddar cheese,
10. Then cover the cheese with the second part of the sliced eggplant.
11. The next step is to make the layer of the ground chicken and all shredded Cheddar cheese,
12. Cover the cheese layer with the last part of the sliced eggplants.
13. Then sprinkle the eggplants with shredded Parmesan cheese.
14. Pour the heavy cream and add butter.
15. Preheat the air fryer to 365 F.
16. Cook the lasagna for 17 minutes.
17. When the time is over – let the lasagna chill gently.
18. Serve it!
Nutrition Info: calories 291, fat 17.6, fiber 4.6, carbs 7.8, protein 27.4

187. Buttered Scallops

Servings: 2
Cooking Time: 4 Minutes
Ingredients:
- ¾ pound sea scallops, cleaned and patted very dry
- 1 tablespoon butter, melted
- ½ tablespoon fresh thyme, minced
- Salt and black pepper, as required

Directions:
1. Preheat the Air fryer to 390 degree F and grease an Air fryer basket.
2. Mix scallops, butter, thyme, salt, and black pepper in a bowl.
3. Arrange scallops in the Air fryer basket and cook for about 4 minutes.
4. Dish out the scallops in a platter and serve hot.
Nutrition Info: Calories: 202, Fat: 7.1g, Carbohydrates: 4.4g, Sugar: 0g, Protein: 28.7g, Sodium: 393mg

188. Broccoli With Olives

Servings: 4
Cooking Time: 19 Minutes
Ingredients:
- 2 pounds broccoli, stemmed and cut into 1-inch florets
- 1/3 cup Kalamata olives, halved and pitted
- ¼ cup Parmesan cheese, grated
- 2 tablespoons olive oil
- Salt and ground black pepper, as required
- 2 teaspoons fresh lemon zest, grated

Directions:
1. Preheat the Air fryer to 400F and grease an Air fryer basket.
2. Boil the broccoli for about 4 minutes and drain well.
3. Mix broccoli, oil, salt, and black pepper in a bowl and toss to coat well.
4. Arrange broccoli into the Air fryer basket and cook for about 15 minutes.
5. Stir in the olives, lemon zest and cheese and dish out to serve.
Nutrition Info: Calories: 169, Fat: 10.2g, Carbohydrates: 16g, Sugar: 3.9g, Protein: 8.5g, Sodium: 254mg

189. Sage Beef

Servings: 4
Cooking Time: 30 Minutes
Ingredients:
- 2 pounds beef stew meat, cubed
- 1 tablespoon sage, chopped
- 2 tablespoons butter, melted
- ½ teaspoon coriander, ground
- ½ tablespoon garlic powder

- 1 teaspoon Italian seasoning
- Salt and black pepper to the taste

Directions:
1. In the air fryer's pan, mix the beef with the sage, melted butter and the other ingredients, introduce the pan in the fryer and cook at 360 degrees F for 30 minutes.
2. Divide everything between plates and serve.

Nutrition Info: Calories 290, Fat 11, Fiber 6, Carbs 20, Protein 29

190. Rich Meatloaf With Mustard And Peppers

Servings: 5
Cooking Time: 20 Minutes
Ingredients:
- 1 pound beef, ground
- 1/2 pound veal, ground
- 1 egg
- 4 tablespoons vegetable juice
- 1/2 cup pork rinds
- 2 bell peppers, chopped
- 1 onion, chopped
- 2 garlic cloves, minced
- 2 tablespoons tomato paste
- 2 tablespoons soy sauce
- 1 (1-ounce package ranch dressing mix
- Sea salt, to taste
- 1/2 teaspoon ground black pepper, to taste
- 7 ounces tomato puree
- 1 tablespoon Dijon mustard

Directions:
1. Start by preheating your Air Fryer to 330 degrees F.
2. In a mixing bowl, thoroughly combine the ground beef, veal, egg, vegetable juice, pork rinds, bell peppers, onion, garlic, tomato paste, soy sauce, ranch dressing mix, salt, and ground black pepper.
3. Mix until everything is well incorporated and press into a lightly greased meatloaf pan.
4. Cook approximately 25 minutes in the preheated Air Fryer. Whisk the tomato puree with the mustard and spread the topping over the top of your meatloaf.
5. Continue to cook 2 minutes more. Let it stand on a cooling rack for 6 minutes before slicing and serving. Enjoy!

Nutrition Info: 398 Calories; 24g Fat; 9g Carbs; 32g Protein; 3g Sugars; 6g Fiber

191. Irish Whisky Steak

Servings: 6
Cooking Time: 20 Minutes
Ingredients:
- 2 pounds sirloin steaks
- 1 ½ tablespoons tamari sauce
- 1/3 teaspoon cayenne pepper
- 1/3 teaspoon ground ginger
- 2 garlic cloves, thinly sliced
- 2 tablespoons Irish whiskey
- 2 tablespoons olive oil
- Fine sea salt, to taste

Directions:
1. Firstly, add all the ingredients, minus the olive oil and the steak, to a resealable plastic bag.
2. Throw in the steak and let it marinate for a couple of hours. After that, drizzle the sirloin steaks with 2 tablespoons olive oil.
3. Roast for approximately 22 minutes at 395 degrees F, turning it halfway through the time.

Nutrition Info: 260 Calories; 17g Fat; 8g Carbs; 35g Protein; 2g Sugars; 1g Fiber

192. Shrimp Casserole Louisiana Style

Servings: 2
Cooking Time: 35 Minutes
Ingredients:
- 3/4 cup uncooked instant rice
- 3/4 cup water
- 1/2 pound small shrimp, peeled and deveined
- 1 tablespoon butter
- 1/2 (4 ounces) can sliced mushrooms, drained
- 1/2 (8 ounces) container sour cream
- 1/3 cup shredded Cheddar cheese

Directions:
1. Place the instant pot air fryer lid on, lightly grease baking pan of the instant pot with cooking spray. Add rice, water, mushrooms, and butter. Cover with foil and place the baking pan in the instant pot.
2. Close the air fryer lid and cook at 360F for 20 minutes.
3. Open foil cover, stir in shrimps, return foil and let it rest for 5 minutes.
4. Remove foil completely and stir in sour cream. Mix well and evenly spread rice. Top with cheese.
5. Cook for 7 minutes at 390F until tops are lightly browned.
6. Serve and enjoy.

Nutrition Info: Calories: 569; Carbs: 38.5g; Protein: 31.8g; Fat: 31.9g

193. Beef, Mushrooms And Noodles Dish

Servings: 5
Cooking Time: 35 Minutes
Ingredients:
- 1½ pounds beef steak
- 1 package egg noodles, cooked
- 1 ounce dry onion soup mix
- 1 can (15 oz cream mushroom soup
- 2 cups mushrooms, sliced
- 1 whole onion, chopped
- ½ cup beef broth

- 3 garlic cloves, minced?

Directions:
1. Preheat your Air Fryer to 360 F. Drizzle onion soup mix all over the meat. In a mixing bowl, mix the sauce, garlic cloves, beef broth, chopped onion, sliced mushrooms and mushroom soup. Top the prepared meat with the prepared sauce mixture. Place the prepared meat in the air fryer's cooking basket and cook for 25 minutes. Serve with cooked egg noodles.

Nutrition Info: 346 Calories; 11g Fat; 4g Carbs; 32g Protein; 1g Sugars; 1g Fiber

194. Sesame Mustard Greens

Servings: 4
Cooking Time: 11 Minutes
Ingredients:
- 2 garlic cloves, minced
- 1 pound mustard greens, torn
- 1 tablespoon olive oil
- ½ cup yellow onion, sliced
- Salt and black pepper to the taste
- 3 tablespoons veggie stock
- ¼ teaspoon dark sesame oil

Directions:
1. Heat up a pan that fits your air fryer with the oil over medium heat, add onions, stir and brown them for 5 minutes.
2. Add garlic, stock, greens, salt and pepper, stir, introduce in your air fryer and cook at 350 °F for 6 minutes.
3. Add sesame oil, toss to coat, divide among plates and serve.

Nutrition Info: Calories: 173; Fat: 6g; Fiber: 2g; Carbs: 4g; Protein: 5g

195. Vegetable Cane

Servings: 4
Cooking Time: More Than 60 Minutes;
Ingredients:
- 2 calf legs
- 4 carrots
- 4 medium potatoes
- 1 clove garlic
- 300ml Broth
- Leave to taste
- Pepper to taste

Directions:
1. Place the ears, garlic, and half of the broth in the greased basket.
2. Set the temperature to 1800C.
3. Cook the stems for 40 minutes, turning them in the middle of cooking.
4. Add the vegetables in pieces, salt, pepper, pour the rest of the broth and cook for another 50 minutes (time may vary depending on the size of the hocks).
5. Mix the vegetables and the ears 2 to 3 times during cooking.

Nutrition Info: Calories 7.9, Fat 0.49g, Carbohydrate 0.77g, Sugar 0.49g, Protein 0.08mg, Cholesterol 0mg

196. Coconut Crusted Shrimp

Servings: 3
Cooking Time: 40 Minutes
Ingredients:
- 8 ounces coconut milk
- ½ cup sweetened coconut, shredded
- ½ cup panko breadcrumbs
- 1 pound large shrimp, peeled and deveined
- Salt and black pepper, to taste

Directions:
1. Preheat the Air fryer to 350-degree F and grease an Air fryer basket.
2. Place the coconut milk in a shallow bowl.
3. Mix coconut, breadcrumbs, salt, and black pepper in another bowl.
4. Dip each shrimp into coconut milk and finally, dredge in the coconut mixture.
5. Arrange half of the shrimps into the Air fryer basket and cook for about 20 minutes.
6. Dish out the shrimps onto serving plates and repeat with the remaining mixture to serve.

Nutrition Info: Calories: 408, Fats: 23.7g, Carbohydrates: 11.7g, Sugar: 3.4g, Proteins: 31g, Sodium: 253mg

197. Almond Pork Bites

Servings: 10
Cooking Time: 40 Minutes
Ingredients:
- 16 oz sausage meat
- 1 whole egg, beaten
- 3 ½ oz onion, chopped
- 2 tbsp dried sage
- 2 tbsp almonds, chopped
- ½ tsp pepper
- 3 ½ oz apple, sliced
- ½ tsp salt

Directions:
1. Preheat your air fryer to 350 f. In a bowl, mix onion, almonds, sliced apples, egg, pepper and salt. Add the almond mixture and sausage in a ziploc bag. Mix to coat well and set aside for 15 minutes.
2. Use the mixture to form cutlets. Add cutlets to your fryer's basket and cook for 25 minutes. Serve with heavy cream and enjoy!

Nutrition Info: Calories: 491.7 Cal Total Fat: 25.9 g Saturated Fat: 4.4 g Cholesterol: 42 mg Sodium: 364.3 mg Total Carbs: 40.4 g Fiber: 3.3 g Sugar: 0.7 g Protein: 21.8 g

198. Greek-style Monkfish With Vegetables

Servings: 2
Cooking Time: 20 Minutes
Ingredients:
- 2 teaspoons olive oil
- 1 cup celery, sliced
- 2 bell peppers, sliced
- 1 teaspoon dried thyme
- 1/2 teaspoon dried marjoram
- 1/2 teaspoon dried rosemary
- 2 monkfish fillets
- 1 tablespoon soy sauce
- 2 tablespoons lime juice
- Coarse salt and ground black pepper, to taste
- 1 teaspoon cayenne pepper
- 1/2 cup Kalamata olives, pitted and sliced

Directions:
1. In a nonstick skillet, heat the olive oil for 1 minute. Once hot, sauté the celery and peppers until tender, about 4 minutes. Sprinkle with thyme, marjoram, and rosemary and set aside.
2. Toss the fish fillets with the soy sauce, lime juice, salt, black pepper, and cayenne pepper. Place the fish fillets in a lightly greased cooking basket and bake at 390 degrees F for 8 minutes.
3. Turn them over, add the olives, and cook an additional 4 minutes. Serve with the sautéed vegetables on the side.

Nutrition Info: 292 Calories; 11g Fat; 1g Carbs; 22g Protein; 9g Sugars; 6g Fiber

199. Almond Asparagus

Servings: 3
Cooking Time: 6 Minutes
Ingredients:
- 1 pound asparagus
- 1/3 cup almonds, sliced
- 2 tablespoons olive oil
- 2 tablespoons balsamic vinegar
- Salt and black pepper, to taste

Directions:
1. Preheat the Air fryer to 400F and grease an Air fryer basket.
2. Mix asparagus, oil, vinegar, salt, and black pepper in a bowl and toss to coat well.
3. Arrange asparagus into the Air fryer basket and sprinkle with the almond slices.
4. Cook for about 6 minutes and dish out to serve hot.

Nutrition Info: Calories: 173, Fat: 14.8g, Carbohydrates: 8.2g, Sugar: 3.3g, Protein: 5.6g, Sodium: 54mg

200. Carrot Beef Cake

Servings: 10
Cooking Time: 60 Minutes
Ingredients:
- 3 eggs, beaten
- 1/2 cup almond milk
- 1-oz. onion soup mix
- 1 cup dry bread crumbs
- 2 cups shredded carrots
- 2 lbs. lean ground beef
- 1/2-lb. ground pork

Directions:
1. Thoroughly mix ground beef with carrots and all other ingredients in a bowl.
2. Grease a meatloaf pan with oil or butter and spread the minced beef in the pan.
3. Press "Power Button" of Air Fry Oven and turn the dial to select the "Bake" mode.
4. Press the Time button and again turn the dial to set the cooking time to 60 minutes.
5. Now push the Temp button and rotate the dial to set the temperature at 350 degrees F.
6. Once preheated, place the beef baking pan in the oven and close its lid.
7. Slice and serve.

Nutrition Info: Calories: 212 Cal Total Fat: 11.8 g Saturated Fat: 2.2 g Cholesterol: 23 mg Sodium: 321 mg Total Carbs: 14.6 g Fiber: 4.4 g Sugar: 8 g Protein: 17.3 g

201. Easy Air Fryed Roasted Asparagus

Servings: 4
Cooking Time: 10 Minutes
Ingredients:
- 1 bunch fresh asparagus
- 1 ½ tsp herbs de provence
- Fresh lemon wedge (optional)
- 1 tablespoon olive oil or cooking spray
- Salt and pepper to taste

Directions:
1. Wash asparagus and trim off hard ends
2. Drizzle asparagus with olive oil and add seasonings
3. Place asparagus in air fryer and cook on 360F for 6 to 10 minutes
4. Drizzle squeezed lemon over roasted asparagus.

Nutrition Info: Calories 46 protein 2g fat 3g net carbs 1g

202. Easy Marinated London Broil

Servings: 4
Cooking Time: 20 Minutes
Ingredients:
- For the marinade:
- 2 tablespoons Worcestershire sauce
- 2 garlic cloves, minced
- 1 tablespoon oil
- 2 tablespoons rice vinegar
- London Broil:

- 2 pounds London broil
- 2 tablespoons tomato paste
- Sea salt and cracked black pepper, to taste
- 1 tablespoon mustard

Directions:
1. Combine all the marinade ingredients in a mixing bowl; add the London boil to the bowl. Cover and let it marinate for 3 hours.
2. Preheat the Air Fryer to 400 degrees F. Spritz the Air Fryer grill pan with cooking oil.
3. Grill the marinated London broil in the preheated Air Fryer for 18 minutes. Turn London broil over, top with the tomato paste, salt, black pepper, and mustard.
4. Continue to grill an additional 10 minutes. Serve immediately.

Nutrition Info: 517 Calories; 21g Fat; 5g Carbs; 70g Protein; 4g Sugars; 7g Fiber

203. Hasselback Potatoes

Servings: 4
Cooking Time: 30 Minutes
Ingredients:
- 4 potatoes
- 2 tablespoons Parmesan cheese, shredded
- 1 tablespoon fresh chives, chopped
- 2 tablespoons olive oil

Directions:
1. Preheat the Air fryer to 355F and grease an Air fryer basket.
2. Cut slits along each potato about ¼-inch apart with a sharp knife, making sure slices should stay connected at the bottom.
3. Coat the potatoes with olive oil and arrange into the Air fryer basket.
4. Cook for about 30 minutes and dish out in a platter.
5. Top with chives and Parmesan cheese to serve.

Nutrition Info: Calories: 218, Fat: 7.9g, Carbohydrates: 33.6g, Sugar: 2.5g, Protein: 4.6g, Sodium: 55mg

204. Mozzarella & Olive Pizza Bagels

Servings: 4
Cooking Time: 10 Minutes
Ingredients:
- 2 whole wheat bagels
- 1/4 cup marinara sauce
- 1/4 teaspoon Italian seasoning
- 1/8 teaspoon red pepper flakes
- 3/4 cup shredded low-moisture mozzarella cheese
- 1/4 cup chopped green pepper
- 3 tablespoons sliced black olives
- Fresh basil
- 1 teaspoon parmesan cheese

Directions:
1. Start by preheating toaster oven to 375°F and lining a pan with parchment paper.
2. Cut bagels in half and lay on pan with inside facing up. Spread sauce over each half.
3. Sprinkle red pepper flakes and 2 tablespoons of mozzarella over each half.
4. Top each half with olives and peppers and then top with another tablespoon of mozzarella.
5. Bake for 8 minutes, then switch to broil setting and broil for another 2 minutes. Top with basil and parmesan and serve.

Nutrition Info: Calories: 222, Sodium: 493 mg, Dietary Fiber: 1.9 g, Total Fat: 6.1 g, Total Carbs: 30.2 g, Protein: 12.1 g.

MEATLESS RECIPES

205. Mushroom Wonton

Ingredients:
- 2 cups cubed mushroom
- 2 tbsp. oil
- 2 tsp. ginger-garlic paste
- 2 tsp. soya sauce
- 2 tsp. vinegar
- 1 ½ cup all-purpose flour
- ½ tsp. salt or to taste
- 5 tbsp. water

Directions:
1. Squeeze the dough and cover it with plastic wrap and set aside. Next, cook the ingredients for the filling and try to ensure that the mushroom is covered well with the sauce.
2. Roll the dough and place the filling in the center. Now, wrap the dough to cover the filling and pinch the edges together.
3. Pre heat the oven at 200° F for 5 minutes. Place the dumplings in the fry basket and close it. Let them cook at the same temperature for another 20 minutes. Recommended sides are chili sauce or ketchup.

206. Bottle Gourd Flat Cakes

Ingredients:
- 2 or 3 green chilies finely chopped
- 1 ½ tbsp. lemon juice
- Salt and pepper to taste
- 2 tbsp. garam masala
- 2 cups sliced bottle gourd
- 3 tsp. ginger finely chopped
- 1-2 tbsp. fresh coriander leaves

Directions:
1. Mix the ingredients in a clean bowl and add water to it. Make sure that the paste is not too watery but is enough to apply on the bottle gourd slices. Pre heat the oven at 160 degrees Fahrenheit for 5 minutes.
2. Place the French Cuisine Galettes in the fry basket and let them cook for another 25 minutes at the same temperature. Keep rolling them over to get a uniform cook. Serve either with mint sauce or ketchup.

207. Roasted Asparagus With Eggs And Tomatoes

Servings: 4
Cooking Time: 12 Minutes

Ingredients:
- 2 pounds (907 g) asparagus, trimmed
- 3 tablespoons extra-virgin olive oil, divided
- 1 teaspoon kosher salt, divided
- 1 pint cherry tomatoes
- 4 large eggs
- ¼ teaspoon freshly ground black pepper

Directions:
1. Put the asparagus in the baking pan and drizzle with 2 tablespoons of olive oil, tossing to coat. Season with ½ teaspoon of kosher salt.
2. Slide the baking pan into Rack Position 2, select Roast, set temperature to 375ºF (190ºC), and set time to 12 minutes.
3. Meanwhile, toss the cherry tomatoes with the remaining 1 tablespoon of olive oil in a medium bowl until well coated.
4. After 6 minutes, remove the pan and toss the asparagus. Evenly spread the asparagus in the middle of the pan. Add the tomatoes around the perimeter of the pan. Return the pan to the oven and continue cooking.
5. After 2 minutes, remove from the oven.
6. Carefully crack the eggs, one at a time, over the asparagus, spacing them out. Season with the remaining ½ teaspoon of kosher salt and the pepper. Return the pan to the oven and continue cooking. Cook for an additional 3 to 7 minutes, or until the eggs are cooked to your desired doneness.
7. When done, divide the asparagus and eggs among four plates. Top each plate evenly with the tomatoes and serve.

208. Tasty Polenta Crisps

Servings: 4
Cooking Time: 25 Minutes + Chilling Time

Ingredients:
- 2 cups milk
- 1 cup instant polenta
- Salt and black pepper to taste
- fresh thyme, chopped

Directions:
1. Fill a saucepan with milk and 2 cups of water and place over low heat. Bring to a simmer. Keep whisking as you pour in the polenta. Continue to whisk until polenta thickens and bubbles; season to taste. Add polenta to a lined with parchment paper baking tray and spread out.
2. Refrigerate for 45 minutes. Slice, set polenta into batons, and spray with olive oil. Arrange polenta chips into the basket and fit in the baking tray; cook for 16 minutes at 380 F on Air Fry function, turning once halfway through. Make sure the fries are golden and crispy. Serve.

209. Pizza

Ingredients:
- 2 tomatoes that have been deseeded and chopped

- 1 tbsp. (optional) mushrooms/corns
- 2 tsp. pizza seasoning
- Some cottage cheese that has been cut into small cubes (optional)
- One pizza base
- Grated pizza cheese (mozzarella cheese preferably) for topping
- Use cooking oil for brushing and topping purposes
- ingredients for topping:
- 2 onions chopped
- 2 capsicums chopped

Directions:
1. Put the pizza base in a pre-heated oven for around 5 minutes. (Pre heated to 340 Fahrenheit). Take out the base.
2. Pour some pizza sauce on top of the base at the center. Using a spoon spread the sauce over the base making sure that you leave some gap around the circumference. Grate some mozzarella cheese and sprinkle it over the sauce layer. Take all the vegetables mentioned in the ingredient list above and mix them in a bowl.
3. Add some oil and seasoning. Also add some salt and pepper according to taste. Mix them properly. Put this topping over the layer of cheese on the pizza. Now sprinkle some more grated cheese and pizza seasoning on top of this layer.
4. Pre heat the oven at 250 Fahrenheit for around 5 minutes. Open the fry basket and place the pizza inside. Close the basket and keep the fryer at 170 degrees for another 10 minutes. If you feel that it is undercooked you may put it at the same temperature for another 2 minutes or so.

210. Amaranthus French Cuisine Galette

Ingredients:
- 1 ½ tbsp. lemon juice
- Salt and pepper to taste
- 2 cups minced Amaranthus
- 3 tsp. ginger finely chopped
- 1-2 tbsp. fresh coriander leaves
- 2 or 3 green chilies finely chopped

Directions:
1. Mix the ingredients in a clean bowl.
2. Mold this mixture into round and flat French Cuisine Galettes.
3. Wet the French Cuisine Galettes slightly with water.
4. Pre heat the oven at 160 degrees Fahrenheit for 5 minutes. Place the French Cuisine Galettes in the fry basket and let them cook for another 25 minutes at the same temperature. Keep rolling them over to get a uniform cook. Serve either with mint sauce or ketchup.

211. Mexican Burritos

Ingredients:
- 1 tbsp. Olive oil
- 1 medium onion finely sliced
- 3 flakes garlic crushed
- 1 tsp. freshly ground peppercorns
- ½ cup pickled jalapenos (Chop them up finely)
- 2 carrots (Cut in to long thin slices)
- 1-2 lettuce leaves shredded.
- 1 or 2 spring onions chopped finely. Also cut the greens.
- Take one tomato. Remove the seeds and chop it into small pieces.
- ½ cup French beans (Slice them lengthwise into thin and long slices)
- ½ cup mushrooms thinly sliced
- 1 cup cottage cheese cut in too long and slightly thick Oregano Fingers
- ½ cup shredded cabbage
- 1 tbsp. coriander, chopped
- 1 tbsp. vinegar
- 1 tsp. white wine
- ½ cup red kidney beans (soaked overnight)
- ½ small onion chopped
- 1 tbsp. olive oil
- 2 tbsp. tomato puree
- ¼ tsp. red chili powder
- 1 tsp. of salt to taste
- 4-5 flour tortillas
- A pinch of salt to taste
- ½ tsp. red chili flakes
- 1 green chili chopped.
- 1 cup of cheddar cheese grated.

Directions:
1. Cook the beans along with the onion and garlic and mash them finely. Now, make the sauce you will need for the burrito. Ensure that you create a slightly thick sauce.
2. For the filling, you will need to cook the ingredients well in a pan and ensure that the vegetables have browned on the outside.
3. To make the salad, toss the ingredients together.

212. Gherkins Flat Cakes

Ingredients:
- 2 or 3 green chilies finely chopped
- 1 ½ tbsp. lemon juice
- Salt and pepper to taste
- 2 tbsp. garam masala
- 2 cups sliced gherkins
- 3 tsp. ginger finely chopped
- 1-2 tbsp. fresh coriander leaves

Directions:
1. Mix the ingredients in a clean bowl and add water to it. Make sure that the paste is not too watery but is enough to apply on the gherkin.

2. Pre heat the oven at 160 degrees Fahrenheit for 5 minutes. Place the French Cuisine Galettes in the fry basket and let them cook for another 25 minutes at the same temperature. Keep rolling them over to get a uniform cook. Serve either with mint sauce or ketchup.

213. Dal Mint Spicy Lemon Kebab

Ingredients:
- 2 tsp. coriander powder
- 1 ½ tbsp. chopped coriander
- ½ tsp. dried mango powder
- 1 cup dry breadcrumbs
- ¼ tsp. black salt
- 1-2 tbsp. all-purpose flour for coating purposes
- 1-2 tbsp. mint (finely chopped)
- 1 cup chickpeas
- Half inch ginger grated or one and a half tsp. of ginger-garlic paste
- 1-2 green chilies chopped finely
- ¼ tsp. red chili powder
- A pinch of salt to taste
- ½ tsp. roasted cumin powder
- 1 onion that has been finely chopped
- ½ cup milk

Directions:
1. Take an open vessel. Boil the chickpeas in the vessel until their texture becomes soft. Make sure that they do not become soggy. Now take this chickpea into another container. Add the grated ginger and the cut green chilies.
2. Grind this mixture until it becomes a thick paste. Keep adding water as and when required. Now add the onions, mint, the breadcrumbs and all the various masalas required. Mix this well until you get a soft dough. Now take small balls of this mixture (about the size of a lemon) and mold them into the shape of flat and round kebabs.
3. Here is where the milk comes into play. Pour a very small amount of milk onto each kebab to wet it. Now roll the kebab in the dry breadcrumbs. Pre heat the oven for 5 minutes at 300 Fahrenheit. Take out the basket.
4. Arrange the kebabs in the basket leaving gaps between them so that no two kebabs are touching each other. Keep the fryer at 340 Fahrenheit for around half an hour. Half way through the cooking process, turn the kebabs over so that they can be cooked properly. Recommended sides for this dish are mint sauce, tomato ketchup or yoghurt sauce.

214. Lemony Wax Beans

Servings: 4
Cooking Time: 12 Minutes
Ingredients:
- 2 pounds (907 g) wax beans
- 2 tablespoons extra-virgin olive oil
- Salt and freshly ground black pepper, to taste
- Juice of ½ lemon, for serving

Directions:
1. Line the air fryer basket with aluminum foil.
2. Toss the wax beans with the olive oil in a large bowl. Lightly season with salt and pepper.
3. Spread out the wax beans in the basket.
4. Put the air fryer basket on the baking pan and slide into Rack Position 2, select Roast, set temperature to 400ºF (205ºC), and set time to 12 minutes.
5. When done, the beans will be caramelized and tender. Remove from the oven to a plate and serve sprinkled with the lemon juice.

215. Snake Gourd French Cuisine Galette

Ingredients:
- 1-2 tbsp. fresh coriander leaves
- 2 or 3 green chilies finely chopped
- 1 ½ tbsp. lemon juice
- Salt and pepper to taste
- 2 tbsp. garam masala
- 1 cup sliced snake gourd
- 1 ½ cup coarsely crushed peanuts
- 3 tsp. ginger finely chopped

Directions:
1. Mix the ingredients in a clean bowl.
2. Mold this mixture into round and flat French Cuisine Galettes.
3. Wet the French Cuisine Galettes slightly with water. Coat each French Cuisine Galette with the crushed peanuts.
4. Pre heat the oven at 160 degrees Fahrenheit for 5 minutes. Place the French Cuisine Galettes in the fry basket and let them cook for another 25 minutes at the same temperature. Keep rolling them over to get a uniform cook. Serve either with mint sauce or ketchup.

216. Honey Chili Potatoes

Ingredients:
- 1 capsicum, cut into thin and long pieces (lengthwise).
- 2 tbsp. olive oil
- 2 onions. Cut them into halves.
- 1 ½ tbsp. sweet chili sauce
- 1 ½ tsp. ginger garlic paste
- ½ tbsp. red chili sauce.
- 2 tbsp. tomato ketchup
- 3 big potatoes (Cut into strips or cubes)
- 2 ½ tsp. ginger-garlic paste
- ¼ tsp. salt
- 1 tsp. red chili sauce
- ¼ tsp. red chili powder/black pepper
- A few drops of edible orange food coloring

- 2 tsp. soya sauce
- 2 tsp. vinegar
- A pinch of black pepper powder
- 1-2 tsp. red chili flakes

Directions:
1. Create the mix for the potato Oregano Fingers and coat the chicken well with it.
2. Pre heat the oven at 250 Fahrenheit for 5 minutes or so. Open the basket of the Fryer. Place the Oregano Fingers inside the basket. Now let the fryer stay at 290 Fahrenheit for another 20 minutes. Keep tossing the Oregano Fingers periodically through the cook to get a uniform cook.
3. Add the ingredients to the sauce and cook it with the vegetables till it thickens. Add the Oregano Fingers to the sauce and cook till the flavors have blended.

217. Zucchini Parmesan Crisps

Servings: 4
Cooking Time: 25 Minutes
Ingredients:
- 4 small zucchini, cut lengthwise
- ½ cup Parmesan cheese, grated
- ½ cup breadcrumbs
- ¼ cup melted butter
- ¼ cup chopped parsley
- 4 garlic cloves, minced
- Salt and black pepper to taste

Directions:
1. Preheat on Air Fry function to 350 F. In a bowl, mix breadcrumbs, Parmesan cheese, garlic, parsley, salt, and pepper. Stir in butter. Place the zucchinis cut-side up in a baking tray.
2. Spread the cheese mixture onto the zucchini evenly. Cook for 13 minutes. Increase the temperature to 370 F and cook for 3 more minutes for extra crunchiness. Serve hot.

218. Cream Cheese Stuffed Bell Peppers

Servings: 2
Cooking Time: 15 Minutes
Ingredients:
- 2 bell peppers, tops and seeds removed
- Salt and pepper, to taste
- ²/₃ cup cream cheese
- 2 tablespoons mayonnaise
- 1 tablespoon chopped fresh celery stalks
- Cooking spray

Directions:
1. Spritz the air fryer basket with cooking spray.
2. Place the peppers in the air fryer basket.
3. Put the air fryer basket on the baking pan and slide into Rack Position 2, select Roast, set temperature to 400ºF (205ºC) and set time to 10 minutes.
4. Flip the peppers halfway through.
5. When cooking is complete, the peppers should be crisp-tender.
6. Remove from the oven to a plate and season with salt and pepper.
7. Mix the cream cheese, mayo, and celery in a small bowl and stir to incorporate. Evenly stuff the roasted peppers with the cream cheese mixture with a spoon. Serve immediately.

219. Panko Green Beans

Servings: 4
Cooking Time: 15 Minutes
Ingredients:
- ½ cup flour
- 2 eggs
- 1 cup panko bread crumbs
- ½ cup grated Parmesan cheese
- 1 teaspoon cayenne pepper
- Salt and black pepper, to taste
- 1½ pounds (680 g) green beans

Directions:
1. In a bowl, place the flour. In a separate bowl, lightly beat the eggs. In a separate shallow bowl, thoroughly combine the bread crumbs, cheese, cayenne pepper, salt, and pepper.
2. Dip the green beans in the flour, then in the beaten eggs, finally in the bread crumb mixture to coat well. Transfer the green beans to the air fryer basket.
3. Put the air fryer basket on the baking pan and slide into Rack Position 2, select Air Fry, set temperature to 400ºF (205ºC), and set time to 15 minutes.
4. Stir the green beans halfway through the cooking time.
5. When cooking is complete, remove from the oven to a bowl and serve.

220. Vegetable Fried Mix Chips

Servings: 4
Cooking Time: 45 Minutes
Ingredients:
- 1 large eggplant
- 4 potatoes
- 3 zucchinis
- ½ cup cornstarch
- ½ cup olive oil
- Salt to season

Directions:
1. Preheat on Air Fry function to 390 F. Cut the eggplant and zucchini in long 3-inch strips. Peel and cut the potatoes into 3-inch strips; set aside.
2. In a bowl, stir in cornstarch, ½ cup of water, salt, pepper, oil, eggplant, zucchini, and potatoes. Place

one-third of the veggie strips in the basket and fit in the baking tray; cook for 12 minutes, shaking once.
3. Once ready, transfer them to a serving platter. Repeat the cooking process for the remaining veggie strips. Serve warm.

221. Feta & Scallion Triangles

Servings: 4
Cooking Time: 20 Minutes
Ingredients:
- 4 oz feta cheese, crumbled
- 2 sheets filo pastry
- 1 egg yolk, beaten
- 2 tbsp fresh parsley, finely chopped
- 1 scallion, finely chopped
- 2 tbsp olive oil
- Salt and black pepper to taste

Directions:
1. In a bowl, mix the yolk with the cheese, parsley, and scallion. Season with salt and black pepper. Cut each filo sheet in 3 strips. Put a teaspoon of the feta mixture on the bottom. Roll the strip in a spinning spiral way until the filling of the inside mixture is completely wrapped in a triangle.
2. Preheat Breville on Bake function to 360 F. Brush the surface of filo with olive oil. Place up to 5 triangles in the oven and press Start. Cook for 5 minutes. Lower the temperature to 330 F, cook for 3 more minutes or until golden brown.

222. French Bean Toast

Ingredients:
- 1 tsp. sugar for every 2 slices
- Crushed cornflakes
- 2 cups baked beans
- Bread slices (brown or white)
- 1 egg white for every 2 slices

Directions:
1. Put two slices together and cut them along the diagonal.
2. In a bowl, whisk the egg whites and add some sugar.
3. Dip the bread triangles into this mixture and then coat them with the crushed cornflakes.
4. Pre heat the oven at 180° C for 4 minutes. Place the coated bread triangles in the fry basket and close it. Let them cook at the same temperature for another 20 minutes at least. Halfway through the process, turn the triangles over so that you get a uniform cook. Top with baked beans and serve.

223. Mushroom Pops

Ingredients:
- 1 tsp. dry basil
- 1 tsp. lemon juice
- 1 tsp. red chili flakes
- 1 cup whole mushrooms
- 1 ½ tsp. garlic paste
- Salt and pepper to taste
- 1 tsp. dry oregano

Directions:
1. Add the ingredients into a separate bowl and mix them well to get a consistent mixture.
2. Dip the mushrooms in the above mixture and leave them aside for some time.
3. Pre heat the oven at 180° C for around 5 minutes. Place the coated cottage cheese pieces in the fry basket and close it properly. Let them cook at the same temperature for 20 more minutes. Keep turning them over in the basket so that they are cooked properly. Serve with tomato ketchup.

224. Baked Chickpea Stars

Ingredients:
- 4 tbsp. roasted sesame seeds
- 2 small onion finely chopped
- ½ tsp. coriander powder
- ½ tsp. cumin powder
- Use olive oil for greasing purposes
- 1 cup white chick peas soaked overnight
- 1 tsp. ginger-garlic paste
- 4 tbsp. chopped coriander leaves
- 2 green chilies finely chopped
- 4 tbsp. thick curd
- Pinches of salt and pepper to taste
- 1 tsp. dry mint

Directions:
1. Since the chickpeas have been soaked you will first have to drain them. Add a pinch of salt and pour water until the chickpeas are submerged. Put this container in a pressure cooker and let the chickpeas cook for around 25 minutes until they turn soft. Remove the cooker from the flame. Now mash the chickpeas.
2. Take another container. Into it add the ginger garlic paste, onions, coriander leaves, coriander powder, cumin powder, green chili, salt and pepper, and 1 tbsp. Use your hands to mix these ingredients Pour this mixture into the container with the mashed chickpeas and mix. Spread this mixture over a flat surface to about a half-inch thickness.
3. Cut star shapes out of this layer. Make a mixture of curd and mint leaves and spread this over the surface of the star shaped cutlets. Coat all the sides with sesame seeds. Pre heat the oven at 200-degree Fahrenheit for 5 minutes. Open the basket of the Fryer and put the stars inside. Close the basket properly. Continue to cook the stars for around half an hour. Periodically turn over the stars in the basket in order to prevent overcooking one side. Serve either with mint sauce or tomato ketchup.

225. Portobello Steaks

Servings: 4
Cooking Time: 20 Minutes
Ingredients:
- Nonstick cooking spray
- ¼ cup olive oil
- 2 tbsp. steak seasoning, unsalted
- 1 rosemary stem
- 4 Portobello mushrooms, large caps with stems removed

Directions:
1. Place baking pan in position 2 and spray with cooking spray.
2. In a large bowl, stir together oil, steak seasoning, and rosemary.
3. Add mushrooms and toss to coat all sides thoroughly.
4. Set oven to bake on 400°F for 25 minutes. After 5 minutes, place the mushrooms on the pan and bake 20 minutes, or until mushrooms are tender. Serve immediately.

Nutrition Info: Calories 142, Total Fat 14g, Saturated Fat 2g, Total Carbs 3g, Net Carbs 2g, Protein 1g, Sugar 1g, Fiber 1g, Sodium 309mg, Potassium 118mg, Phosphorus 20mg

226. Barbeque Corn Sandwich

Ingredients:
- ½ flake garlic crushed
- ¼ cup chopped onion
- ¼ tbsp. red chili sauce
- ½ cup water
- 2 slices of white bread
- 1 tbsp. softened butter
- 1 cup sweet corn kernels
- 1 small capsicum
- ¼ tbsp. Worcestershire sauce
- ½ tsp. olive oil

Directions:
1. Take the slices of bread and remove the edges. Now cut the slices horizontally.
2. Cook the ingredients for the sauce and wait till it thickens. Now, add the corn to the sauce and stir till it obtains the flavors. Roast the capsicum and peel the skin off. Cut the capsicum into slices. Apply the sauce on the slices.
3. Pre-heat the oven for 5 minutes at 300 Fahrenheit. Open the basket of the Fryer and place the prepared Classic Sandwiches in it such that no two Classic Sandwiches are touching each other. Now keep the fryer at 250 degrees for around 15 minutes. Turn the Classic Sandwiches in between the cooking process to cook both slices. Serve the Classic Sandwiches with tomato ketchup or mint sauce.

227. Cornflakes French Toast

Ingredients:
- 1 tsp. sugar for every 2 slices
- Crushed cornflakes
- Bread slices (brown or white)
- 1 egg white for every 2 slices

Directions:
1. Put two slices together and cut them along the diagonal.
2. In a bowl, whisk the egg whites and add some sugar.
3. Dip the bread triangles into this mixture and then coat them with the crushed cornflakes.
4. Pre heat the oven at 180° C for 4 minutes. Place the coated bread triangles in the fry basket and close it. Let them cook at the same temperature for another 20 minutes at least. Halfway through the process, turn the triangles over so that you get a uniform cook. Serve these slices with chocolate sauce.

228. Simple Polenta Crisps

Servings: 4
Cooking Time: 25 Minutes + Chilling Time
Ingredients:
- 2 cups milk
- 1 cup instant polenta
- Salt and black pepper
- Fresh thyme, chopped

Directions:
1. Line a tray with parchment paper. Pour milk and 2 cups of water into a saucepan and simmer. Keep whisking as you pour in the polenta. Continue to whisk until polenta thickens and bubbles; season to taste. Add polenta to the lined tray and spread out. Refrigerate for 45 minutes.
2. Slice the polenta into batons and spray with oil. Arrange the polenta chips on the basket and press Start. Cook for 16 minutes at 380 F on AirFry function until golden and crispy.

229. Hearty Roasted Veggie Salad

Servings: 2
Cooking Time: 20 Minutes
Ingredients:
- 1 potato, chopped
- 1 carrot, sliced diagonally
- 1 cup cherry tomatoes
- ½ small beetroot, sliced
- ¼ onion, sliced
- ½ teaspoon turmeric
- ½ teaspoon cumin
- ¼ teaspoon sea salt
- 2 tablespoons olive oil, divided
- A handful of arugula
- A handful of baby spinach

- Juice of 1 lemon
- 3 tablespoons canned chickpeas, for serving
- Parmesan shavings, for serving

Directions:
1. Combine the potato, carrot, cherry tomatoes, beetroot, onion, turmeric, cumin, salt, and 1 tablespoon of olive oil in a large bowl and toss until well coated.
2. Arrange the veggies in the air fryer basket.
3. Put the air fryer basket on the baking pan and slide into Rack Position 2, select Roast, set temperature to 370ºF (188ºC) and set time to 20 minutes.
4. Stir the vegetables halfway through.
5. When cooking is complete, the potatoes should be golden brown.
6. Let the veggies cool for 5 to 10 minutes in the oven.
7. Put the arugula, baby spinach, lemon juice, and remaining 1 tablespoon of olive oil in a salad bowl and stir to combine. Mix in the roasted veggies and toss well.
8. Scatter the chickpeas and Parmesan shavings on top and serve immediately.

230. Asparagus French Cuisine Galette

Ingredients:
- 1 ½ tbsp. lemon juice
- Salt and pepper to taste
- 2 cups minced asparagus
- 3 tsp. ginger finely chopped
- 1-2 tbsp. fresh coriander leaves
- 2 or 3 green chilies finely chopped

Directions:
1. Mix the ingredients in a clean bowl.
2. Mold this mixture into round and flat French Cuisine Galettes.
3. Wet the French Cuisine Galettes slightly with water.
4. Pre heat the oven at 160 degrees Fahrenheit for 5 minutes. Place the French Cuisine Galettes in the fry basket and let them cook for another 25 minutes at the same temperature. Keep rolling them over to get a uniform cook. Serve either with mint sauce or ketchup.

231. Yam French Cuisine Galette

Ingredients:
- 1 ½ tbsp. lemon juice
- Salt and pepper to taste
- 2 cups minced yam
- 3 tsp. ginger finely chopped
- 1-2 tbsp. fresh coriander leaves
- 2 or 3 green chilies finely chopped

Directions:
1. Mix the ingredients in a clean bowl.
2. Mold this mixture into round and flat French Cuisine Galettes.
3. Wet the French Cuisine Galettes slightly with water.
4. Pre heat the oven at 160 degrees Fahrenheit for 5 minutes. Place the French Cuisine Galettes in the fry basket and let them cook for another 25 minutes at the same temperature. Keep rolling them over to get a uniform cook. Serve either with mint sauce or ketchup.

232. Eggplant Patties With Mozzarella

Servings: 1
Cooking Time: 10 Minutes
Ingredients:
- 1 hamburger bun
- 2-inch eggplant slices, cut along the round axis
- 1 mozzarella cheese slice
- 3 red onion rings
- 1 lettuce leaf
- ½ tbsp tomato sauce
- 1 pickle, sliced

Directions:
1. Preheat Breville on Bake function to 330 F. Cook in the eggplant slices to roast for 6 minutes. Place the mozzarella slice on top of the eggplant and cook for 30 more seconds. Spread tomato sauce on one half of the bun.
2. Place the lettuce leaf on top of the sauce. Place the cheesy eggplant on top of the lettuce. Top with onion rings and pickles, and then with the other bun half and enjoy.

233. Green Chili Taquitos

Servings: 3
Cooking Time: 10 Minutes
Ingredients:
- Nonstick cooking spray
- 6 corn tortillas
- ¾ cup vegan cream cheese
- 1 cup vegan cheddar cheese, grated
- 4 oz. green chilies, diced & drained

Directions:
1. Place baking pan in position 2. Lightly spray fryer basket with cooking spray.
2. Wrap tortillas in paper towels and microwave 1 minute.
3. Spread the cream cheese over tortillas. Top with cheddar cheese and chilies. Roll up tightly. Place, seam side down, in fryer basket.
4. Place the basket on the baking pan and set oven to air fry on 350°F for 10 minutes or until tortillas are browned and crispy. Turn taquitos over halfway through cooking time. Serve immediately.

Nutrition Info: Calories 706, Total Fat 34g, Saturated Fat 18g, Total Carbs 51g, Net Carbs 35g,

Protein 24g, Sugar 11g, Fiber 16g, Sodium 2371mg, Potassium 1074mg, Phosphorus 850mg

234. Spicy Sweet Potato Friespotato Fries

Servings: 4
Cooking Time: 37 Minutes
Ingredients:
- 2 tbsp. sweet potato fry seasoning mix
- 2 tbsp. olive oil
- 2 sweet potatoes
- Seasoning Mix:
- 2 tbsp. salt
- 1 tbsp. cayenne pepper
- 1 tbsp. dried oregano
- 1 tbsp. fennel
- 2 tbsp. coriander

Directions:
1. Preparing the Ingredients. Slice both ends off sweet potatoes and peel. Slice lengthwise in half and again crosswise to make four pieces from each potato.
2. Slice each potato piece into 2-3 slices, then slice into fries.
3. Grind together all of seasoning mix ingredients and mix in the salt.
4. Ensure the air fryer oven is preheated to 350 degrees.
5. Toss potato pieces in olive oil, sprinkling with seasoning mix and tossing well to coat thoroughly.
6. Air Frying. Add fries to air fryer rack/basket. Set temperature to 350°F, and set time to 27 minutes. Select START/STOP to begin.
7. Take out the basket and turn fries. Turn off air fryer oven and let cook 10-12 minutes till fries are golden.

Nutrition Info: CALORIES: 89; FAT: 14G; PROTEIN: 8Gs; SUGAR:3

235. Veg Momo's Recipe

Ingredients:
- 2 tsp. ginger-garlic paste
- 2 tsp. soya sauce
- 2 tsp. vinegar
- 1 ½ cup all-purpose flour
- ½ tsp. salt or to taste
- 5 tbsp. water
- 2 cup carrots grated
- 2 cup cabbage grated
- 2 tbsp. oil

Directions:
1. Squeeze the dough and cover it with plastic wrap and set aside. Next, cook the ingredients for the filling and try to ensure that the vegetables are covered well with the sauce.
2. Roll the dough and cut it into a square. Place the filling in the center. Now, wrap the dough to cover the filling and pinch the edges together.
3. Pre heat the oven at 200° F for 5 minutes. Place the gnocchi's in the fry basket and close it. Let them cook at the same temperature for another 20 minutes. Recommended sides are chili sauce or ketchup.

236. Masala Potato Wedges

Ingredients:
- 1 tsp. mixed herbs
- ½ tsp. red chili flakes
- A pinch of salt to taste
- 1 tbsp. lemon juice
- 2 medium sized potatoes (Cut into wedges)
- ingredients for the marinade:
- 1 tbsp. olive oil
- 1 tsp. garam masala

Directions:
1. Boil the potatoes and blanch them. Mix the ingredients for the marinade and add the potato Oregano Fingers to it making sure that they are coated well.
2. Pre heat the oven for around 5 minutes at 300 Fahrenheit. Take out the basket of the fryer and place the potato Oregano Fingers in them. Close the basket.
3. Now keep the fryer at 200 Fahrenheit for 20 or 25 minutes. In between the process, toss the fries twice or thrice so that they get cooked properly.

237. Cauliflower Spicy Lemon Kebab

Ingredients:
- 3 tsp. lemon juice
- 2 tsp. garam masala
- 3 eggs
- 2 ½ tbsp. white sesame seeds
- 2 cups cauliflower florets
- 3 onions chopped
- 5 green chilies-roughly chopped
- 1 ½ tbsp. ginger paste
- 1 ½ tsp. garlic paste
- 1 ½ tsp. salt

Directions:
1. Grind the ingredients except for the egg and form a smooth paste. Coat the florets in the paste. Now, beat the eggs and add a little salt to it.
2. Dip the coated florets in the egg mixture and then transfer to the sesame seeds and coat the florets well. Place the vegetables on a stick.
3. Pre heat the oven at 160 degrees Fahrenheit for around 5 minutes. Place the sticks in the basket and let them cook for another 25 minutes at the same temperature. Turn the sticks over in between the cooking process to get a uniform cook.

238. Mushroom Homemade Fried Sticks

Ingredients:
- One or two poppadums'
- 4 or 5 tbsp. corn flour
- 1 cup of water
- 2 cups whole mushrooms
- 1 big lemon-juiced
- 1 tbsp. ginger-garlic paste
- For seasoning, use salt and red chili powder in small amounts
- ½ tsp. carom

Directions:
1. Make a mixture of lemon juice, red chili powder, salt, ginger garlic paste and carom to use as a marinade. Let the cottage cheese pieces marinate in the mixture for some time and then roll them in dry corn flour. Leave them aside for around 20 minutes.
2. Take the poppadum into a pan and roast them. Once they are cooked, crush them into very small pieces. Now take another container and pour around 100 ml of water into it. Dissolve 2 tbsp. of corn flour in this water. Dip the cottage cheese pieces in this solution of corn flour and roll them on to the pieces of crushed poppadum so that the poppadum sticks to the cottage cheese.
3. Pre heat the oven for 10 minutes at 290 Fahrenheit. Then open the basket of the fryer and place the cottage cheese pieces inside it. Close the basket properly. Let the fryer stay at 160 degrees for another 20 minutes. Halfway through, open the basket and toss the cottage cheese around a bit to allow for uniform cooking. Once they are done, you can serve it either with ketchup or mint sauce. Another recommended side is mint sauce.

239. Russian-style Eggplant Caviar

Servings: 3
Cooking Time: 20 Minutes
Ingredients:
- 3 medium eggplants
- ½ red onion, chopped and blended
- 2 tbsp balsamic vinegar
- 1 tbsp olive oil
- Salt to taste

Directions:
1. Arrange the eggplants on the AirFryer basket and fit in the baking tray. Cook them in your for 15 minutes at 380 F on Bake function. Let cool.
2. Peel the cooled eggplants and chop them. Process the onion and eggplant in a blender. Add in the vinegar, olive oil, and salt, then blend again. Serve cool with bread and tomato sauce.

240. Parmesan Coated Green Beans

Servings: 4
Cooking Time: 20 Minutes
Ingredients:
- 1 cup panko breadcrumbs
- 2 whole eggs, beaten
- ½ cup Parmesan cheese, grated
- ½ cup flour
- 1 tsp cayenne pepper powder
- 1 ½ pounds green beans
- Salt to taste

Directions:
1. Preheat Breville on AirFry function to 380 F. In a bowl, mix breadcrumbs, Parmesan cheese, cayenne pepper powder, salt, and pepper. Flour the green beans and dip them in eggs. Dredge beans in the Parmesan-panko mix. Place in the cooking basket and cook for 15 minutes Serve.

241. Stuffed Peppers With Beans And Rice

Servings: 4
Cooking Time: 18 Minutes
Ingredients:
- 4 medium red, green, or yellow bell peppers, halved and deseeded
- 4 tablespoons extra-virgin olive oil, divided
- ½ teaspoon kosher salt, divided
- 1 (15-ounce / 425-g) can chickpeas
- 1½ cups cooked white rice
- ½ cup diced roasted red peppers
- ¼ cup chopped parsley
- ½ small onion, finely chopped
- 3 garlic cloves, minced
- ½ teaspoon cumin
- ¼ teaspoon freshly ground black pepper
- ¾ cup panko bread crumbs

Directions:
1. Brush the peppers inside and out with 1 tablespoon of olive oil. Season the insides with ¼ teaspoon of kosher salt. Arrange the peppers in the air fryer basket, cut side up.
2. Place the chickpeas with their liquid into a large bowl. Lightly mash the beans with a potato masher. Sprinkle with the remaining ¼ teaspoon of kosher salt and 1 tablespoon of olive oil. Add the rice, red peppers, parsley, onion, garlic, cumin, and black pepper to the bowl and stir to incorporate.
3. Divide the mixture among the bell pepper halves.
4. Stir together the remaining 2 tablespoons of olive oil and panko in a small bowl. Top the pepper halves with the panko mixture.
5. Put the air fryer basket on the baking pan and slide into Rack Position 2, select Roast, set temperature to 375ºF (190ºC), and set time to 18 minutes.
6. When done, the peppers should be slightly wrinkled, and the panko should be golden brown.
7. Remove from the oven and serve on a plate.

242. Tortellini With Veggies And Parmesan

Servings: 4
Cooking Time: 16 Minutes
Ingredients:
- 8 ounces (227 g) sugar snap peas, trimmed
- ½ pound (227 g) asparagus, trimmed and cut into 1-inch pieces
- 2 teaspoons kosher salt or 1 teaspoon fine salt, divided
- 1 tablespoon extra-virgin olive oil
- 1½ cups water
- 1 (20-ounce / 340-g) package frozen cheese tortellini
- 2 garlic cloves, minced
- 1 cup heavy (whipping) cream
- 1 cup cherry tomatoes, halved
- ½ cup grated Parmesan cheese
- ¼ cup chopped fresh parsley or basil
- Add the peas and asparagus to a large bowl. Add ½ teaspoon of kosher salt and the olive oil and toss until well coated. Place the veggies in the baking pan.

Directions:
1. Slide the baking pan into Rack Position 1, select Convection Bake, set the temperature to 450ºF (235ºC), and set the time for 4 minutes.
2. Meanwhile, dissolve 1 teaspoon of kosher salt in the water.
3. Once cooking is complete, remove the pan from the oven and place the tortellini in the pan. Pour the salted water over the tortellini. Put the pan back to the oven.
4. Slide the baking pan into Rack Position 1, select Convection Bake, set temperature to 450ºF (235ºC), and set time for 7 minutes.
5. Meantime, stir together the garlic, heavy cream, and remaining ½ teaspoon of kosher salt in a small bowl.
6. Once cooking is complete, remove the pan from the oven. Blot off any remaining water with a paper towel. Gently stir the ingredients. Drizzle the cream over and top with the tomatoes.
7. Slide the baking pan into Rack Position 2, select Roast, set the temperature to 375ºF (190ºC), and set the time for 5 minutes.
8. After 4 minutes, remove from the oven.
9. Add the Parmesan cheese and stir until the cheese is melted
10. Serve topped with the parsley.

243. Tofu & Pea Cauli Rice

Servings: 4
Cooking Time: 30 Minutes
Ingredients:
- Tofu:
- ½ block tofu
- ½ cup onions, chopped
- 2 tbsp soy sauce
- 1 tsp turmeric
- 1 cup carrots, chopped
- Cauliflower:
- 3 cups cauliflower rice
- 2 tbsp soy sauce
- ½ cup broccoli, chopped
- 2 garlic cloves, minced
- 1 ½ tsp toasted sesame oil
- 1 tbsp fresh ginger, minced
- ½ cup frozen peas
- 1 tbsp rice vinegar

Directions:
1. Preheat Breville on AirFry function to 370 F. Crumble the tofu and combine it with all tofu ingredients. Place in a baking dish and cook for 10 minutes.
2. Meanwhile, place all cauliflower ingredients in a large bowl; mix to combine. Add the cauliflower mixture to the tofu and stir to combine. Press Start and cook for 12 minutes. Serve.

244. Black Gram French Cuisine Galette

Ingredients:
- 2 or 3 green chilies finely chopped
- 1 ½ tbsp. lemon juice
- Salt and pepper to taste
- 2 cup black gram
- 2 medium potatoes boiled and mashed
- 1 ½ cup coarsely crushed peanuts
- 3 tsp. ginger finely chopped
- 1-2 tbsp. fresh coriander leaves

Directions:
1. Mix the ingredients in a clean bowl.
2. Mold this mixture into round and flat French Cuisine Galettes.
3. Wet the French Cuisine Galettes slightly with water.
4. Pre heat the oven at 160 degrees Fahrenheit for 5 minutes. Place the French Cuisine Galettes in the fry basket and let them cook for another 25 minutes at the same temperature. Keep rolling them over to get a uniform cook. Serve either with mint sauce or ketchup.

245. Cabbage Steaks With Fennel Seeds

Servings: 3
Cooking Time: 25 Minutes
Ingredients:
- 1 cabbage head
- 1 tbsp garlic paste
- Salt and black pepper to taste
- 2 tbsp olive oil
- 2 tsp fennel seeds

Directions:
1. Preheat Breville on AirFry function to 350 F. Slice the cabbage into 1 ½-inch slice. In a small bowl,

combine all the other ingredients; brush cabbage with the mixture. Arrange the steaks on a greased baking dish and press Start. Cook for 15 minutes.

246. Gorgonzola Cheese & Pumpkin Salad

Servings: 2
Cooking Time: 30 Minutes + Chilling Time
Ingredients:
- ½ lb pumpkin
- 2 oz gorgonzola cheese, crumbled
- 2 tbsp pine nuts, toasted
- 1 tbsp olive oil
- ½ cup baby spinach
- 1 spring onion, sliced
- 2 radishes, thinly sliced
- 1 tsp apple cider vinegar

Directions:
1. Preheat Breville on Bake function to 360 F. Peel the pumpkin and chop it into small pieces. Place in a greased baking dish and bake for 20 minutes. Let cool.
2. Add baby spinach, radishes, and spring onion in a serving bowl and toss with olive oil and vinegar. Top with the pumpkin and gorgonzola cheese and sprinkle with the pine nuts to serve.

247. Rosemary Butternut Squash Roast

Servings: 2
Cooking Time: 30 Minutes
Ingredients:
- 1 butternut squash
- 1 tbsp dried rosemary
- 2 tbsp maple syrup
- Salt to taste

Directions:
1. Place the squash on a cutting board and peel. Cut in half and remove the seeds and pulp. Slice into wedges and season with salt. Preheat on Air Fry function to 350 F. Spray the wedges with cooking spray and sprinkle with rosemary. Place the wedges in the basket without overlapping and fit in the baking tray. Cook for 20 minutes, flipping once halfway through. Serve with maple syrup and goat cheese.

248. Rosemary Roasted Squash With Cheese

Servings: 2
Cooking Time: 20 Minutes
Ingredients:
- 1 pound (454 g) butternut squash, cut into wedges
- 2 tablespoons olive oil
- 1 tablespoon dried rosemary
- Salt, to salt
- 1 cup crumbled goat cheese
- 1 tablespoon maple syrup

Directions:
1. Toss the squash wedges with the olive oil, rosemary, and salt in a large bowl until well coated.
2. Transfer the squash wedges to the air fryer basket, spreading them out in as even a layer as possible.
3. Put the air fryer basket on the baking pan and slide into Rack Position 2, select Air Fry, set temperature to 350ºF (180ºC), and set time to 20 minutes.
4. After 10 minutes, remove from the oven and flip the squash. Return the pan to the oven and continue cooking for 10 minutes.
5. When cooking is complete, the squash should be golden brown. Remove from the oven. Sprinkle the goat cheese on top and serve drizzled with the maple syrup.

249. Veggie Mix Fried Chips

Servings: 4
Cooking Time: 45 Minutes
Ingredients:
- 1 large eggplant, cut into strips
- 5 potatoes, peeled and cut into strips
- 3 zucchinis, cut into strips
- ½ cup cornstarch
- ½ cup olive oil
- Salt to taste

Directions:
1. Preheat Breville on AirFry function to 390 F. In a bowl, stir cornstarch, ½ cup of water, salt, pepper, olive oil, eggplants, zucchini, and potatoes. Place the veggie mixture in the basket and press Start. Cook for 12 minutes. Serve warm.

250. Zucchini Fried Baked Pastry

Ingredients:
- 1 or 2 green chilies that are finely chopped or mashed
- ½ tsp. cumin
- 1 tsp. coarsely crushed coriander
- 1 dry red chili broken into pieces
- A small amount of salt (to taste)
- ½ tsp. dried mango powder
- ½ tsp. red chili power.
- 2 tbsp. unsalted butter
- 1 ½ cup all-purpose flour
- A pinch of salt to taste
- Add as much water as required to make the dough stiff and firm
- 3 medium zucchinis (mashed)
- ¼ cup boiled peas
- 1 tsp. powdered ginger

- 1-2 tbsp. coriander.

Directions:
1. Mix the dough for the outer covering and make it stiff and smooth. Leave it to rest in a container while making the filling.
2. Cook the ingredients in a pan and stir them well to make a thick paste. Roll the paste out.
3. Roll the dough into balls and flatten them. Cut them in halves and add the
4. filling. Use water to help you fold the edges to create the shape of a cone.
5. Pre-heat the oven for around 5 to 6 minutes at 300 Fahrenheit. Place all the samosas in the fry basket and close the basket properly. Keep the oven at 200 degrees for another 20 to 25 minutes. Around the halfway point, open the basket and turn the samosas over for uniform cooking. After this, fry at 250 degrees for around 10 minutes in order to give them the desired golden-brown color. Serve hot. Recommended sides are tamarind or mint sauce.

251. Cottage Cheese And Mushroom Mexican Burritos

Ingredients:
- ½ cup mushrooms thinly sliced
- 1 cup cottage cheese cut in too long and slightly thick Oregano Fingers
- A pinch of salt to taste
- ½ tsp. red chili flakes
- 1 tsp. freshly ground peppercorns
- ½ cup pickled jalapenos
- 1-2 lettuce leaves shredded.
- ½ cup red kidney beans (soaked overnight)
- ½ small onion chopped
- 1 tbsp. olive oil
- 2 tbsp. tomato puree
- ¼ tsp. red chili powder
- 1 tsp. of salt to taste
- 4-5 flour tortillas
- 1 or 2 spring onions chopped finely. Also cut the greens.
- Take one tomato. Remove the seeds and chop it into small pieces.
- 1 green chili chopped.
- 1 cup of cheddar cheese grated.
- 1 cup boiled rice (not necessary).
- A few flour tortillas to put the filing in.

Directions:
1. Cook the beans along with the onion and garlic and mash them finely.
2. Now, make the sauce you will need for the burrito. Ensure that you create a slightly thick sauce.
3. For the filling, you will need to cook the ingredients well in a pan and ensure that the vegetables have browned on the outside.
4. To make the salad, toss the ingredients together. Place the tortilla and add a layer of sauce, followed by the beans and the filling at the center. Before you roll it, you will need to place the salad on top of the filling.
5. Pre-heat the oven for around 5 minutes at 200 Fahrenheit. Open the fry basket and keep the burritos inside. Close the basket properly. Let the Air
6. Fryer remain at 200 Fahrenheit for another 15 minutes or so. Halfway through, remove the basket and turn all the burritos over in order to get a uniform cook.

252. Herby Tofu

Servings: 2
Cooking Time: 30 Minutes
Ingredients:
- 6 oz extra firm tofu
- Black pepper to taste
- 1 tbsp vegetable broth
- 1 tbsp soy sauce
- ⅓ tsp dried oregano
- ⅓ tsp garlic powder
- ⅓ tsp dried basil
- ⅓ tsp onion powder

Directions:
1. Place the tofu on a cutting board and cut it into 3 lengthwise slices with a knife. Line a side of the cutting board with paper towels, place the tofu on it, and cover with a paper towel. Use your hands to press the tofu gently until as much liquid has been extracted from it. Chop the tofu into 8 cubes; set aside.
2. In another bowl, add the soy sauce, vegetable broth, oregano, basil, garlic powder, onion powder, and black pepper and mix well with a spoon. Rub the spice mixture on the tofu. Let it marinate for 10 minutes.
3. Preheat on Air Fry function to 390 F. Place the tofu in the fryer's basket in a single layer and fit in the baking tray. Cook for 10 minutes, flipping it at the 6-minute mark. Remove to a plate and serve with green salad.

253. Jalapeño & Tomato Gratin

Servings: 4
Cooking Time: 35 Minutes
Ingredients:
- 1 (16 oz) can jalapeño peppers
- 1 cup cheddar cheese, shredded
- 1 cup Monterey Jack cheese, shredded
- 2 tbsp all-purpose flour
- 2 large eggs, beaten
- ½ cup milk
- 1 can tomato sauce

Directions:

1. Preheat on Air Fry function to 380 F. Arrange the jalapeño peppers on the greased Air Fryer baking pan and top with half of the cheese.
2. In a medium bowl, combine the eggs, milk, and flour and pour the mixture over the chilies. Cook in your for 20 minutes. Take out the chilies and pour the tomato sauce over them. Return and cook for 15 more minutes. Sprinkle with the remaining cheese and serve.

254. Easy Cheesy Vegetable Quesadilla

Servings: 1
Cooking Time: 10 Minutes
Ingredients:
- 1 teaspoon olive oil
- 2 flour tortillas
- ¼ zucchini, sliced
- ¼ yellow bell pepper, sliced
- ¼ cup shredded gouda cheese
- 1 tablespoon chopped cilantro
- ½ green onion, sliced

Directions:
1. Coat the air fryer basket with 1 teaspoon of olive oil.
2. Arrange a flour tortilla in the basket and scatter the top with zucchini, bell pepper, gouda cheese, cilantro, and green onion. Place the other flour tortilla on top.
3. Put the air fryer basket on the baking pan and slide into Rack Position 2, select Air Fry, set temperature to 390ºF (199ºC), and set time to 10 minutes.
4. When cooking is complete, the tortillas should be lightly browned and the vegetables should be tender. Remove from the oven and cool for 5 minutes before slicing into wedges.

255. Caramelized Eggplant With Yogurt Sauce

Servings: 2
Cooking Time: 15 Minutes
Ingredients:
- 1 medium eggplant, quartered and cut crosswise into ½-inch-thick slices
- 2 tablespoons vegetable oil
- Kosher salt and freshly ground black pepper, to taste
- ½ cup plain yogurt (not Greek)
- 2 tablespoons harissa paste
- 1 garlic clove, grated
- 2 teaspoons honey

Directions:
1. Toss the eggplant slices with the vegetable oil, salt, and pepper in a large bowl until well coated.
2. Lay the eggplant slices in the air fryer basket.
3. Put the air fryer basket on the baking pan and slide into Rack Position 2, select Air Fry, set temperature to 400ºF (205ºC), and set time to 15 minutes.
4. Stir the slices two to three times during cooking.
5. Meanwhile, make the yogurt sauce by whisking together the yogurt, harissa paste, and garlic in a small bowl.
6. When cooking is complete, the eggplant slices should be golden brown. Spread the yogurt sauce on a platter, and pile the eggplant slices over the top. Serve drizzled with the honey.

256. Cauliflower Rice With Tofu & Peas

Servings: 4
Cooking Time: 30 Minutes
Ingredients:
- Tofu:
- ½ block tofu, crumbled
- ½ cup diced onion
- 2 tbsp soy sauce
- 1 tsp turmeric
- 1 cup diced carrot
- Cauliflower:
- 3 cups cauliflower rice
- 2 tbsp soy sauce
- ½ cup chopped broccoli
- 2 garlic cloves, minced
- 1 ½ tsp toasted sesame oil
- 1 tbsp minced ginger
- ½ cup frozen peas
- 1 tbsp rice vinegar

Directions:
1. Preheat on Air Fry function to 370 F. Combine all the tofu ingredients in a greased baking dish. Cook for 10 minutes.
2. Meanwhile, place all cauliflower ingredients in a large bowl and mix to combine. Stir the cauliflower mixture in the tofu baking dish and return to the oven; cook for 12 minutes. Serve.

257. Baked Turnip And Zucchini

Servings: 4
Cooking Time: 18 Minutes
Ingredients:
- 3 turnips, sliced
- 1 large zucchini, sliced
- 1 large red onion, cut into rings
- 2 cloves garlic, crushed
- 1 tablespoon olive oil
- Salt and black pepper, to taste

Directions:
1. Put the turnips, zucchini, red onion, and garlic in the baking pan. Drizzle the olive oil over the top and sprinkle with the salt and pepper.
2. Slide the baking pan into Rack Position 1, select Convection Bake, set temperature to 330ºF (166ºC), and set time to 18 minutes.

3. When cooking is complete, the vegetables should be tender. Remove from the oven and serve on a plate.

258. Cottage Cheese Best Homemade Croquette(2)

Ingredients:
- 1 big capsicum (Cut this capsicum into big cubes)
- 1 onion (Cut it into quarters. Now separate the layers carefully.)
- 5 tbsp. gram flour
- A pinch of salt to taste
- 2 cup fresh green coriander
- ½ cup mint leaves
- 4 tsp. fennel
- 1 small onion
- 2 tbsp. ginger-garlic paste
- 6-7 garlic flakes (optional)
- 3 tbsp. lemon juice
- 2 cups cottage cheese cut into slightly thick and long pieces (similar to
- French fries)
- Salt

Directions:
1. Take a clean and dry container. Put into it the coriander, mint, fennel, and ginger, onion/garlic, salt and lemon juice. Mix them.
2. Pour the mixture into a grinder and blend until you get a thick paste. Now move on to the cottage cheese pieces.
3. Slit these pieces almost till the end and leave them aside. Now stuff all the pieces with the paste that was obtained from the previous step. Now leave the stuffed cottage cheese aside. Take the sauce and add to it the gram flour and some salt.
4. Mix them together properly. Rub this mixture all over the stuffed cottage cheese pieces. Now leave the cottage cheese aside. Now, to the leftover sauce, add the capsicum and onions. Apply the sauce generously on each of the pieces of capsicum and onion.
5. Now take satay sticks and arrange the cottage cheese pieces and vegetables on separate sticks. Pre heat the oven at 290 Fahrenheit for around 5 minutes. Open the basket. Arrange the satay sticks properly. Close the basket.
6. Keep the sticks with the cottage cheese at 180 degrees for around half an hour while the sticks with the vegetables are to be kept at the same temperature for only 7 minutes. Turn the sticks in between so that one side does not get burnt and also to provide a uniform cook.

259. Cheesy Ravioli Lunch

Servings: 6
Cooking Time: 15 Minutes
Ingredients:
- 1 package cheese ravioli
- 2 cup Italian breadcrumbs
- ¼ cup Parmesan cheese, grated
- 1 cup buttermilk
- 1 tsp olive oil
- ¼ tsp garlic powder

Directions:
1. Preheat Breville on AirFry function to 390 F. In a bowl, combine breadcrumbs, Parmesan cheese, garlic, and olive oil. Dip the ravioli in the buttermilk and coat with the breadcrumb mixture.
2. Line a baking sheet with parchment paper and arrange the ravioli on it. Press Start and cook for 5 minutes. Serve with marinara jar sauce.

260. Cheese And Garlic French Fries

Ingredients:
- 1 cup molten cheese
- 2 tsp. garlic powder
- 1 tbsp. lemon juice
- 2 medium sized potatoes peeled and cut into thick pieces lengthwise
- ingredients for the marinade:
- 1 tbsp. olive oil
- 1 tsp. mixed herbs
- ½ tsp. red chili flakes
- A pinch of salt to taste

Directions:
1. Boil the potatoes and blanch them. Cut the potato into Oregano Fingers. Mix the ingredients for the marinade and add the potato Oregano Fingers to it making sure that they are coated well.
2. Pre heat the oven for around 5 minutes at 300 Fahrenheit. Take out the basket of the fryer and place the potato Oregano Fingers in them. Close the basket.
3. Now keep the fryer at 200 Fahrenheit for 20 or 25 minutes. In between the process, toss the fries twice or thrice so that they get cooked properly.

261. Cheesy Broccoli Tots

Servings: 4
Cooking Time: 15 Minutes
Ingredients:
- 12 ounces (340 g) frozen broccoli, thawed, drained, and patted dry
- 1 large egg, lightly beaten
- ½ cup seasoned whole-wheat bread crumbs
- ¼ cup shredded reduced-fat sharp Cheddar cheese
- ¼ cup grated Parmesan cheese
- 1½ teaspoons minced garlic
- Salt and freshly ground black pepper, to taste
- Cooking spray

Directions:
1. Spritz the air fryer basket lightly with cooking spray.
2. Place the remaining ingredients into a food processor and process until the mixture resembles a coarse meal. Transfer the mixture to a bowl.

3. Using a tablespoon, scoop out the broccoli mixture and form into 24 oval "tater tot" shapes with your hands.
4. Put the tots in the prepared basket in a single layer, spacing them 1 inch apart. Mist the tots lightly with cooking spray.
5. Put the air fryer basket on the baking pan and slide into Rack Position 2, select Air Fry, set temperature to 375ºF (190ºC), and set time to 15 minutes.
6. Flip the tots halfway through the cooking time.
7. When done, the tots will be lightly browned and crispy. Remove from the oven and serve on a plate.

262. Stuffed Portobellos With Peppers And Cheese

Servings: 4
Cooking Time: 15 Minutes
Ingredients:
- 4 tablespoons sherry vinegar or white wine vinegar
- 6 garlic cloves, minced, divided
- 1 tablespoon fresh thyme leaves
- 1 teaspoon Dijon mustard
- 1 teaspoon kosher salt, divided
- ¼ cup plus 3¼ teaspoons extra-virgin olive oil, divided
- 8 portobello mushroom caps, each about 3 inches across, patted dry
- 1 small red or yellow bell pepper, thinly sliced
- 1 small green bell pepper, thinly sliced
- 1 small onion, thinly sliced
- ¼ teaspoon red pepper flakes
- Freshly ground black pepper, to taste
- 4 ounces (113 g) shredded Fontina cheese

Directions:
1. Stir together the vinegar, 4 minced garlic cloves, thyme, mustard, and ½ teaspoon of kosher salt in a small bowl. Slowly pour in ¼ cup of olive oil, whisking constantly, or until an emulsion is formed. Reserve 2 tablespoons of the marinade and set aside.
2. Put the mushrooms in a resealable plastic bag and pour in the marinade. Seal and shake the bag, coating the mushrooms in the marinade. Transfer the mushrooms to the baking pan, gill-side down.
3. Put the remaining 2 minced garlic cloves, bell peppers, onion, red pepper flakes, remaining ½ teaspoon of salt, and black pepper in a medium bowl. Drizzle with the remaining 3¼ teaspoons of olive oil and toss well. Transfer the bell pepper mixture to the pan.
4. Slide the baking pan into Rack Position 2, select Roast, set temperature to 375ºF (190ºC), and set time to 12 minutes.
5. After 7 minutes, remove the pan and stir the peppers and flip the mushrooms. Return the pan to the oven and continue cooking for 5 minutes.
6. Remove from the oven and place the pepper mixture onto a cutting board and coarsely chop.
7. Brush both sides of the mushrooms with the reserved 2 tablespoons marinade. Stuff the caps evenly with the pepper mixture. Scatter the cheese on top.
8. Select Convection Broil, set temperature to High, and set time to 3 minutes.
9. When done, the mushrooms should be tender and the cheese should be melted.
10. Serve warm.

263. Zucchini Parmesan Chips

Servings: 10
Cooking Time: 8 Minutes
Ingredients:
- ½ tsp. paprika
- ½ C. grated parmesan cheese
- ½ C. Italian breadcrumbs
- 1 lightly beaten egg
- 2 thinly sliced zucchinis

Directions:
1. Preparing the Ingredients. Use a very sharp knife or mandolin slicer to slice zucchini as thinly as you can. Pat off extra moisture.
2. Beat egg with a pinch of pepper and salt and a bit of water.
3. Combine paprika, cheese, and breadcrumbs in a bowl.
4. Dip slices of zucchini into the egg mixture and then into breadcrumb mixture. Press gently to coat.
5. Air Frying. With olive oil cooking spray, mist coated zucchini slices. Place into your air fryer oven in a single layer. Set temperature to 350°F, and set time to 8 minutes.
6. Sprinkle with salt and serve with salsa.

Nutrition Info: CALORIES: 211; FAT: 16G; PROTEIN:8G; SUGAR:0G

264. Cheese & Vegetable Pizza

Servings: 1
Cooking Time: 15 Minutes
Ingredients:
- 1 tbsp tomato paste
- ¼ cup mozzarella cheese, grated
- 1 tbsp sweet corn, cooked
- 4 zucchini slices
- 4 eggplant slices
- 4 red onion rings
- ½ green bell pepper, chopped
- 3 cherry tomatoes, quartered
- 1 tortilla
- ¼ tsp oregano

Directions:
1. Preheat Breville on Pizza function to 350 F. Spread the tomato paste on the tortilla. Top with zucchini and eggplant slices first, then green peppers, and onion rings.
2. Arrange the cherry tomatoes on top and scatter the corn. Sprinkle with oregano and top with

mozzarella cheeses. Press Start and cook for 10-12 minutes. Serve warm.

265. Potato Club Barbeque Sandwich

Ingredients:
- ½ flake garlic crushed
- ¼ cup chopped onion
- ¼ tbsp. red chili sauce
- 2 slices of white bread
- 1 tbsp. softened butter
- 1 cup boiled potato
- 1 small capsicum
- ¼ tbsp. Worcestershire sauce
- ½ tsp. olive oil

Directions:
1. Take the slices of bread and remove the edges. Now cut the slices horizontally.
2. Cook the ingredients for the sauce and wait till it thickens. Now, add the potato to the sauce and stir till it obtains the flavors. Roast the capsicum and peel the skin off. Cut the capsicum into slices. Mix the ingredients together and apply it to the bread slices.
3. Pre-heat the oven for 5 minutes at 300 Fahrenheit. Open the basket of the Fryer and place the prepared Classic Sandwiches in it such that no two Classic Sandwiches are touching each other. Now keep the fryer at 250 degrees for around 15 minutes. Turn the Classic Sandwiches in between the cooking process to cook both slices. Serve the Classic Sandwiches with tomato ketchup or mint sauce.

266. Carrot & Chickpea Oat Balls With Cashews

Servings: 4
Cooking Time: 30 Minutes
Ingredients:
- 2 tbsp olive oil
- 2 tbsp soy sauce
- 1 tbsp flax meal
- 2 cups canned chickpeas, drained
- ½ cup sweet onions, diced
- ½ cup carrots, grated
- ½ cup cashews, toasted
- Juice of 1 lemon
- ½ tsp turmeric
- 1 tsp cumin
- 1 tsp garlic powder
- 1 cup rolled oats

Directions:
1. Preheat Breville on AirFry function to 380 F. Heat olive oil in a skillet and sauté onions and carrots for 5 minutes. Ground the oats and cashews in a food processor. Transfer to a bowl.
2. Place the chickpeas, lemon juice, and soy sauce in the food processor and process until smooth. Add them to the bowl as well. Mix in the onions and carrots.
3. Stir in the remaining ingredients until fully incorporated. Make balls out of the mixture. Place them in the frying basket and press Start. Cook for 12 minutes. Serve warm.

267. Tofu, Carrot And Cauliflower Rice

Servings: 4
Cooking Time: 22 Minutes
Ingredients:
- ½ block tofu, crumbled
- 1 cup diced carrot
- ½ cup diced onions
- 2 tablespoons soy sauce
- 1 teaspoon turmeric
- Cauliflower:
- 3 cups cauliflower rice
- ½ cup chopped broccoli
- ½ cup frozen peas
- 2 tablespoons soy sauce
- 1 tablespoon minced ginger
- 2 garlic cloves, minced
- 1 tablespoon rice vinegar
- 1½ teaspoons toasted sesame oil

Directions:
1. Mix the tofu, carrot, onions, soy sauce, and turmeric in a baking pan and stir until well incorporated.
2. Slide the baking pan into Rack Position 2, select Roast, set temperature to 370ºF (188ºC) and set time to 10 minutes.
3. Flip the tofu and carrot halfway through the cooking time.
4. When cooking is complete, the tofu should be crisp.
5. Meanwhile, in a large bowl, combine all the ingredients for the cauliflower and toss well.
6. Remove the pan from the oven and add the cauliflower mixture to the tofu and stir to combine.
7. Return to the oven and set time to 12 minutes on Roast.
8. When cooking is complete, the vegetables should be tender.
9. Cool for 5 minutes before serving.

268. Spinach Enchiladas With Mozzarella

Servings: 4
Cooking Time: 20 Minutes
Ingredients:
- 8 corn tortillas, warm
- 2 cups mozzarella cheese, shredded
- 1 cup ricotta cheese, crumbled
- 1 package frozen spinach
- 1 garlic clove, minced
- ½ cup sliced onions
- ½ cup sour cream
- 1 tbsp butter
- 1 can enchilada sauce

Directions:

1. In a saucepan, heat oil and sauté garlic and onion for 3 minutes. Stir in the spinach and cook for 5 more minutes. Remove and stir in the ricotta cheese, sour cream and some mozzarella.
2. Spoon ¼ cup of spinach mixture in the middle of a tortilla. Roll up and place seam side down in the basket. Repeat the process with the remaining tortillas.
3. Pour the enchilada sauce all over and sprinkle with the remaining mozzarella. Cook for 15 minutes at 380 F on AirFry function.

269. Grandma's Ratatouille

Servings: 2
Cooking Time: 30 Minutes
Ingredients:
- 1 tbsp olive oil
- 3 Roma tomatoes, thinly sliced
- 2 garlic cloves, minced
- 1 zucchini, thinly sliced
- 2 yellow bell peppers, sliced
- 1 tbsp vinegar
- 2 tbsp herbs de Provence
- Salt and black pepper to taste

Directions:
1. Preheat Breville on AirFry function to 390 F. Place all ingredients in a bowl. Season with salt and pepper and stir to coat. Arrange the vegetable on a baking dish and place in the Breville oven. Cook for 15 minutes, shaking occasionally. Let sit for 5 more minutes after the timer goes off.

270. Crispy Fried Okra With Chili

Servings: 4
Cooking Time: 10 Minutes
Ingredients:
- 3 tablespoons sour cream
- 2 tablespoons flour
- 2 tablespoons semolina
- ½ teaspoon red chili powder
- Salt and black pepper, to taste
- 1 pound (454 g) okra, halved
- Cooking spray

Directions:
1. Spray the air fryer basket with cooking spray. Set aside.
2. In a shallow bowl, place the sour cream. In another shallow bowl, thoroughly combine the flour, semolina, red chili powder, salt, and pepper.
3. Dredge the okra in the sour cream, then roll in the flour mixture until evenly coated. Transfer the okra to the air fryer basket.
4. Put the air fryer basket on the baking pan and slide into Rack Position 2, select Air Fry, set temperature to 400ºF (205ºC), and set time to 10 minutes.
5. Flip the okra halfway through the cooking time.
6. When cooking is complete, the okra should be golden brown and crispy. Remove from the oven and cool for 5 minutes before serving.

271. Asparagus Flat Cakes

Ingredients:
- 2 or 3 green chilies finely chopped
- 1 ½ tbsp. lemon juice
- Salt and pepper to taste
- 2 tbsp. garam masala
- 2 cups sliced asparagus
- 3 tsp. ginger finely chopped
- 1-2 tbsp. fresh coriander leaves

Directions:
1. Mix the ingredients in a clean bowl and add water to it. Make sure that the paste is not too watery but is enough to apply on the asparagus.
2. Pre heat the oven at 160 degrees Fahrenheit for 5 minutes. Place the French Cuisine Galettes in the fry basket and let them cook for another 25 minutes at the same temperature. Keep rolling them over to get a uniform cook. Serve either with mint sauce or ketchup.

272. Parmesan Cabbage With Blue Cheese Sauce

Servings: 4
Cooking Time: 25 Minutes
Ingredients:
- ½ head cabbage, cut into wedges
- 2 cups Parmesan cheese, chopped
- 4 tbsp butter, melted
- Salt and black pepper to taste
- ½ cup blue cheese sauce

Directions:
1. Drizzle cabbage wedges with butter and coat with Parmesan cheese. Place them in the frying basket and cook for 20 minutes at 380 F on AirFry setting. Serve topped with blue cheese sauce.

FISH & SEAFOOD RECIPES

273. Party Cod Nuggets

Servings: 4
Cooking Time: 25 Minutes
Ingredients:
- 1 ¼ lb cod fillets, cut into 4 chunks each
- ½ cup flour
- 1 egg
- 1 cup cornflakes
- 1 tbsp olive oil
- Salt and black pepper to taste

Directions:
1. Place the oil and cornflakes in a food processor and process until crumbed. Season the fish chunks with salt and pepper. In a bowl, beat the egg with 1 tbsp of water.
2. Dredge the chunks in flour first, then dip in the egg, and finally coat with cornflakes. Arrange on a lined sheet and press Start. Cook on AirFry function at 350 F for 15 minutes until crispy. Serve.

274. Thyme Rosemary Shrimp

Servings: 4
Cooking Time: 10 Minutes
Ingredients:
- 1 lb shrimp, peeled and deveined
- 1/2 tbsp fresh rosemary, chopped
- 1 tbsp olive oil
- 2 garlic cloves, minced
- 1/2 tbsp fresh thyme, chopped
- Pepper
- Salt

Directions:
1. Fit the oven with the rack in position
2. Add shrimp and remaining ingredients in a large bowl and toss well.
3. Pour shrimp mixture into the baking dish.
4. Set to bake at 400 F for 15 minutes. After 5 minutes place the baking dish in the preheated oven.
5. Serve and enjoy.

Nutrition Info: Calories 169 Fat 5.5 g Carbohydrates 2.7 g Sugar 0 g Protein 26 g Cholesterol 239 mg

275. Panko-crusted Tilapia

Servings: 3
Cooking Time: 10 Minutes
Ingredients:
- 2 tsp. Italian seasoning
- 2 tsp. lemon pepper
- 1/3 C. panko breadcrumbs
- 1/3 C. egg whites
- 1/3 C. almond flour
- 3 tilapia fillets
- Olive oil

Directions:
1. Preparing the Ingredients. Place panko, egg whites, and flour into separate bowls. Mix lemon pepper and Italian seasoning in with breadcrumbs.
2. Pat tilapia fillets dry. Dredge in flour, then egg, then breadcrumb mixture.
3. Air Frying. Add to the Oven rack/basket and spray lightly with olive oil. Place the Rack on the middle-shelf of the air fryer oven.
4. Cook 10-11 minutes at 400 degrees, making sure to flip halfway through cooking.

Nutrition Info: CALORIES: 256; FAT: 9G; PROTEIN:39G; SUGAR:5G

276. Old Bay Crab Cakes

Servings: 4
Cooking Time: 20 Minutes
Ingredients:
- 2 slices dried bread, crusts removed
- Small amount of milk
- 1 tablespoon mayonnaise
- 1 tablespoon Worcestershire sauce
- 1 tablespoon baking powder
- 1 tablespoon parsley flakes
- 1 teaspoon Old Bay® Seasoning
- 1/4 teaspoon salt
- 1 egg
- 1 pound lump crabmeat

Directions:
1. Preparing the Ingredients. Crush your bread over a large bowl until it is broken down into small pieces. Add milk and stir until bread crumbs are moistened. Mix in mayo and Worcestershire sauce. Add remaining ingredients and mix well. Shape into 4 patties.
2. Air Frying. Cook at 360 degrees for 20 minutes, flip half way through.

Nutrition Info: CALORIES: 165; CARBS:5.8; FAT: 4.5G; PROTEIN:24G; FIBER:0G

277. Air Fryer Salmon

Servings: 2
Cooking Time: 10 Minutes
Ingredients:
- ½ tsp. salt
- ½ tsp. garlic powder
- ½ tsp. smoked paprika
- Salmon

Directions:
1. Preparing the Ingredients. Mix spices and sprinkle onto salmon.
2. Place seasoned salmon into the air fryer oven.
3. Air Frying. Set temperature to 400°F, and set time to 10 minutes.

Nutrition Info: CALORIES: 185; FAT: 11G; PROTEIN:21G; SUGAR:0G

278. Parmesan Fish Fillets

Servings: 4
Cooking Time: 17 Minutes
Ingredients:
- ⅓ cup grated Parmesan cheese
- ½ teaspoon fennel seed
- ½ teaspoon tarragon
- ⅓ teaspoon mixed peppercorns
- 2 eggs, beaten
- 4 (4-ounce / 113-g) fish fillets, halved
- 2 tablespoons dry white wine
- 1 teaspoon seasoned salt

Directions:
1. Place the grated Parmesan cheese, fennel seed, tarragon, and mixed peppercorns in a food processor and pulse for about 20 seconds until well combined. Transfer the cheese mixture to a shallow dish.
2. Place the beaten eggs in another shallow dish.
3. Drizzle the dry white wine over the top of fish fillets. Dredge each fillet in the beaten eggs on both sides, shaking off any excess, then roll them in the cheese mixture until fully coated. Season with the salt.
4. Arrange the fillets in the air fryer basket.
5. Put the air fryer basket on the baking pan and slide into Rack Position 2, select Air Fry, set temperature to 345ºF (174ºC), and set time to 17 minutes.
6. Flip the fillets once halfway through the cooking time.
7. When cooking is complete, the fish should be cooked through no longer translucent. Remove from the oven and cool for 5 minutes before serving.

279. Spicy Lemon Cod

Servings: 2
Cooking Time: 10 Minutes
Ingredients:
- 1 lb cod fillets
- 1/4 tsp chili powder
- 1 tbsp fresh parsley, chopped
- 1 1/2 tbsp olive oil
- 1 tbsp fresh lemon juice
- 1/8 tsp cayenne pepper
- 1/4 tsp salt

Directions:
1. Fit the oven with the rack in position
2. Arrange fish fillets in a baking dish. Drizzle with oil and lemon juice.
3. Sprinkle with chili powder, salt, and cayenne pepper.
4. Set to bake at 400 F for 15 minutes. After 5 minutes place the baking dish in the preheated oven.
5. Garnish with parsley and serve.

Nutrition Info: Calories 276 Fat 12.7 g Carbohydrates 0.5 g Sugar 0.2 g Protein 40.7 g Cholesterol 111 mg

280. Salmon Fries

Ingredients:
- 1 lb. boneless salmon filets
- 2 cup dry breadcrumbs
- 2 tsp. oregano
- 2 tsp. red chili flakes
- 1 ½ tbsp. ginger-garlic paste
- 4 tbsp. lemon juice
- 2 tsp. salt
- 1 tsp. pepper powder
- 1 tsp. red chili powder
- 6 tbsp. corn flour
- 4 eggs

Directions:
1. Mix all the ingredients for the marinade and put the salmon filets inside and let it rest overnight. Mix the breadcrumbs, oregano and red chili flakes well and place the marinated Oregano Fingers on this mixture. Cover it with plastic wrap and leave it till right before you serve to cook.
2. Pre heat the oven at 160 degrees Fahrenheit for 5 minutes.
3. Place the Oregano Fingers in the fry basket and close it. Let them cook at the same temperature for another 15 minutes or so. Toss the Oregano Fingers well so that they are cooked uniformly.

281. Crispy Cheesy Fish Fingers

Servings: 4
Cooking Time: 20 Minutes
Ingredients:
- Large codfish filet, approximately 6-8 ounces, fresh or frozen and thawed, cut into 1 ½-inch strips
- 2 raw eggs
- ½ cup of breadcrumbs (we like Panko, but any brand or home recipe will do)
- 2 tablespoons of shredded or powdered parmesan cheese
- 1 tablespoons of shredded cheddar cheese
- Pinch of salt and pepper

Directions:
1. Preparing the Ingredients. Cover the basket of the air fryer oven with a lining of tin foil, leaving the edges uncovered to allow air to circulate through the basket.
2. Preheat the air fryer oven to 350 degrees.
3. In a large mixing bowl, beat the eggs until fluffy and until the yolks and whites are fully combined.
4. Dunk all the fish strips in the beaten eggs, fully submerging.

5. In a separate mixing bowl, combine the bread crumbs with the parmesan, cheddar, and salt and pepper, until evenly mixed.
6. One by one, coat the egg-covered fish strips in the mixed dry ingredients so that they're fully covered, and place on the foil-lined Oven rack/basket. Place the Rack on the middle-shelf of the air fryer oven.
7. Air Frying. Set the air-fryer timer to 20 minutes.
8. Halfway through the cooking time, shake the handle of the air-fryer so that the breaded fish jostles inside and fry-coverage is even.
9. After 20 minutes, when the fryer shuts off, the fish strips will be perfectly cooked and their breaded crust golden-brown and delicious! Using tongs, remove from the air fryer oven and set on a serving dish to cool.

282. Smoked Paprika Tiger Shrimp

Servings: 4
Cooking Time: 10 Minutes
Ingredients:
- 1 lb tiger shrimp
- 2 tbsp olive oil
- ¼ tbsp garlic powder
- 1 tbsp smoked paprika
- 2 tbsp fresh parsley, chopped
- Sea salt to taste

Directions:
1. Preheat Breville on AirFry function to 380 F. Mix garlic powder, smoked paprika, salt, parsley, and olive oil in a large bowl. Add in the shrimp and toss to coat. Place the shrimp in the frying basket press Start. Fry for 6-7 minutes. Serve with salad.

283. Fried Cod Nuggets

Servings: 4
Cooking Time: 25 Minutes
Ingredients:
- 1 ¼ lb cod fillets, cut into 4 to 6 chunks each
- ½ cup flour
- 1 egg
- 1 cup cornflakes
- 1 tbsp olive oil
- Salt and black pepper to taste

Directions:
1. Place the olive oil and cornflakes in a food processor and process until crumbed. Season the fish chunks with salt and pepper. In a bowl, beat the egg along with 1 tbsp of water. Dredge the chunks in flour first, then dip in the egg, and finally coat with cornflakes. Arrange the fish pieces on a lined sheet and cook in your on Air Fry at 350 F for 15 minutes until crispy.

284. Roasted Salmon With Asparagus

Servings: 4
Cooking Time: 15 Minutes
Ingredients:
- 4 (6-ounce / 170 g) salmon fillets, patted dry
- 1 teaspoon kosher salt, divided
- 1 tablespoon honey
- 2 tablespoons unsalted butter, melted
- 2 teaspoons Dijon mustard
- 2 pounds (907 g) asparagus, trimmed
- Lemon wedges, for serving

Directions:
1. Season both sides of the salmon fillets with ½ teaspoon of kosher salt.
2. Whisk together the honey, 1 tablespoon of butter, and mustard in a small bowl. Set aside.
3. Arrange the asparagus in the baking pan. Drizzle the remaining 1 tablespoon of butter all over and season with the remaining ½ teaspoon of salt, tossing to coat. Move the asparagus to the outside of the pan.
4. Put the salmon fillets in the pan, skin-side down. Brush the fillets generously with the honey mixture.
5. Slide the baking pan into Rack Position 2, select Roast, set temperature to 375ºF (190ºC), and set time to 15 minutes.
6. Toss the asparagus once halfway through the cooking time.
7. When done, transfer the salmon fillets and asparagus to a plate. Serve warm with a squeeze of lemon juice.

285. Parmesan-crusted Hake With Garlic Sauce

Servings: 3
Cooking Time: 10 Minutes
Ingredients:
- Fish:
- 6 tablespoons mayonnaise
- 1 tablespoon fresh lime juice
- 1 teaspoon Dijon mustard
- 1 cup grated Parmesan cheese
- Salt, to taste
- ¼ teaspoon ground black pepper, or more to taste
- 3 hake fillets, patted dry
- Nonstick cooking spray
- Garlic Sauce:
- ¼ cup plain Greek yogurt
- 2 tablespoons olive oil
- 2 cloves garlic, minced
- ½ teaspoon minced tarragon leaves

Directions:
1. Mix the mayo, lime juice, and mustard in a shallow bowl and whisk to combine. In another shallow bowl, stir together the grated Parmesan cheese, salt, and pepper.

2. Dredge each fillet in the mayo mixture, then roll them in the cheese mixture until they are evenly coated on both sides.
3. Spray the air fryer basket with nonstick cooking spray. Place the fillets in the pan.
4. Put the air fryer basket on the baking pan and slide into Rack Position 2, select Air Fry, set temperature to 395ºF (202ºC), and set time to 10 minutes.
5. Flip the fillets halfway through the cooking time.
6. Meanwhile, in a small bowl, whisk all the ingredients for the sauce until well incorporated.
7. When cooking is complete, the fish should flake apart with a fork. Remove the fillets from the oven and serve warm alongside the sauce.

286. Garlic Butter Shrimp Scampi

Servings: 4
Cooking Time: 8 Minutes
Ingredients:
- Sauce:
- ¼ cup unsalted butter
- 2 tablespoons fish stock or chicken broth
- 2 cloves garlic, minced
- 2 tablespoons chopped fresh basil leaves
- 1 tablespoon lemon juice
- 1 tablespoon chopped fresh parsley, plus more for garnish
- 1 teaspoon red pepper flakes
- Shrimp:
- 1 pound (454 g) large shrimp, peeled and deveined, tails removed
- Fresh basil sprigs, for garnish

Directions:
1. Put all the ingredients for the sauce in the baking pan and stir to incorporate.
2. Put the air fryer basket on the baking pan and slide into Rack Position 2, select Air Fry, set temperature to 350ºF (180ºC), and set time to 8 minutes.
3. After 3 minutes, remove from the oven and add the shrimp to the baking pan, flipping to coat in the sauce. Return to the oven and continue cooking for 5 minutes until the shrimp are pink and opaque. Stir the shrimp twice during cooking.
4. When cooking is complete, remove from the oven. Serve garnished with the parsley and basil sprigs.

287. Sweet And Savory Breaded Shrimp

Servings: 2
Cooking Time: 20 Minutes
Ingredients:
- ½ pound of fresh shrimp, peeled from their shells and rinsed
- 2 raw eggs
- ½ cup of breadcrumbs (we like Panko, but any brand or home recipe will do)
- ½ white onion, peeled and rinsed and finely chopped
- 1 teaspoon of ginger-garlic paste
- ½ teaspoon of turmeric powder
- ½ teaspoon of red chili powder
- ½ teaspoon of cumin powder
- ½ teaspoon of black pepper powder
- ½ teaspoon of dry mango powder
- Pinch of salt

Directions:
1. Preparing the Ingredients. Cover the basket of the air fryer oven with a lining of tin foil, leaving the edges uncovered to allow air to circulate through the basket.
2. Preheat the air fryer oven to 350 degrees.
3. In a large mixing bowl, beat the eggs until fluffy and until the yolks and whites are fully combined.
4. Dunk all the shrimp in the egg mixture, fully submerging.
5. In a separate mixing bowl, combine the bread crumbs with all the dry ingredients until evenly blended.
6. One by one, coat the egg-covered shrimp in the mixed dry ingredients so that fully covered, and place on the foil-lined air-fryer basket.
7. Air Frying. Set the air-fryer timer to 20 minutes.
8. Halfway through the cooking time, shake the handle of the air-fryer so that the breaded shrimp jostles inside and fry-coverage is even.
9. After 20 minutes, when the fryer shuts off, the shrimp will be perfectly cooked and their breaded crust golden-brown and delicious! Using tongs, remove from the air fryer oven and set on a serving dish to cool.

288. Flavorful Herb Salmon

Servings: 4
Cooking Time: 15 Minutes
Ingredients:
- 1 lb salmon fillets
- 1/2 tbsp dried rosemary
- 1 tbsp olive oil
- 1/4 tsp dried basil
- 1 tbsp dried chives
- 1/4 tsp dried thyme
- Pepper
- Salt

Directions:
1. Fit the oven with the rack in position 2.
2. Place salmon skin side down in air fryer basket then place an air fryer basket in baking pan.
3. Mix olive oil, thyme, basil, chives, and rosemary in a small bowl.
4. Brush salmon with oil mixture.
5. Place a baking pan on the oven rack. Set to air fry at 400 F for 15 minutes.

6. Serve and enjoy.
Nutrition Info: Calories 182 Fat 10.6 g Carbohydrates 0.4 g Sugar 0 g Protein 22.1 g Cholesterol 50 mg

289. Air Fry Prawns

Servings: 4
Cooking Time: 6 Minutes
Ingredients:
- 24 prawns
- 6 tbsp mayonnaise
- 1 1/2 tsp chili powder
- 2 tbsp vinegar
- 2 tbsp ketchup
- 1 tsp red chili flakes
- 1/2 tsp sea salt

Directions:
1. Fit the oven with the rack in position 2.
2. In a bowl, toss prawns with chili flakes, chili powder, and salt.
3. Add shrimp to the air fryer basket then place an air fryer basket in the baking pan.
4. Place a baking pan on the oven rack. Set to air fry at 350 F for 6 minutes.
5. In a small bowl, mix mayonnaise, vinegar, and ketchup and serve with shrimp.

Nutrition Info: Calories 255 Fat 9.8 g Carbohydrates 9.8 g Sugar 3.2 g Protein 30.5 g Cholesterol 284 mg

290. Baked Tilapia

Servings: 4
Cooking Time: 10 Minutes
Ingredients:
- 1 1/4 lbs tilapia fillets
- 2 tsp onion powder
- 2 tbsp olive oil
- 1/2 tsp garlic powder
- 1/2 tsp dried thyme
- 1/2 tsp oregano
- 1/2 tsp chili powder
- 2 tbsp sweet paprika
- 1 tsp pepper
- 1/2 tsp salt

Directions:
1. Fit the oven with the rack in position
2. Brush fish fillets with oil and place in baking dish.
3. Mix together spices and sprinkle over the fish fillets.
4. Set to bake at 425 F for 15 minutes. After 5 minutes place the baking dish in the preheated oven.
5. Serve and enjoy.

Nutrition Info: Calories 195 Fat 8.9 g Carbohydrates 3.9 g Sugar 0.9 g Protein 27.2 g Cholesterol 69 mg

291. Tasty Lemon Pepper Basa

Servings: 4
Cooking Time: 12 Minutes
Ingredients:
- 4 basa fish fillets
- 8 tsp olive oil
- 2 tbsp fresh parsley, chopped
- 1/4 cup green onion, sliced
- 1/2 tsp garlic powder
- 1/4 tsp lemon pepper seasoning
- 4 tbsp fresh lemon juice
- Pepper
- Salt

Directions:
1. Fit the oven with the rack in position
2. Place fish fillets in a baking dish.
3. Pour remaining ingredients over fish fillets.
4. Set to bake at 425 F for 12 minutes. After 5 minutes place the baking dish in the preheated oven.
5. Serve and enjoy.

Nutrition Info: Calories 308 Fat 21.4 g Carbohydrates 5.5 g Sugar 3.4 g Protein 24.1 g Cholesterol 0 mg

292. Herbed Salmon With Asparagus

Servings: 2
Cooking Time: 12 Minutes
Ingredients:
- 2 teaspoons olive oil, plus additional for drizzling
- 2 (5-ounce / 142-g) salmon fillets, with skin
- Salt and freshly ground black pepper, to taste
- 1 bunch asparagus, trimmed
- 1 teaspoon dried tarragon
- 1 teaspoon dried chives
- Fresh lemon wedges, for serving

Directions:
1. Rub the olive oil all over the salmon fillets. Sprinkle with salt and pepper to taste.
2. Put the asparagus on the foil-lined baking pan and place the salmon fillets on top, skin-side down.
3. Slide the baking pan into Rack Position 1, select Convection Bake, set temperature to 350ºF (180ºC), and set time to 12 minutes.
4. When cooked, the fillets should register 145ºF (63ºC) on an instant-read thermometer. Remove from the oven and cut the salmon fillets in half crosswise, then use a metal spatula to lift flesh from skin and transfer to a serving plate. Discard the skin and drizzle the salmon fillets with additional olive oil. Scatter with the herbs.
5. Serve the salmon fillets with asparagus spears and lemon wedges on the side.

293. Lemon Tilapia

Servings: 4

Cooking Time: 12 Minutes
Ingredients:
- 1 tablespoon olive oil
- 1 tablespoon lemon juice
- 1 teaspoon minced garlic
- ½ teaspoon chili powder
- 4 tilapia fillets

Directions:
1. Line the baking pan with parchment paper.
2. In a shallow bowl, stir together the olive oil, lemon juice, garlic, and chili powder to make a marinade. Put the tilapia fillets in the bowl, turning to coat evenly.
3. Place the fillets in the baking pan in a single layer.
4. Put the air fryer basket on the baking pan and slide into Rack Position 2, select Air Fry, set temperature to 375ºF (190ºC), and set time to 12 minutes.
5. When cooked, the fish will flake apart with a fork. Remove from the oven to a plate and serve hot.

294. Cheesy Tuna Patties

Servings: 4
Cooking Time: 17 To 18 Minutes
Ingredients:
- Tuna Patties:
- 1 pound (454 g) canned tuna, drained
- 1 egg, whisked
- 2 tablespoons shallots, minced
- 1 garlic clove, minced
- 1 cup grated Romano cheese
- Sea salt and ground black pepper, to taste
- 1 tablespoon sesame oil
- Cheese Sauce:
- 1 tablespoon butter
- 1 cup beer
- 2 tablespoons grated Colby cheese

Directions:
1. Mix together the canned tuna, whisked egg, shallots, garlic, cheese, salt, and pepper in a large bowl and stir to incorporate.
2. Divide the tuna mixture into four equal portions and form each portion into a patty with your hands. Refrigerate the patties for 2 hours.
3. When ready, brush both sides of each patty with sesame oil, then place in the baking pan.
4. Slide the baking pan into Rack Position 1, select Convection Bake, set temperature to 360ºF (182ºC), and set time to 14 minutes.
5. Flip the patties halfway through the cooking time.
6. Meanwhile, melt the butter in a saucepan over medium heat.
7. Pour in the beer and whisk constantly, or until it begins to bubble. Add the grated Colby cheese and mix well. Continue cooking for 3 to 4 minutes, or until the cheese melts. Remove from the heat.
8. When cooking is complete, the patties should be lightly browned and cooked through. Remove the patties from the oven to a plate. Drizzle them with the cheese sauce and serve immediately.

295. Baked Lemon Swordfish

Servings: 2
Cooking Time: 10 Minutes
Ingredients:
- 12 oz swordfish fillets
- 1/8 tsp crushed red pepper
- 1 garlic clove, minced
- 2 tsp fresh parsley, chopped
- 3 tbsp olive oil
- 1/2 tsp lemon zest, grated
- 1/2 tsp ginger, grated

Directions:
1. Fit the oven with the rack in position
2. In a small bowl, mix 2 tbsp oil, lemon zest, red pepper, ginger, garlic, and parsley.
3. Season fish fillets with salt.
4. Heat remaining oil in a pan over medium-high heat.
5. Place fish fillets in the pan and cook until browned, about 2-3 minutes.
6. Transfer fish fillets in a baking dish.
7. Set to bake at 400 F for 15 minutes. After 5 minutes place the baking dish in the preheated oven.
8. Pour oil mixture over fish fillets and serve.

Nutrition Info: Calories 449 Fat 29.8 g Carbohydrates 1.1 g Sugar 0.1 g Protein 43.4 g Cholesterol 85 mg

296. Crispy Crab And Fish Cakes

Servings: 4
Cooking Time: 12 Minutes
Ingredients:
- 8 ounces (227 g) imitation crab meat
- 4 ounces (113 g) leftover cooked fish (such as cod, pollock, or haddock)
- 2 tablespoons minced celery
- 2 tablespoons minced green onion
- 2 tablespoons light mayonnaise
- 1 tablespoon plus 2 teaspoons Worcestershire sauce
- ¾ cup crushed saltine cracker crumbs
- 2 teaspoons dried parsley flakes
- 1 teaspoon prepared yellow mustard
- ½ teaspoon garlic powder
- ½ teaspoon dried dill weed, crushed
- ½ teaspoon Old Bay seasoning
- ½ cup panko bread crumbs
- Cooking spray

Directions:
1. Pulse the crab meat and fish in a food processor until finely chopped.

2. Transfer the meat mixture to a large bowl, along with the celery, green onion, mayo, Worcestershire sauce, cracker crumbs, parsley flakes, mustard, garlic powder, dill weed, and Old Bay seasoning. Stir to mix well.
3. Scoop out the meat mixture and form into 8 equal-sized patties with your hands.
4. Place the panko bread crumbs on a plate. Roll the patties in the bread crumbs until they are evenly coated on both sides. Put the patties in the baking pan and spritz them with cooking spray.
5. Slide the baking pan into Rack Position 1, select Convection Bake, set temperature to 390ºF (199ºC), and set time to 12 minutes.
6. Flip the patties halfway through the cooking time.
7. When cooking is complete, they should be golden brown and cooked through. Remove the pan from the oven. Divide the patties among four plates and serve.

297. Spiced Red Snapper

Servings: 4
Cooking Time: 10 Minutes
Ingredients:
- 1 teaspoon olive oil
- 1½ teaspoons black pepper
- ¼ teaspoon garlic powder
- ¼ teaspoon thyme
- ⅛ teaspoon cayenne pepper
- 4 (4-ounce / 113-g) red snapper fillets, skin on
- 4 thin slices lemon
- Nonstick cooking spray

Directions:
1. Spritz the baking pan with nonstick cooking spray.
2. In a small bowl, stir together the olive oil, black pepper, garlic powder, thyme, and cayenne pepper. Rub the mixture all over the fillets until completely coated.
3. Lay the fillets, skin-side down, in the baking pan and top each fillet with a slice of lemon.
4. Slide the baking pan into Rack Position 1, select Convection Bake, set temperature to 390ºF (199ºC), and set time to 10 minutes.
5. Flip the fillets halfway through the cooking time.
6. When cooking is complete, the fish should be cooked through. Let the fish cool for 5 minutes and serve.

298. Lobster Grandma's Easy To Cook Wontons

Ingredients:
- 1 ½ cup all-purpose flour
- ½ tsp. salt
- 5 tbsp. water
- For filling:
- 2 cups minced lobster
- 2 tbsp. oil
- 2 tsp. ginger-garlic paste
- 2 tsp. soya sauce
- 2 tsp. vinegar

Directions:
1. Squeeze the dough and cover it with plastic wrap and set aside. Next, cook the ingredients for the filling and try to ensure that the lobster is covered well with the sauce.
2. Roll the dough and place the filling in the center. Now, wrap the dough to cover the filling and pinch the edges together.
3. Pre heat the oven at 200° F for 5 minutes. Place the wontons in the fry basket and close it. Let them cook at the same temperature for another 20 minutes. Recommended sides are chili sauce or ketchup.

299. Mediterranean Sole

Servings: 6
Cooking Time: 20 Minutes
Ingredients:
- Nonstick cooking spray
- 2 tbsp. olive oil
- 8 scallions, sliced thin
- 2 cloves garlic, diced fine
- 4 tomatoes, chopped
- ½ cup dry white wine
- 2 tbsp. fresh parsley, chopped fine
- 1 tsp oregano
- 1 tsp pepper
- 2 lbs. sole, cut in 6 pieces
- 4 oz. feta cheese, crumbled

Directions:
1. Place the rack in position 1 of the oven. Spray an 8x11-inch baking dish with cooking spray.
2. Heat the oil in a medium skillet over medium heat. Add scallions and garlic and cook until tender, stirring frequently.
3. Add the tomatoes, wine, parsley, oregano, and pepper. Stir to mix. Simmer for 5 minutes, or until sauce thickens. Remove from heat.
4. Pour half the sauce on the bottom of the prepared dish. Lay fish on top then pour remaining sauce over the top. Sprinkle with feta.
5. Set the oven to bake on 400°F for 25 minutes. After 5 minutes, place the baking dish on the rack and cook 15-18 minutes or until fish flakes easily with a fork. Serve immediately.

Nutrition Info: Calories 220, Total Fat 12g, Saturated Fat 4g, Total Carbs 6g, Net Carbs 4g, Protein 22g, Sugar 4g, Fiber 2g, Sodium 631mg, Potassium 540mg, Phosphorus 478mg

300. Parmesan-crusted Halibut Fillets

Servings: 4
Cooking Time: 10 Minutes
Ingredients:
- 2 medium-sized halibut fillets
- Dash of tabasco sauce
- 1 teaspoon curry powder
- ½ teaspoon ground coriander
- ½ teaspoon hot paprika
- Kosher salt and freshly cracked mixed peppercorns, to taste
- 2 eggs
- 1½ tablespoons olive oil
- ½ cup grated Parmesan cheese

Directions:
1. On a clean work surface, drizzle the halibut fillets with the tabasco sauce. Sprinkle with the curry powder, coriander, hot paprika, salt, and cracked mixed peppercorns. Set aside.
2. In a shallow bowl, beat the eggs until frothy. In another shallow bowl, combine the olive oil and Parmesan cheese.
3. One at a time, dredge the halibut fillets in the beaten eggs, shaking off any excess, then roll them over the Parmesan cheese until evenly coated.
4. Arrange the halibut fillets in the air fryer basket in a single layer.
5. Put the air fryer basket on the baking pan and slide into Rack Position 2, select Roast, set temperature to 365ºF (185ºC), and set time to 10 minutes.
6. When cooking is complete, the fish should be golden brown and crisp. Cool for 5 minutes before serving.

301. Dill Salmon Patties

Servings: 2
Cooking Time: 10 Minutes
Ingredients:
- 14 oz can salmon, drained and discard bones
- 1 tsp dill, chopped
- 1 egg, lightly beaten
- 1/4 tsp garlic powder
- 1/2 cup breadcrumbs
- 1/4 cup onion, diced
- Pepper
- Salt

Directions:
1. Fit the oven with the rack in position 2.
2. Add all ingredients into the large bowl and mix well.
3. Make equal shapes of patties from mixture and place in the air fryer basket then place the air fryer basket in the baking pan.
4. Place a baking pan on the oven rack. Set to air fry at 370 F for 10 minutes.
5. Serve and enjoy.

Nutrition Info: Calories 422 Fat 15.7 g Carbohydrates 21.5 g Sugar 2.5 g Protein 46 g Cholesterol 191 mg

302. Seafood Pizza

Ingredients:
- One pizza base
- Grated pizza cheese (mozzarella cheese preferably) for topping
- Some pizza topping sauce
- Use cooking oil for brushing and topping purposes
- ingredients for topping:
- 2 onions chopped
- 2 cups mixed seafood
- 2 capsicums chopped
- 2 tomatoes that have been deseeded and chopped
- 1 tbsp. (optional) mushrooms/corns
- 2 tsp. pizza seasoning
- Some cottage cheese that has been cut into small cubes (optional)

Directions:
1. Put the pizza base in a pre-heated oven for around 5 minutes. (Pre heated to 340 Fahrenheit). Take out the base. Pour some pizza sauce on top of the base at the center. Using a spoon spread the sauce over the base making sure that you leave some gap around the circumference. Grate some mozzarella cheese and sprinkle it over the sauce layer. Take all the vegetables and the seafood and mix them in a bowl. Add some oil and seasoning.
2. Also add some salt and pepper according to taste. Mix them properly. Put this topping over the layer of cheese on the pizza. Now sprinkle some more grated cheese and pizza seasoning on top of this layer. Pre heat the oven at 250 Fahrenheit for around 5 minutes.
3. Open the fry basket and place the pizza inside. Close the basket and keep the fryer at 170 degrees for another 10 minutes. If you feel that it is undercooked you may put it at the same temperature for another 2 minutes or so.

303. Rosemary Garlic Shrimp

Servings: 4
Cooking Time: 10 Minutes
Ingredients:
- 1 lb shrimp, peeled and deveined
- 2 garlic cloves, minced
- 1/2 tbsp fresh rosemary, chopped
- 1 tbsp olive oil
- Pepper
- Salt

Directions:
1. Fit the oven with the rack in position

2. Add shrimp and remaining ingredients in a large bowl and toss well.
3. Pour shrimp mixture into the baking dish.
4. Set to bake at 400 F for 15 minutes. After 5 minutes place the baking dish in the preheated oven.
5. Serve and enjoy.
Nutrition Info: Calories 168 Fat 5.5 g Carbohydrates 2.5 g Sugar 0 g Protein 26 g Cholesterol 239 mg

304. Baked Halibut Steaks With Parsley

Servings: 4
Cooking Time: 10 Minutes
Ingredients:
- 1 pound (454 g) halibut steaks
- ¼ cup vegetable oil
- 2½ tablespoons Worcester sauce
- 2 tablespoons honey
- 2 tablespoons vermouth
- 1 tablespoon freshly squeezed lemon juice
- 1 tablespoon fresh parsley leaves, coarsely chopped
- Salt and pepper, to taste
- 1 teaspoon dried basil

Directions:
1. Put all the ingredients in a large mixing dish and gently stir until the fish is coated evenly. Transfer the fish to the baking pan.
2. Slide the baking pan into Rack Position 1, select Convection Bake, set temperature to 375ºF (190ºC), and set time to 10 minutes.
3. Flip the fish halfway through cooking time.
4. When cooking is complete, the fish should reach an internal temperature of at least 145ºF (63ºC) on a meat thermometer. Remove from the oven and let the fish cool for 5 minutes before serving.

305. Sweet & Spicy Lime Salmon

Servings: 6
Cooking Time: 15 Minutes
Ingredients:
- 1 1/2 lbs salmon fillets
- 3 tbsp brown sugar
- 2 tbsp fresh lime juice
- 1/3 cup olive oil
- 1/2 tsp red pepper flakes
- 2 garlic cloves, minced
- Pepper
- Salt

Directions:
1. Fit the oven with the rack in position
2. Place salmon on a prepared baking sheet and season with pepper and salt.
3. In a small bowl, whisk oil, red pepper flakes, garlic, brown sugar, and lime juice.
4. Pour oil mixture over salmon.
5. Set to bake at 350 F for 20 minutes. After 5 minutes place the baking dish in the preheated oven.
6. Serve and enjoy.
Nutrition Info: Calories 269 Fat 18.3 g Carbohydrates 6.1 g Sugar 4.7 g Protein 22.2 g Cholesterol 50 mg

306. Rosemary Buttered Prawns

Servings: 2
Cooking Time: 15 Minutes + Marinating Time
Ingredients:
- 8 large prawns
- 1 rosemary sprig, chopped
- ½ tbsp melted butter
- Salt and black pepper to taste

Directions:
1. Combine butter, rosemary, salt, and pepper in a bowl. Add in the prawns and mix to coat. Cover the bowl and refrigerate for 1 hour.
2. Preheat on Air Fry function to 350 F Remove the prawns from the fridge and place them in the basket. Fit in the baking tray and cook for 10 minutes, flipping once. Serve.

307. Sweet Cajun Salmon

Servings: 1
Cooking Time: 10 Minutes
Ingredients:
- 1 salmon fillet
- ¼ tsp brown sugar
- Juice of ½ lemon
- 1 tbsp cajun seasoning
- 2 lemon wedges
- 1 tbsp chopped parsley

Directions:
1. Preheat on Bake function to 350 F. Combine sugar and lemon juice; coat the salmon with this mixture. Coat with the Cajun seasoning as well. Place a parchment paper on a baking tray and cook the fish in your for 10 minutes. Serve with lemon wedges and parsley.

308. Golden Beer-battered Cod

Servings: 4
Cooking Time: 15 Minutes
Ingredients:
- 2 eggs
- 1 cup malty beer
- 1 cup all-purpose flour
- ½ cup cornstarch
- 1 teaspoon garlic powder
- Salt and pepper, to taste
- 4 (4-ounce / 113-g) cod fillets
- Cooking spray

Directions:

1. In a shallow bowl, beat together the eggs with the beer. In another shallow bowl, thoroughly combine the flour and cornstarch. Sprinkle with the garlic powder, salt, and pepper.
2. Dredge each cod fillet in the flour mixture, then in the egg mixture. Dip each piece of fish in the flour mixture a second time.
3. Spritz the air fryer basket with cooking spray. Arrange the cod fillets in the pan in a single layer.
4. Put the air fryer basket on the baking pan and slide into Rack Position 2, select Air Fry, set temperature to 400ºF (205ºC), and set time to 15 minutes.
5. Flip the fillets halfway through the cooking time.
6. When cooking is complete, the cod should reach an internal temperature of 145ºF (63ºC) on a meat thermometer and the outside should be crispy. Let the fish cool for 5 minutes and serve.

309. Breaded Scallops

Servings: 4
Cooking Time: 7 Minutes
Ingredients:
- 1 egg
- 3 tablespoons flour
- 1 cup bread crumbs
- 1 pound (454 g) fresh scallops
- 2 tablespoons olive oil
- Salt and black pepper, to taste

Directions:
1. In a bowl, lightly beat the egg. Place the flour and bread crumbs into separate shallow dishes.
2. Dredge the scallops in the flour and shake off any excess. Dip the flour-coated scallops in the beaten egg and roll in the bread crumbs.
3. Brush the scallops generously with olive oil and season with salt and pepper, to taste. Transfer the scallops to the air fryer basket.
4. Put the air fryer basket on the baking pan and slide into Rack Position 2, select Air Fry, set temperature to 360ºF (182ºC), and set time to 7 minutes.
5. Flip the scallops halfway through the cooking time.
6. When cooking is complete, the scallops should reach an internal temperature of just 145ºF (63ºC) on a meat thermometer. Remove from the oven. Let the scallops cool for 5 minutes and serve.

310. Easy Shrimp And Vegetable Paella

Servings: 4
Cooking Time: 16 Minutes
Ingredients:
- 1 (10-ounce / 284-g) package frozen cooked rice, thawed
- 1 (6-ounce / 170-g) jar artichoke hearts, drained and chopped
- ¼ cup vegetable broth
- ½ teaspoon dried thyme
- ½ teaspoon turmeric
- 1 cup frozen cooked small shrimp
- ½ cup frozen baby peas
- 1 tomato, diced

Directions:
1. Mix together the cooked rice, chopped artichoke hearts, vegetable broth, thyme, and turmeric in the baking pan and stir to combine.
2. Slide the baking pan into Rack Position 1, select Convection Bake, set temperature to 340ºF (171ºC), and set time to 16 minutes.
3. After 9 minutes, remove from the oven and add the shrimp, baby peas, and diced tomato to the baking pan. Mix well. Return the pan to the oven and continue cooking for 7 minutes more, or until the shrimp are done and the paella is bubbling.
4. When cooking is complete, remove from the oven. Cool for 5 minutes before serving.

311. Firecracker Shrimp

Servings: 4
Cooking Time: 8 Minutes
Ingredients:
- For the shrimp
- 1 pound raw shrimp, peeled and deveined
- Salt
- Pepper
- 1 egg
- ½ cup all-purpose flour
- ¾ cup panko bread crumbs
- Cooking oil
- For the firecracker sauce
- ⅓ cup sour cream
- 2 tablespoons Sriracha
- ¼ cup sweet chili sauce

Directions:
1. Preparing the Ingredients. Season the shrimp with salt and pepper to taste. In a small bowl, beat the egg. In another small bowl, place the flour. In a third small bowl, add the panko bread crumbs.
2. Spray the Oven rack/basket with cooking oil. Dip the shrimp in the flour, then the egg, and then the bread crumbs. Place the shrimp in the Oven rack/basket. It is okay to stack them. Spray the shrimp with cooking oil. Place the Rack on the middle-shelf of the air fryer oven.
3. Air Frying. Cook for 4 minutes. Open the air fryer oven and flip the shrimp. I recommend flipping individually instead of shaking to keep the breading intact. Cook for an additional 4 minutes or until crisp.
4. While the shrimp is cooking, make the firecracker sauce: In a small bowl, combine the sour cream, Sriracha, and sweet chili sauce. Mix well. Serve with the shrimp.

Nutrition Info: CALORIES: 266; CARBS:23g; FAT:6G; PROTEIN:27G; FIBER:1G

312. Prawn Grandma's Easy To Cook Wontons

Ingredients:
- 1 ½ cup all-purpose flour
- ½ tsp. salt
- 5 tbsp. water
- 2 cups minced prawn
- 2 tbsp. oil
- 2 tsp. ginger-garlic paste
- 2 tsp. soya sauce
- 2 tsp. vinegar

Directions:
1. Squeeze the dough and cover it with plastic wrap and set aside. Next, cook the ingredients for the filling and try to ensure that the prawn is covered well with the sauce. Roll the dough and place the filling in the center.
2. Now, wrap the dough to cover the filling and pinch the edges together. Pre heat the oven at 200° F for 5 minutes. Place the wontons in the fry basket and close it. Let them cook at the same temperature for another 20 minutes. Recommended sides are chili sauce or ketchup.

313. Herbed Scallops With Vegetables

Servings: 4
Cooking Time: 9 Minutes

Ingredients:
- 1 cup frozen peas
- 1 cup green beans
- 1 cup frozen chopped broccoli
- 2 teaspoons olive oil
- ½ teaspoon dried oregano
- ½ teaspoon dried basil
- 12 ounces (340 g) sea scallops, rinsed and patted dry

Directions:
1. Put the peas, green beans, and broccoli in a large bowl. Drizzle with the olive oil and toss to coat well. Transfer the vegetables to the air fryer basket.
2. Put the air fryer basket on the baking pan and slide into Rack Position 2, select Air Fry, set temperature to 400ºF (205ºC), and set time to 5 minutes.
3. When cooking is complete, the vegetables should be fork-tender. Transfer the vegetables to a serving bowl. Scatter with the oregano and basil and set aside.
4. Place the scallops in the basket.
5. Put the air fryer basket on the baking pan and slide into Rack Position 2, select Air Fry, set temperature to 400ºF (205ºC), and set time to 4 minutes.
6. When cooking is complete, the scallops should be firm and just opaque in the center. Remove from the oven to the bowl of vegetables and toss well. Serve warm.

314. Old Bay Tilapia Fillets

Servings: 4
Cooking Time: 15 Minutes

Ingredients:
- 1 pound tilapia fillets
- 1 tbsp old bay seasoning
- 2 tbsp canola oil
- 2 tbsp lemon pepper
- Salt to taste
- 2-3 butter buds

Directions:
1. Preheat your oven to 400 F on Bake function. Drizzle tilapia fillets with canola oil. In a bowl, mix salt, lemon pepper, butter buds, and seasoning; spread on the fish. Place the fillet on the basket and fit in the baking tray. Cook for 10 minutes, flipping once until tender and crispy.

315. Prawn French Cuisine Galette

Ingredients:
- 2 tbsp. garam masala
- 1 lb. minced prawn
- 3 tsp ginger finely chopped
- 1-2 tbsp. fresh coriander leaves
- 2 or 3 green chilies finely chopped
- 1 ½ tbsp. lemon juice
- Salt and pepper to taste

Directions:
1. Mix the ingredients in a clean bowl.
2. Mold this mixture into round and flat French Cuisine Galettes.
3. Wet the French Cuisine Galettes slightly with water.
4. Pre heat the oven at 160 degrees Fahrenheit for 5 minutes. Place the French Cuisine Galettes in the fry basket and let them cook for another 25 minutes at the same temperature. Keep rolling them over to get a uniform cook. Serve either with mint sauce or ketchup.

316. Basil White Fish

Servings: 4
Cooking Time: 20 Minutes

Ingredients:
- 2 tbsp fresh basil, chopped
- 2 garlic cloves, minced
- 1 tbsp Parmesan cheese, grated
- Salt and black pepper to taste
- 2 tbsp pine nuts
- 4 white fish fillets
- 2 tbsp olive oil

Directions:
1. Preheat Breville on AirFry function to 350 F. Season the fillets with salt and pepper and place in the basket. Drizzle with some olive oil and press Start. Cook for 12-14 minutes. In a bowl, mix basil,

remaining olive oil, pine nuts, garlic, and Parmesan cheese and spread on the fish. Serve.

317. Cajun And Lemon Pepper Cod
Servings: 2 Cod Fillets
Cooking Time: 12 Minutes
Ingredients:
- 1 tablespoon Cajun seasoning
- 1 teaspoon salt
- ½ teaspoon lemon pepper
- ½ teaspoon freshly ground black pepper
- 2 (8-ounce / 227-g) cod fillets, cut to fit into the air fryer basket
- Cooking spray
- 2 tablespoons unsalted butter, melted
- 1 lemon, cut into 4 wedges

Directions:
1. Spritz the baking pan with cooking spray.
2. Thoroughly combine the Cajun seasoning, salt, lemon pepper, and black pepper in a small bowl. Rub this mixture all over the cod fillets until completely coated.
3. Put the fillets in the prepared pan and brush the melted butter over both sides of each fillet.
4. Slide the baking pan into Rack Position 1, select Convection Bake, set temperature to 360ºF (182ºC), and set time to 12 minutes.
5. Flip the fillets halfway through the cooking time.
6. When cooking is complete, the fish should flake apart with a fork. Remove the fillets from the oven and serve with fresh lemon wedges.

318. Old Bay Seasoned Scallops
Servings: 4
Cooking Time: 4 Minutes
Ingredients:
- 1 lb sea scallops
- 1/2 tsp garlic powder
- 1/2 cup crushed crackers
- 2 tbsp butter, melted
- 1/2 tsp old bay seasoning

Directions:
1. Fit the oven with the rack in position 2.
2. In a shallow dish, mix crushed crackers, garlic powder, and old bay seasoning.
3. Add melted butter in a separate shallow dish.
4. Dip scallops in melted butter and coat with crushed crackers.
5. Place coated scallops in air fryer basket then place air fryer basket in baking pan.
6. Place a baking pan on the oven rack. Set to air fry at 390 F for 4 minutes.
7. Serve and enjoy.

Nutrition Info: Calories 167 Fat 7.4 g Carbohydrates 4.8 g Sugar 0.5 g Protein 19.5 g Cholesterol 53 mg

319. Spicy Baked Shrimp
Servings: 4
Cooking Time: 8 Minutes
Ingredients:
- 2 lbs shrimp, peeled & deveined
- 1/4 tsp cayenne pepper
- 1 tsp garlic powder
- 2 tbsp chili powder
- 2 tbsp olive oil
- 1 tsp kosher salt

Directions:
1. Fit the oven with the rack in position
2. Toss shrimp with remaining ingredients.
3. Transfer shrimp into the baking pan.
4. Set to bake at 400 F for 13 minutes. After 5 minutes place the baking pan in the preheated oven.
5. Serve and enjoy.

Nutrition Info: Calories 344 Fat 11.5 g Carbohydrates 6.1 g Sugar 0.5 g Protein 52.3 g Cholesterol 478 mg

320. Lemony Tuna
Servings: 4
Cooking Time: 10 Minutes
Ingredients:
- 2 (6-ounce) cans water packed plain tuna
- 2 teaspoons Dijon mustard
- ½ cup breadcrumbs
- 1 tablespoon fresh lime juice
- 2 tablespoons fresh parsley, chopped
- 1 egg
- Chefman of hot sauce
- 3 tablespoons canola oil
- Salt and freshly ground black pepper, to taste

Directions:
1. Preparing the Ingredients. Drain most of the liquid from the canned tuna.
2. In a bowl, add the fish, mustard, crumbs, citrus juice, parsley, and hot sauce and mix till well combined. Add a little canola oil if it seems too dry. Add egg, salt and stir to combine. Make the patties from tuna mixture. Refrigerate the tuna patties for about 2 hours.
3. Air Frying. Preheat the air fryer oven to 355 degrees F. Cook for about 10-12 minutes.

321. Maryland Crab Cakes
Servings: 6
Cooking Time: 10 Minutes
Ingredients:
- Nonstick cooking spray
- 2 eggs
- 1 cup Panko bread crumbs
- 1 stalk celery, chopped
- 3 tbsp. mayonnaise
- 1 tsp Worcestershire sauce
- ¼ cup mozzarella cheese, grated

- 1 tsp Italian seasoning
- 1 tbsp. fresh parsley, chopped
- 1 tsp pepper
- ¾ lb. lump crabmeat, drained

Directions:
1. Place baking pan in position 2 of the oven. Lightly spray the fryer basket with cooking spray.
2. In a large bowl, combine all ingredients except crab meat, mix well.
3. Fold in crab carefully so it retains some chunks. Form mixture into 12 patties.
4. Place patties in a single layer in the fryer basket. Place the basket on the baking pan.
5. Set oven to air fryer on 350°F for 10 minutes. Cook until golden brown, turning over halfway through cooking time. Serve immediately.

Nutrition Info: Calories 172, Total Fat 8g, Saturated Fat 2g, Total Carbs 14g, Net Carbs 13g, Protein 16g, Sugar 1g, Fiber 1g, Sodium 527mg, Potassium 290mg, Phosphorus 201mg

322. Basil Tomato Salmon

Servings: 2
Cooking Time: 20 Minutes
Ingredients:
- 2 salmon fillets
- 1 tomato, sliced
- 1 tbsp dried basil
- 2 tbsp parmesan cheese, grated
- 1 tbsp olive oil

Directions:
1. Fit the oven with the rack in position
2. Place salmon fillets in a baking dish.
3. Sprinkle basil on top of salmon fillets.
4. Arrange tomato slices on top of salmon fillets. Drizzle with oil and top with cheese.
5. Set to bake at 375 F for 25 minutes. After 5 minutes place the baking dish in the preheated oven.
6. Serve and enjoy.

Nutrition Info: Calories 324 Fat 19.6 g Carbohydrates 1.5 g Sugar 0.8 g Protein 37.1 g Cholesterol 83 mg

323. Prawn Momo's Recipe

Ingredients:
- 1 ½ cup all-purpose flour
- ½ tsp. salt
- 5 tbsp. water
- For filling:
- 2 cups minced prawn
- 2 tbsp. oil
- 2 tsp. ginger-garlic paste
- 2 tsp. soya sauce
- 2 tsp. vinegar

Directions:
1. Squeeze the dough and cover it with plastic wrap and set aside. Next, cook the ingredients for the filling and try to ensure that the prawn is covered well with the sauce. Roll the dough and cut it into a square.
2. Place the filling in the center. Now, wrap the dough to cover the filling and pinch the edges together. Pre heat the oven at 200° F for 5 minutes. Place the wontons in the fry basket and close it. Let them cook at the same temperature for another 20 minutes. Recommended sides are chili sauce or ketchup.

324. Crispy Fish Sticks

Servings: 8
Cooking Time: 6 Minutes
Ingredients:
- 8 ounces (227 g) fish fillets (pollock or cod), cut into ½ × 3 inches strips
- Salt, to taste (optional)
- ½ cup plain bread crumbs
- Cooking spray

Directions:
1. Season the fish strips with salt to taste, if desired.
2. Place the bread crumbs on a plate, then roll the fish in the bread crumbs until well coated. Spray all sides of the fish with cooking spray. Transfer to the air fryer basket in a single layer.
3. Put the air fryer basket on the baking pan and slide into Rack Position 2, select Air Fry, set temperature to 400ºF (205ºC), and set time to 6 minutes.
4. When cooked, the fish sticks should be golden brown and crispy. Remove from the oven to a plate and serve hot.

325. Panko Crab Sticks With Mayo Sauce

Servings: 4
Cooking Time: 12 Minutes
Ingredients:
- Crab Sticks:
- 2 eggs
- 1 cup flour
- $1/3$ cup panko bread crumbs
- 1 tablespoon old bay seasoning
- 1 pound (454 g) crab sticks
- Cooking spray
- Mayo Sauce:
- ½ cup mayonnaise
- 1 lime, juiced
- 2 garlic cloves, minced

Directions:
1. In a bowl, beat the eggs. In a shallow bowl, place the flour. In another shallow bowl, thoroughly combine the panko bread crumbs and old bay seasoning.
2. Dredge the crab sticks in the flour, shaking off any excess, then in the beaten eggs, finally press them in the bread crumb mixture to coat well.
3. Arrange the crab sticks in the air fryer basket and spray with cooking spray.

4. Put the air fryer basket on the baking pan and slide into Rack Position 2, select Air Fry, set temperature to 390ºF (199ºC), and set time to 12 minutes.
5. Flip the crab sticks halfway through the cooking time.
6. Meanwhile, make the sauce by whisking together the mayo, lime juice, and garlic in a small bowl.
7. When cooking is complete, remove from the oven. Serve the crab sticks with the mayo sauce on the side.

326. Easy Baked Fish Fillet

Servings: 4
Cooking Time: 15 Minutes
Ingredients:
- 1 lb white fish fillets
- 2 tbsp dried parsley
- 1/4 tsp red chili flakes
- 2 tbsp garlic, minced
- 2 tbsp olive oil
- Pepper
- Salt

Directions:
1. Fit the oven with the rack in position
2. Place fish fillets in a baking dish and drizzle with oil.
3. Sprinkle with chili flakes, parsley, and garlic. Season with pepper and salt.
4. Set to bake at 400 F for 20 minutes. After 5 minutes place the baking dish in the preheated oven.
5. Serve and enjoy.

Nutrition Info: Calories 262 Fat 15.6 g Carbohydrates 1.5 g Sugar 0.1 g Protein 28.1 g Cholesterol 87 mg

327. Sticky Hoisin Tuna

Servings: 4
Cooking Time: 5 Minutes
Ingredients:
- ½ cup hoisin sauce
- 2 tablespoons rice wine vinegar
- 2 teaspoons sesame oil
- 2 teaspoons dried lemongrass
- 1 teaspoon garlic powder
- ¼ teaspoon red pepper flakes
- ½ small onion, quartered and thinly sliced
- 8 ounces (227 g) fresh tuna, cut into 1-inch cubes
- Cooking spray
- 3 cups cooked jasmine rice

Directions:
1. In a small bowl, whisk together the hoisin sauce, vinegar, sesame oil, lemongrass, garlic powder, and red pepper flakes.
2. Add the sliced onion and tuna cubes and gently toss until the fish is evenly coated.
3. Arrange the coated tuna cubes in the air fryer basket in a single layer.
4. Put the air fryer basket on the baking pan and slide into Rack Position 2, select Air Fry, set temperature to 390ºF (199ºC), and set time to 5 minutes.
5. Flip the fish halfway through the cooking time.
6. When cooking is complete, the fish should begin to flake. Continue cooking for 1 minute, if necessary. Remove from the oven and serve over hot jasmine rice.

328. Glazed Tuna And Fruit Kebabs

Servings: 4
Cooking Time: 10 Minutes
Ingredients:
- Kebabs:
- 1 pound (454 g) tuna steaks, cut into 1-inch cubes
- ½ cup canned pineapple chunks, drained, juice reserved
- ½ cup large red grapes
- Marinade:
- 1 tablespoon honey
- 1 teaspoon olive oil
- 2 teaspoons grated fresh ginger
- Pinch cayenne pepper
- Special Equipment:
- 4 metal skewers

Directions:
1. Make the kebabs: Thread, alternating tuna cubes, pineapple chunks, and red grapes, onto the metal skewers.
2. Make the marinade: Whisk together the honey, olive oil, ginger, and cayenne pepper in a small bowl. Brush generously the marinade over the kebabs and allow to sit for 10 minutes.
3. When ready, transfer the kebabs to the air fryer basket.
4. Put the air fryer basket on the baking pan and slide into Rack Position 2, select Air Fry, set temperature to 370ºF (188ºC), and set time to 10 minutes.
5. After 5 minutes, remove from the oven and flip the kebabs and brush with the remaining marinade. Return the pan to the oven and continue cooking for an additional 5 minutes.
6. When cooking is complete, the kebabs should reach an internal temperature of 145ºF (63ºC) on a meat thermometer. Remove from the oven and discard any remaining marinade. Serve hot.

329. Citrus Cilantro Catfish

Servings: 2
Cooking Time: 20 Minutes
Ingredients:
- 2 catfish fillets
- 2 tsp blackening seasoning

- Juice of 1 lime
- 2 tbsp butter, melted
- 1 garlic clove, mashed
- 2 tbsp fresh cilantro, chopped

Directions:
1. In a bowl, blend garlic, lime juice, cilantro, and butter. Pour half of the mixture over the fillets and sprinkle with blackening seasoning. Place the fillets in the basket and press Start. Cook for 15 minutes at 360 F on AirFry function. Serve the fish topped with the remaining sauce.

330. Tomato Garlic Shrimp

Servings: 4
Cooking Time: 25 Minutes
Ingredients:
- 1 lb shrimp, peeled
- 1 tbsp garlic, sliced
- 2 cups cherry tomatoes
- 1 tbsp olive oil
- Pepper
- Salt

Directions:
1. Fit the oven with the rack in position
2. Add shrimp, oil, garlic, tomatoes, pepper, and salt into the large bowl and toss well.
3. Transfer shrimp mixture into the baking dish.
4. Set to bake at 400 F for 30 minutes. After 5 minutes place the baking dish in the preheated oven.
5. Serve and enjoy.

Nutrition Info: Calories 184 Fat 5.6 g Carbohydrates 5.9 g Sugar 2.4 g Protein 26.8 gCholesterol 239 mg

331. Salmon Tandoor

Ingredients:
- 2 lb. boneless salmon filets
- 1st Marinade:
- 3 tbsp. vinegar or lemon juice
- 2 or 3 tsp. paprika
- 1 tsp. black pepper
- 1 tsp. salt
- 3 tsp. ginger-garlic paste
- 2nd Marinade:
- 1 cup yogurt
- 4 tsp. tandoori masala
- 2 tbsp. dry fenugreek leaves
- 1 tsp. black salt
- 1 tsp. chat masala
- 1 tsp. garam masala powder
- 1 tsp. red chili powder
- 1 tsp. salt
- 3 drops of red color

Directions:
1. Make the first marinade and soak the fileted salmon in it for four hours. While this is happening, make the second marinade and soak the salmon in it overnight to let the flavors blend. Pre heat the oven at 160 degrees Fahrenheit for 5 minutes.

2. Place the Oregano Fingers in the fry basket and close it. Let them cook at the same temperature for another 15 minutes or so. Toss the Oregano Fingers well so that they are cooked uniformly. Serve them with mint sauce.

332. Crispy Crab Legs

Servings: 4
Cooking Time: 15 Minutes
Ingredients:
- 3 pounds crab legs
- ½ cup butter, melted

Directions:
1. Preheat on Air Fry function to 380 F. Cover the crab legs with salted water and let them stay for a few minutes. Drain, pat them dry, and place the legs in the basket. Fit in the baking tray and brush with some butter; cook for 10 minutes, flipping once. Drizzle with the remaining butter and serve.

333. Fish Cakes With Mango Relish

Servings: 4
Cooking Time: 10 Minutes
Ingredients:
- 1 lb White Fish Fillets
- 3 Tbsps Ground Coconut
- 1 Ripened Mango
- ½ Tsps Chili Paste
- Tbsps Fresh Parsley
- 1 Green Onion
- 1 Lime
- 1 Tsp Salt
- 1 Egg

Directions:
1. Preparing the Ingredients. To make the relish, peel and dice the mango into cubes. Combine with a half teaspoon of chili paste, a tablespoon of parsley, and the zest and juice of half a lime.
2. In a food processor, pulse the fish until it forms a smooth texture. Place into a bowl and add the salt, egg, chopped green onion, parsley, two tablespoons of the coconut, and the remainder of the chili paste and lime zest and juice. Combine well
3. Portion the mixture into 10 equal balls and flatten them into small patties. Pour the reserved tablespoon of coconut onto a dish and roll the patties over to coat.
4. Preheat the Air fryer oven to 390 degrees
5. Air Frying. Place the fish cakes into the air fryer oven and cook for 8 minutes. They should be crisp and lightly browned when ready
6. Serve hot with mango relish

334. Cheesy Tilapia Fillets

Servings: 4
Cooking Time: 15 Minutes
Ingredients:

- ¾ cup grated Parmesan cheese
- 1 tbsp olive oil
- 2 tsp paprika
- 1 tbsp chopped parsley
- ¼ tsp garlic powder
- 4 tilapia fillets

Directions:
1. Preheat on Air Fry function to 350 F. Mix parsley, Parmesan cheese, garlic, and paprika in a bowl. Brush the olive oil over the fillets and then coat with the Parmesan mixture. Place the tilapia onto a lined baking sheet and cook for 8-10 minutes, turning once. Serve.

335. Quick Shrimp Bowl

Servings: 4
Cooking Time: 15 Minutes
Ingredients:
- 1 ¼ pounds tiger shrimp
- ¼ tsp cayenne pepper
- ½ tsp old bay seasoning
- ¼ tsp smoked paprika
- A pinch of salt
- 1 tbsp olive oil

Directions:
1. Preheat your oven to 390 F on Air Fry function. In a bowl, mix all the ingredients. Place the mixture in your the cooking basket and fit in the baking tray; cook for 5 minutes, flipping once. Serve drizzled with lemon juice.

336. Paprika Cod

Servings: 4
Cooking Time: 15 Minutes
Ingredients:
- 4 cod fillets
- 1 tsp smoked paprika
- 1/2 cup parmesan cheese, grated
- 1/2 tbsp olive oil
- 1 tsp parsley
- Pepper
- Salt

Directions:
1. Fit the oven with the rack in position
2. Brush fish fillets with oil and season with pepper and salt.
3. In a shallow dish, mix parmesan cheese, paprika, and parsley.
4. Coat fish fillets with cheese mixture and place into the baking dish.
5. Set to bake at 400 F for 20 minutes. After 5 minutes place the baking dish in the preheated oven.
6. Serve and enjoy.

Nutrition Info: Calories 125 Fat 5 g Carbohydrates 0.7 g Sugar 0.1 g Protein 19.8 g Cholesterol 52 mg

337. Roasted Nicoise Salad

Servings: 4
Cooking Time: 15 Minutes
Ingredients:
- 10 ounces (283 g) small red potatoes, quartered
- 8 tablespoons extra-virgin olive oil, divided
- 1 teaspoon kosher salt, divided
- ½ pound (227 g) green beans, trimmed
- 1 pint cherry tomatoes
- 1 teaspoon Dijon mustard
- 3 tablespoons red wine vinegar
- Freshly ground black pepper, to taste
- 1 (9-ounce / 255-g) bag spring greens, washed and dried if needed
- 2 (5-ounce / 142-g) cans oil-packed tuna, drained
- 2 hard-cooked eggs, peeled and quartered
- 1/3 cup kalamata olives, pitted

Directions:
1. In a large bowl, drizzle the potatoes with 1 tablespoon of olive oil and season with ¼ teaspoon of kosher salt. Transfer to the baking pan.
2. Slide the baking pan into Rack Position 2, select Roast, set temperature to 375ºF (190ºC), and set time to 15 minutes.
3. Meanwhile, in a mixing bowl, toss the green beans and cherry tomatoes with 1 tablespoon of olive oil and ¼ teaspoon of kosher salt until evenly coated.
4. After 10 minutes, remove the pan and fold in the green beans and cherry tomatoes. Return the pan to the oven and continue cooking.
5. Meanwhile, make the vinaigrette by whisking together the remaining 6 tablespoons of olive oil, mustard, vinegar, the remaining ½ teaspoon of kosher salt, and black pepper in a small bowl. Set aside.
6. When done, remove from the oven. Allow the vegetables to cool for 5 minutes.
7. Spread out the spring greens on a plate and spoon the tuna into the center of the greens. Arrange the potatoes, green beans, cheery tomatoes, and eggs around the tuna. Serve drizzled with the vinaigrette and scattered with the olives.

338. Paprika Basil Baked Basa

Servings: 2
Cooking Time: 30 Minutes
Ingredients:
- 2 basa fish fillets
- 4 lemon slices
- 1/8 tsp lemon juice
- 1/2 tbsp dried basil
- 1/2 tbsp sweet paprika
- 4 tbsp butter, melted
- 1/8 tsp salt

Directions:
1. Fit the oven with the rack in position
2. Place fish fillets into the baking dish.
3. Pour remaining ingredients over fish fillets.

4. Set to bake at 350 F for 30 minutes. After 5 minutes place the baking dish in the preheated oven.
5. Serve and enjoy.
Nutrition Info: Calories 433 Fat 35.2 g Carbohydrates 6.5 g Sugar 3.4 g Protein 24.4 g Cholesterol 61 mg

339. Tuna Lettuce Wraps

Servings: 4
Cooking Time: 4 To 7 Minutes
Ingredients:
- 1 pound (454 g) fresh tuna steak, cut into 1-inch cubes
- 2 garlic cloves, minced
- 1 tablespoon grated fresh ginger
- ½ teaspoon toasted sesame oil
- 4 low-sodium whole-wheat tortillas
- 2 cups shredded romaine lettuce
- 1 red bell pepper, thinly sliced
- ¼ cup low-fat mayonnaise

Directions:
1. Combine the tuna cubes, garlic, ginger, and sesame oil in a medium bowl and toss until well coated. Allow to sit for 10 minutes.
2. When ready, place the tuna cubes in the air fryer basket.
3. Put the air fryer basket on the baking pan and slide into Rack Position 2, select Air Fry, set temperature to 390ºF (199ºC), and set time to 6 minutes.
4. When cooking is complete, the tuna cubes should be cooked through and golden brown. Remove the tuna cubes from the oven to a plate.
5. Make the wraps: Place the tortillas on a flat work surface and top each tortilla evenly with the cooked tuna, lettuce, bell pepper, and finish with the mayonnaise. Roll them up and serve immediately.

340. Caesar Shrimp Salad

Servings: 4
Cooking Time: 15 Minutes
Ingredients:
- ½ baguette, cut into 1-inch cubes (about 2½ cups)
- 4 tablespoons extra-virgin olive oil, divided
- ¼ teaspoon granulated garlic
- ¼ teaspoon kosher salt
- ¾ cup Caesar dressing, divided
- 2 romaine lettuce hearts, cut in half lengthwise and ends trimmed
- 1 pound (454 g) medium shrimp, peeled and deveined
- 2 ounces (57 g) Parmesan cheese, coarsely grated

Directions:
1. Make the croutons: Put the bread cubes in a medium bowl and drizzle 3 tablespoons of olive oil over top. Season with granulated garlic and salt and toss to coat. Transfer to the air fryer basket in a single layer.
2. Put the air fryer basket on the baking pan and slide into Rack Position 2, select Air Fry, set temperature to 400ºF (205ºC), and set time to 4 minutes.
3. Toss the croutons halfway through the cooking time.
4. When done, remove from the oven and set aside.
5. Brush 2 tablespoons of Caesar dressing on the cut side of the lettuce. Set aside.
6. Toss the shrimp with the ¼ cup of Caesar dressing in a large bowl until well coated. Set aside.
7. Coat the baking pan with the remaining 1 tablespoon of olive oil. Arrange the romaine halves on the coated pan, cut side down. Brush the tops with the remaining 2 tablespoons of Caesar dressing.
8. Slide the baking pan into Rack Position 2, select Roast, set temperature to 375ºF (190ºC), and set time to 10 minutes.
9. After 5 minutes, remove from the oven and flip the romaine halves. Spoon the shrimp around the lettuce. Return the pan to the oven and continue cooking.
10. When done, remove from the oven. If they are not quite cooked through, roast for another 1 minute.
11. On each of four plates, put a romaine half. Divide the shrimp among the plates and top with croutons and grated Parmesan cheese. Serve immediately.

APPETIZERS AND SIDE DISHES

341. Paprika Pickle Chips
Servings: 3
Cooking Time: 20 Minutes
Ingredients:
- 36 sweet pickle chips
- 1 cup buttermilk
- 3 tbsp smoked paprika
- 2 cups flour
- ¼ cup cornmeal
- Salt and black pepper to taste

Directions:
1. Preheat Breville on Air Fryer function to 400 F. In a bowl, mix flour, paprika, pepper, salt, and cornmeal. Place pickles in buttermilk and let sit for 5 minutes. Drain and dip in the spice mixture. Place them in the cooking basket. Cook for 10 minutes until brown and crispy.

342. Creamy Fennel(3)
Servings: 4
Cooking Time: 20 Minutes
Ingredients:
- 2 big fennel bulbs; sliced
- ½ cup coconut cream
- 2 tbsp. butter; melted
- Salt and black pepper to taste.

Directions:
1. In a pan that fits the air fryer, combine all the ingredients, toss, introduce in the machine and cook at 370°F for 12 minutes
2. Divide between plates and serve as a side dish.

Nutrition Info: Calories: 151; Fat: 3g; Fiber: 2g; Carbs: 4g; Protein: 6g

343. Homemade Cheddar Biscuits
Servings: 8
Cooking Time: 35 Minutes
Ingredients:
- ½ cup + 1 tbsp butter
- 2 tbsp sugar
- 3 cups flour
- 1 ⅓ cups buttermilk
- ½ cup cheddar cheese, grated

Directions:
1. Preheat on Bake function to 380 F. Lay a parchment paper on a baking plate. In a bowl, mix sugar, flour, ½ cup of butter, half of the cheddar cheese, and buttermilk to form a batter. Make 8 balls from the batter and roll in flour.
2. Place the balls in your Air Fryer baking tray and flatten into biscuit shapes. Sprinkle the remaining cheddar cheese and remaining butter on top. Cook for 30 minutes, tossing every 10 minutes. Serve.

344. Chili Endives
Servings: 4
Cooking Time: 20 Minutes
Ingredients:
- 2 scallions; chopped.
- 4 endives; trimmed and roughly shredded
- 3 garlic cloves; minced
- 1 tbsp. olive oil
- 1 tsp. chili sauce
- Salt and black pepper to taste.

Directions:
1. Grease a pan that fits your air fryer with the oil, add all the ingredients, toss, introduce in the air fryer and cook at 370°F for 20 minutes
2. Divide everything between plates and serve.

Nutrition Info: Calories: 184; Fat: 2g; Fiber: 2g; Carbs: 3g; Protein: 5g

345. Delicious Mac And Cheese
Servings: 6
Cooking Time: 30 Minutes
Ingredients:
- 2 ½ cups pasta, uncooked
- 1/2 cup cream
- 1 cup vegetable broth
- 2 tbsp flour
- 1/2 cup parmesan cheese, grated
- 1/2 cup Velveeta cheese, cut into small cubes
- 2 cups Colby cheese, shredded
- 2 tbsp butter
- 1 tsp salt

Directions:
1. Fit the oven with the rack in position
2. Cook pasta according to the packet instructions. Drain well.
3. Melt butter in a pan over medium heat. Slowly whisk in flour.
4. Whisk constantly and slowly add the broth.
5. Slowly pour the cream and whisk constantly.
6. Slowly add parmesan cheese, Velveeta cheese, and Colby cheese and whisk until smooth.
7. Add cooked pasta to the sauce and stir well to coat.
8. Transfer pasta into the greased casserole dish.
9. Set to bake at 350 F for 35 minutes. After 5 minutes place the casserole dish in the preheated oven.
10. Serve and enjoy.

Nutrition Info: Calories 410 Fat 21.8 g Carbohydrates 34 g Sugar 1.3 g Protein 20 g Cholesterol 99 mg

346. Spicy Pumpkin-ham Fritters

Servings: 4
Cooking Time: 10 Minutes
Ingredients:
- 1 oz ham, chopped
- 1 cup dry pancake mix
- 1 egg
- 2 tbsp canned puree pumpkin
- 1 oz cheddar, shredded
- ½ tsp chili powder
- 3 tbsp of flour
- 1 oz beer
- 2 tbsp scallions, chopped

Directions:
1. Preheat on Air Fry function to 370 F. In a bowl, combine the pancake mix and chili powder. Mix in the egg, puree pumpkin, beer, shredded cheddar, ham and scallions. Form balls and roll them in the flour.
2. Arrange the balls into the basket and fit in the baking tray. Cook for 8 minutes. Drain on paper towel before serving.

347. Zucchini Spaghetti

Servings: 4
Cooking Time: 20 Minutes
Ingredients:
- 1 lb. zucchinis, cut with a spiralizer
- 1 cup parmesan; grated
- ¼ cup parsley; chopped.
- ¼ cup olive oil
- 6 garlic cloves; minced
- ½ tsp. red pepper flakes
- Salt and black pepper to taste.

Directions:
1. In a pan that fits your air fryer, mix all the ingredients, toss, introduce in the fryer and cook at 370°F for 15 minutes.
2. Divide between plates and serve as a side dish.

Nutrition Info: Calories: 200; Fat: 6g; Fiber: 3g; Carbs: 4g; Protein: 5g

348. Spicy Broccoli With Hot Sauce

Servings: 6
Cooking Time: 14 Minutes
Ingredients:
- Broccoli:
- 1 medium-sized head broccoli, cut into florets
- 1½ tablespoons olive oil
- 1 teaspoon shallot powder
- 1 teaspoon porcini powder
- ½ teaspoon freshly grated lemon zest
- ½ teaspoon hot paprika
- ½ teaspoon granulated garlic
- $1/3$ teaspoon fine sea salt
- $1/3$ teaspoon celery seeds
- Hot Sauce:
- ½ cup tomato sauce
- 1 tablespoon balsamic vinegar
- ½ teaspoon ground allspice

Directions:
1. In a mixing bowl, combine all the ingredients for the broccoli and toss to coat. Transfer the broccoli to the air fryer basket.
2. Put the air fryer basket on the baking pan and slide into Rack Position 2, select Air Fry, set temperature to 360ºF (182ºC), and set time to 14 minutes.
3. Meanwhile, make the hot sauce by whisking together the tomato sauce, balsamic vinegar, and allspice in a small bowl.
4. When cooking is complete, remove the broccoli from the oven and serve with the hot sauce.

349. Air Fry Garlic Baby Potatoes

Servings: 4
Cooking Time: 20 Minutes
Ingredients:
- 1 lb baby potatoes, cut into quarters
- 1/2 tsp granulated garlic
- 1 tbsp olive oil
- 1/2 tsp dried parsley
- 1/4 tsp salt

Directions:
1. Fit the oven with the rack in position 2.
2. In a mixing bowl, toss baby potatoes with oil, garlic, parsley, and salt.
3. Transfer potatoes in air fryer basket then place air fryer basket in baking pan.
4. Place a baking pan on the oven rack. Set to air fry at 350 F for 20 minutes.
5. Serve and enjoy.

Nutrition Info: Calories 97 Fat 3.6 g Carbohydrates 14.4 g Sugar 0.1 g Protein 3 g Cholesterol 0 mg

350. Pineapple Pork Ribs

Servings: 4
Cooking Time: 30 Minutes
Ingredients:
- 2 lb cut spareribs
- 7 oz salad dressing
- 1 (5-oz) can pineapple juice
- 2 cups water
- Salt and black pepper to taste

Directions:
1. Preheat your to 390 F on Bake function. Sprinkle the ribs with salt and pepper and place them in a greased baking dish. Cook for 15 minutes. Prepare the sauce by combining the salad dressing and the pineapple juice. Serve the ribs drizzled with the sauce.

351. Creamy Corn Casserole

Servings: 4
Cooking Time: 15 Minutes
Ingredients:
- 2 cups frozen yellow corn
- 1 egg, beaten
- 3 tablespoons flour
- ½ cup grated Swiss or Havarti cheese
- ½ cup light cream
- ¼ cup milk
- Pinch salt
- Freshly ground black pepper, to taste
- 2 tablespoons butter, cut into cubes
- Nonstick cooking spray

Directions:
1. Spritz the baking pan with nonstick cooking spray.
2. Stir together the remaining ingredients except the butter in a medium bowl until well incorporated. Transfer the mixture to the prepared baking pan and scatter with the butter cubes.
3. Slide the baking pan into Rack Position 1, select Convection Bake, set temperature to 320ºF (160ºC), and set time to 15 minutes.
4. When cooking is complete, the top should be golden brown and a toothpick inserted in the center should come out clean. Remove from the oven. Let the casserole cool for 5 minutes before slicing into wedges and serving.

352. Herbed Radish Sauté(1)

Servings: 4
Cooking Time: 20 Minutes
Ingredients:
- 2 bunches red radishes; halved
- 2 tbsp. parsley; chopped.
- 2 tbsp. balsamic vinegar
- 1 tbsp. olive oil
- Salt and black pepper to taste.

Directions:
1. Take a bowl and mix the radishes with the remaining ingredients except the parsley, toss and put them in your air fryer's basket.
2. Cook at 400°F for 15 minutes, divide between plates, sprinkle the parsley on top and serve as a side dish

Nutrition Info: Calories: 180; Fat: 4g; Fiber: 2g; Carbs: 3g; Protein: 5g

353. Cheese Biscuits

Servings: 6
Cooking Time: 35 Minutes
Ingredients:
- ½ cup + 1 tbsp butter
- 2 tbsp sugar
- 3 cups flour
- 1 ⅓ cups buttermilk
- ½ cup cheddar cheese, grated

Directions:
1. Preheat Breville on AirFry function to 380 F. Lay a parchment paper on a baking plate. In a bowl, mix sugar, flour, ½ cup butter, cheese, and buttermilk to form a batter. Make balls from the batter and roll in the flour. Place the balls in the baking plate and flatten into biscuit shapes. Sprinkle with cheese and the remaining butter. Place in the oven and press Start. Cook for 30 minutes, tossing every 10 minutes. Serve chilled.

354. Easy Broccoli Bread

Servings: 6
Cooking Time: 30 Minutes
Ingredients:
- 5 eggs, lightly beaten
- 3/4 cup broccoli florets, chopped
- 2 tsp baking powder
- 3 1/1 tbsp coconut flour
- 1 cup cheddar cheese, shredded

Directions:
1. Fit the oven with the rack in position
2. Add all ingredients into the bowl and mix well.
3. Pour egg mixture into the greased loaf pan.
4. Set to bake at 350 F for 35 minutes. After 5 minutes place the loaf pan in the preheated oven.
5. Cut the loaf into the slices and serve.

Nutrition Info: Calories 174 Fat 11.3 g Carbohydrates 7.4 g Sugar 1.2 g Protein 11 g Cholesterol 156 mg

355. Herby Carrot Cookies

Servings: 6
Cooking Time: 30 Minutes
Ingredients:
- 6 carrots, sliced
- Salt and black pepper to taste
- 1 tbsp parsley
- ½ cup oats
- 1 whole egg, beaten
- 1 tbsp thyme

Directions:
1. Preheat Breville on Air Fryer function to 360 F. In a saucepan over medium heat, add carrots and cover with water. Cook for 10 minutes until tender. Remove to a plate. Season with salt, pepper, and parsley and mash using a fork.
2. Add in egg, oats, and thyme as you continue mashing to mix well. Form the batter into cookie shapes. Place in the frying basket and press Start. Cook for 15 minutes until edges are browned.

356. Potato Chips With Lemony Dip

Servings: 3
Cooking Time: 25 Minutes
Ingredients:
- 3 large potatoes, sliced
- 1 cup sour cream
- 2 scallions, white part minced
- 3 tbsp olive oil.
- ½ tsp lemon juice
- salt and black pepper

Directions:
1. Preheat on Air Fry function to 350 F. Place the potatoes into the AirFryer basket and fit in the baking tray. Cook for 15 minutes, flipping once. Season with salt and pepper. Mix sour cream, olive oil, scallions, lemon juice, salt, and pepper and serve with chips.

357. Classic Cauliflower Hash Browns

Servings: 2
Cooking Time: 20 Minutes
Ingredients:
- 2/3 pound cauliflower, peeled and grated
- 2 eggs, whisked
- 1/4 cup scallions, chopped
- 1 teaspoon fresh garlic, minced
- Sea salt and ground black pepper, to taste
- 1/4 teaspoon ground allspice
- 1/2 teaspoon cinnamon
- 1 tablespoon peanut oil

Directions:
1. Boil cauliflower over medium-low heat until fork-tender, 5 to 7 minutes Drain the water; pat cauliflower dry with a kitchen towel.
2. Now, add the remaining ingredients; stir to combine well.
3. Cook in the preheated Air Fryer at 395 degrees F for 20 minutes. Shake the basket once or twice. Serve with low-carb tomato sauce.
Nutrition Info: 157 Calories; 12g Fat; 3g Carbs; 8g Protein; 6g Sugars; 6g Fiber

358. Crunchy Cheese Twists

Servings: 8
Cooking Time: 45 Minutes
Ingredients:
- 2 cups cauliflower florets, steamed
- 1 egg
- 3 ½ oz oats
- 1 red onion, diced
- 1 tsp mustard
- 5 oz cheddar cheese, shredded
- Salt and black pepper to taste

Directions:
1. Preheat on Air Fry function to 350 F. Place the oats in a food processor and pulse until they are the consistency of breadcrumbs.
2. Place the cauliflower florets in a large bowl. Add in the rest of the ingredients and mix to combine. Take a little bit of the mixture and twist it into a straw.
3. Place onto a lined baking tray and repeat the process with the rest of the mixture. Cook for 10 minutes, turn over, and cook for an additional 10 minutes. Serve.

359. Pineapple & Mozzarella Tortillas

Servings: 2
Cooking Time: 15 Minutes
Ingredients:
- 2 tortillas
- 8 ham slices
- 8 mozzarella slices
- 8 thin pineapple slices
- 2 tbsp tomato sauce
- ½ tsp dried parsley

Directions:
1. Preheat on Air Fry function to 330 F. Spread the tomato sauce onto the tortillas. Arrange 4 ham slices on each tortilla. Top the ham with the pineapple and sprinkle with mozzarella and parsley. Cook for 10 minutes and enjoy.

360. Creamy Fennel(1)

Servings: 4
Cooking Time: 20 Minutes
Ingredients:
- 2 big fennel bulbs; sliced
- ½ cup coconut cream
- 2 tbsp. butter; melted
- Salt and black pepper to taste.

Directions:
1. In a pan that fits the air fryer, combine all the ingredients, toss, introduce in the machine and cook at 370°F for 12 minutes
2. Divide between plates and serve as a side dish.
Nutrition Info: Calories: 151; Fat: 3g; Fiber: 2g; Carbs: 4g; Protein: 6g

361. Garlic Lemon Roasted Chicken

Servings: 4
Cooking Time: 60 Minutes
Ingredients:
- 1 (3 ½ pounds) whole chicken
- 2 tbsp olive oil
- Salt and black pepper to taste
- 1 lemon, cut into quarters
- 5 garlic cloves

Directions:
1. Preheat on Air Fry function to 360 F. Brush the chicken with olive oil and season with salt and pepper. Stuff with lemon and garlic cloves into the cavity.
2. Place the chicken breast-side down onto the Air Fryer basket. Tuck the legs and wings tips under. Fit in the baking tray and cook for 45 minutes at 350 F on Bake function. Let rest for 5-6 minutes, then carve and serve.

362. Creamy Eggplant Cakes

Servings: 4
Cooking Time: 20 Minutes
Ingredients:
- 1 ½ cups flour
- 1 tsp cinnamon
- 3 eggs
- 2 tsp baking powder
- 2 tbsp sugar
- 1 cup milk
- 2 tbsp butter, melted
- 1 tbsp yogurt
- ½ cup shredded eggplant
- Pinch of salt
- 2 tbsp cream cheese

Directions:
1. Preheat on Air Fry function to 350 F. In a bowl, whisk the eggs along with the sugar, salt, cinnamon, cream cheese, flour, and baking powder. In another bowl, combine all of the liquid ingredients. Gently combine the dry and liquid mixtures; stir in eggplant.
2. Line the muffin tins and pour the batter inside; cook for 12 minutes. Check with a toothpick: you may need to cook them for an additional 2 to 3 minutes. Serve chilled.

363. Healthy Spinach Muffins

Servings: 12
Cooking Time: 15 Minutes
Ingredients:
- 10 eggs
- 2 cups spinach, chopped
- 1/2 tsp dried basil
- 1 1/2 cups parmesan cheese, grated
- 1/4 tsp garlic powder
- 1/4 tsp onion powder
- Salt

Directions:
1. Fit the oven with the rack in position
2. Spray 12-cups muffin tin with cooking spray and set aside.
3. In a large bowl, whisk eggs with basil, garlic powder, onion powder, and salt.
4. Add cheese and spinach and stir well.
5. Pour egg mixture into the prepared muffin tin.
6. Set to bake at 400 F for 20 minutes. After 5 minutes place muffin tin in the preheated oven.
7. Serve and enjoy.

Nutrition Info: Calories 90 Fat 6.1 g Carbohydrates 0.9 g Sugar 0.3 g Protein 8.4 g Cholesterol 144 mg

364. Sausage Mushroom Caps(2)

Servings: 2
Cooking Time: 20 Minutes
Ingredients:
- ½ lb. Italian sausage
- 6 large Portobello mushroom caps
- ¼ cup grated Parmesan cheese.
- ¼ cup chopped onion
- 2 tbsp. blanched finely ground almond flour
- 1 tsp. minced fresh garlic

Directions:
1. Use a spoon to hollow out each mushroom cap, reserving scrapings.
2. In a medium skillet over medium heat, brown the sausage about 10 minutes or until fully cooked and no pink remains. Drain and then add reserved mushroom scrapings, onion, almond flour, Parmesan and garlic.
3. Gently fold ingredients together and continue cooking an additional minute, then remove from heat
4. Evenly spoon the mixture into mushroom caps and place the caps into a 6-inch round pan. Place pan into the air fryer basket
5. Adjust the temperature to 375 Degrees F and set the timer for 8 minutes. When finished cooking, the tops will be browned and bubbling. Serve warm.

Nutrition Info: Calories: 404; Protein: 24.3g; Fiber: 4.5g; Fat: 25.8g; Carbs: 18.2g

365. Cheddar Broccoli Fritters

Servings: 4
Cooking Time: 30 Minutes
Ingredients:
- 3 cups broccoli florets, steam & chopped
- 2 cups cheddar cheese, shredded
- 1/4 cup breadcrumbs
- 2 eggs, lightly beaten
- 2 garlic cloves, minced
- Pepper
- Salt

Directions:
1. Fit the oven with the rack in position
2. Add all ingredients into the large bowl and mix until well combined.
3. Make patties from broccoli mixture and place in baking pan.
4. Set to bake at 375 F for 35 minutes. After 5 minutes place the baking pan in the preheated oven.
5. Serve and enjoy.

Nutrition Info: Calories 311 Fat 21.5 g Carbohydrates 10.8 g Sugar 2.1 g Protein 19.8 g Cholesterol 141 mg

366. Dijon Zucchini Patties

Servings: 6
Cooking Time: 30 Minutes
Ingredients:
- 1 cup zucchini, shredded and squeeze out all liquid
- 2 tbsp onion, minced
- 1 egg, lightly beaten
- 1/4 tsp red pepper flakes
- 1/4 cup parmesan cheese, grated
- 1/2 tbsp Dijon mustard
- 1/2 tbsp mayonnaise
- 1/2 cup breadcrumbs
- Pepper
- Salt

Directions:
1. Fit the oven with the rack in position
2. Add all ingredients into the bowl and mix until well combined.
3. Make small patties from the zucchini mixture and place it in a parchment-lined baking pan.
4. Set to bake at 400 F for 35 minutes. After 5 minutes place the baking pan in the preheated oven.
5. Serve and enjoy.

Nutrition Info: Calories 69 Fat 2.5 g Carbohydrates 8 g Sugar 1.2 g Protein 3.7 g Cholesterol 30 mg

367. Green Beans

Servings: 4
Cooking Time: 20 Minutes
Ingredients:
- 6 cups green beans; trimmed
- 1 tbsp. hot paprika
- 2 tbsp. olive oil
- A pinch of salt and black pepper

Directions:
1. Take a bowl and mix the green beans with the other ingredients, toss, put them in the air fryer's basket and cook at 370°F for 20 minutes
2. Divide between plates and serve as a side dish.

Nutrition Info: Calories: 120; Fat: 5g; Fiber: 1g; Carbs: 4g; Protein: 2g

368. Butternut And Apple Mash

Servings: 4
Cooking Time: 15 Minutes
Ingredients:
- 1 butternut squash, peeled and cut into medium chunks
- 2 apples, cored and sliced
- 1 cup water
- ½ teaspoon apple pie spice
- Salt, to taste
- 2 tablespoons butter, browned
- 1 yellow onion, thinly sliced

Directions:
1. Place the pieces of pumpkin, onion and apple in the steam basket of the Instant Pot, add the water to the Instant Pot, cover and cook for 8 minutes in manual setting.
2. Quickly release the pressure and transfer the pumpkin, onion and apple to a bowl. Smash everything with a potato masher, add salt, apple pie spices and brown butter, mix well and serve hot.

Nutrition Info: Calories: 140, Fat: 2.3, Fiber: 6.5, Carbohydrate: 24, Proteins: 2.5

369. Crunchy Mozzarella Sticks With Sweet Thai Sauce

Servings: 4
Cooking Time: 20 Minutes
Ingredients:
- 12 mozzarella string cheese
- 2 cups breadcrumbs
- 3 eggs
- 1 cup sweet Thai sauce
- 4 tbsp skimmed milk

Directions:
1. Pour the crumbs in a bowl. Crack the eggs into another bowl and beat with the milk. One after the other, dip cheese sticks in the egg mixture, in the crumbs, then egg mixture again and then in the crumbs again. Place the coated cheese sticks on a cookie sheet and freeze for 1 hour.
2. Preheat Breville on AirFry function to 380 F. Arrange the sticks in the frying basket without overcrowding. Press Start and cook for 8 minutes until brown. Serve with sweet Thai sauce.

370. Delicious Chicken Wings With Alfredo Sauce

Servings: 4
Cooking Time: 60 Minutes
Ingredients:
- 1 ½ pounds chicken wings
- Salt and black pepper to taste
- ½ cup Alfredo sauce

Directions:
1. Preheat on Air Fry function to 370 F. Season the wings with salt and pepper. Arrange them on the greased basket without touching. Fit in the baking tray and cook for 20 minutes until no longer pink in the center. Work in batches if needed. Increase the heat to 390 F and cook for 5 minutes more. Remove to a large bowl and drizzle with the Alfredo sauce. Serve.

371. Savory Chicken Nuggets With Parmesan Cheese

Servings: 4
Cooking Time: 25 Minutes
Ingredients:
- 1 lb chicken breasts, cubed
- Salt and black pepper to taste
- 2 tbsp olive oil
- 5 tbsp plain breadcrumbs
- 2 tbsp panko breadcrumbs
- 2 tbsp grated Parmesan cheese

Directions:
1. Preheat on Air Fry function to 380 F. Season the chicken with salt and pepper; set aside. In a bowl, mix the breadcrumbs with the Parmesan cheese.
2. Brush the chicken pieces with the olive oil, then dip into breadcrumb mixture, and transfer to the Air Fryer basket. Fit in the baking tray and lightly spray chicken with cooking spray. Cook for 10 minutes, flipping once halfway through until golden brown on the outside and no more pink on the inside. Serve warm.

372. Balsamic Keto Vegetables

Servings: 3
Cooking Time: 20 Minutes
Ingredients:
- 1/2-pound cauliflower florets
- 1/2-pound button mushrooms, whole
- 1 cup pearl onions, whole
- Pink Himalayan salt and ground black pepper, to taste
- 1/4 teaspoon smoked paprika
- 1 teaspoon garlic powder
- 1/2 teaspoon dried thyme
- 1/2 teaspoon dried marjoram
- 3 tablespoons olive oil
- 2 tablespoons balsamic vinegar

Directions:
1. Toss all ingredients in a large mixing dish.
2. Roast in the preheated Air Fryer at 400 degrees F for 5 minutes. Shake the basket and cook for 7 minutes more.
3. Serve with some extra fresh herbs if desired.

Nutrition Info: 170 Calories; 14g Fat; 7g Carbs; 2g Protein; 5g Sugars; 9g Fiber

373. Pineapple Spareribs

Servings: 4
Cooking Time: 35 Minutes
Ingredients:
- 2 lb cut spareribs
- 7 oz salad dressing
- 1 (5-oz) can pineapple juice
- 2 cups water
- 1 tsp garlic powder
- Salt and black pepper

Directions:
1. Sprinkle the ribs with garlic powder, salt, and pepper. Arrange them on the frying basket. sprinkle with garlic salt. Select AirFry function, adjust the temperature to 400 F, and press Start. Cook for 20-25 minutes until golden brown. Prepare the sauce by combining the salad dressing and the pineapple juice. Serve the ribs drizzled with the sauce.

374. Baked Potatoes & Carrots

Servings: 2
Cooking Time: 40 Minutes
Ingredients:
- 1/2 lb potatoes, cut into 1-inch cubes
- 1/2 onion, diced
- 1/2 tsp Italian seasoning
- 1/4 tsp garlic powder
- 1/2 lb carrots, peeled & cut into chunks
- 1 tbsp olive oil
- Pepper
- Salt

Directions:
1. Fit the oven with the rack in position
2. In a large bowl, toss carrots, potatoes, garlic powder, Italian seasoning, oil, onion, pepper, and salt.
3. Transfer carrot potato in baking pan.
4. Set to bake at 400 F for 45 minutes. After 5 minutes place the baking pan in the preheated oven.
5. Serve and enjoy.

Nutrition Info: Calories 201 Fat 7.5 g Carbohydrates 32 g Sugar 8.2 g Protein 3.2 g Cholesterol 1 mg

375. Rice And Artichokes

Servings: 4
Cooking Time: 20 Minutes
Ingredients:
- 2 garlic cloves, peeled and crushed
- 1¼ cups chicken broth
- 1 tablespoon extra-virgin olive oil
- 5 ounces Arborio rice
- 1 tablespoon white wine
- 15 ounces canned artichoke hearts, chopped
- 16 ounces cream cheese
- 1 tablespoon grated Parmesan cheese
- 1½ tablespoons fresh thyme, chopped
- Salt and ground black pepper, to taste
- 6 ounces graham cracker crumbs
- 1¼ cups water

Directions:
1. Put the Instant Pot in the sauté mode, add the oil, heat, add the rice and cook for 2 minutes. Add the garlic, mix and cook for 1 minute.

2. Transfer to a heat-resistant plate. Add the stock, crumbs, salt, pepper and wine, mix and cover the plate with aluminum foil.
3. Place the dish in the basket to cook the Instant Pot, add water, cover and cook for 8 minutes on rice. Release the pressure, remove the dish, uncover, add cream cheese, parmesan, artichoke hearts and thyme.
4. Mix well and serve.
Nutrition Info: Calories: 240, Fat: 7.2, Fiber: 5.1, Carbohydrate: 34, Proteins: 6

376. Whole Chicken With Bbq Sauce
Servings: 3
Cooking Time: 25 Minutes
Ingredients:
- 1 whole small chicken, cut into pieces
- 1 tsp salt
- 1 tsp smoked paprika
- 1 tsp garlic powder
- 1 cup BBQ sauce

Directions:
1. Coat the chicken with salt, paprika, and garlic. Place the chicken pieces skin-side down in the greased baking tray. Cook in the oven for around 15 minutes at 400 F on Bake function until slightly golden. Remove to a plate and brush with barbecue sauce. Return the chicken to the oven skin-side up and cook for 5 minutes at 340 F. Serve with more barbecue sauce.

377. Poached Fennel
Servings: 3
Cooking Time: 6 Minutes
Ingredients:
- Ground nutmeg
- 1 tablespoon white flour
- 2 cups milk
- Salt, to taste
- 2 big fennel bulbs, sliced
- 2 tablespoons butter

Directions:
1. Put the Instant Pot in Saute mode, add the butter and melt. Add the fennel slices, mix and cook until lightly browned.
2. Add the flour, salt, pepper, nutmeg and milk, mix, cover and cook in the manual for 6 minutes. Relieve the pressure, transfer the fennel to the dishes and serve.
Nutrition Info: Calories: 140, Fat: 5, Fiber: 4.7, Carbohydrate: 12, Proteins: 4.4

378. Rosemary Potato Chips
Servings: 4
Cooking Time: 30 Minutes
Ingredients:

- 1 pound potatoes, cut into thin slices
- ¼ cup olive oil
- 1 tbsp garlic puree
- ½ cup heavy cream
- 2 tbsp fresh rosemary, chopped

Directions:
1. Preheat Breville on AirFry function to 390 F. In a bowl, mix oil, garlic puree, and salt. Add in the potato slices and toss to coat. Lay the potato slices onto the frying basket and place in the oven. Press Start and cook for 20-25 minutes. Sprinkle with rosemary and serve.

379. Brussels Sprouts With Garlic
Servings: 2
Cooking Time: 25 Minutes
Ingredients:
- 1 lb Brussels sprouts, trimmed
- ½ tsp garlic, chopped
- 2 tbsp olive oil
- Salt and black pepper to taste

Directions:
1. In a bowl, mix olive oil, garlic, salt, and pepper. Stir in the Brussels sprouts and let rest for 5 minutes. Place the coated sprouts in the Air Fryer basket and fit in the baking tray. Cook for 15 minutes at 380 F, shaking once. Serve warm.

380. Garlic Asparagus
Servings: 4
Cooking Time: 10 Minutes
Ingredients:
- 1 pound (454 g) asparagus, woody ends trimmed
- 2 tablespoons olive oil
- 1 tablespoon balsamic vinegar
- 2 teaspoons minced garlic
- Salt and freshly ground black pepper, to taste
- In a large shallow bowl, toss the asparagus with the olive oil, balsamic vinegar, garlic, salt, and pepper until thoroughly coated. Put the asparagus in the baking pan.
- Slide the baking pan into Rack Position 1, select Convection Bake, set temperature to 350ºF (180ºC), and set time to 10 minutes.
- Flip the asparagus with tongs halfway through the cooking time.
- When cooking is complete, the asparagus should be crispy. Remove from the oven and serve warm.

Directions:
1. Spicy Cabbage
2. Prep time: 5 minutes | Cooking Time: 7 minutes | Servings: 4
3. head cabbage, sliced into 1-inch-thick ribbons
4. tablespoon olive oil
5. teaspoon garlic powder

6. teaspoon red pepper flakes
7. teaspoon salt
8. teaspoon freshly ground black pepper
9. Toss the cabbage with the olive oil, garlic powder, red pepper flakes, salt, and pepper in a large mixing bowl until well coated.
10. Transfer the cabbage to the baking pan.
11. Slide the baking pan into Rack Position 1, select Convection Bake, set temperature to 350ºF (180ºC), and set time to 7 minutes.
12. Flip the cabbage with tongs halfway through the cooking time.
13. When cooking is complete, the cabbage should be crisp. Remove from the oven to a plate and serve warm.

381. Traditional Indian Kofta

Servings: 4
Cooking Time: 20 Minutes
Ingredients:
- Veggie Balls:
- 3/4-pound zucchini, grated and well drained
- 1/4-pound kohlrabi, grated and well drained
- 2 cloves garlic, minced
- 1 tablespoon Garam masala
- 1 cup paneer, crumbled
- 1/4 cup coconut flour
- 1/2 teaspoon chili powder
- Himalayan pink salt and ground black pepper, to taste
- Sauce:
- 1 tablespoon sesame oil
- 1/2 teaspoon cumin seeds
- 2 cloves garlic, roughly chopped
- 1 onion, chopped
- 1 Kashmiri chili pepper, seeded and minced
- 1 (1-inchpiece ginger, chopped
- 1 teaspoon paprika
- 1 teaspoon turmeric powder
- 2 ripe tomatoes, pureed
- 1/2 cup vegetable broth
- 1/4 full fat coconut milk

Directions:
1. Start by preheating your Air Fryer to 360 degrees F. Thoroughly combine the zucchini, kohlrabi, garlic, Garam masala, paneer, coconut flour, chili powder, salt and ground black pepper.
2. Shape the vegetable mixture into small balls and arrange them in the lightly greased cooking basket.
3. Cook in the preheated Air Fryer at 360 degrees F for 15 minutes or until thoroughly cooked and crispy. Repeat the process until you run out of ingredients.
4. Heat the sesame oil in a saucepan over medium heat and add the cumin seeds. Once the cumin seeds turn brown, add the garlic, onions, chili pepper, and ginger. Sauté for 2 to 3 minutes.
5. Add the paprika, turmeric powder, tomatoes, and broth; let it simmer, covered, for 4 to 5 minutes, stirring occasionally.
6. Add the coconut milk. Heat off; add the veggie balls and gently stir to combine.

Nutrition Info: 259 Calories; 11g Fat; 1g Carbs; 19g Protein; 3g Sugars; 4g Fiber

382. Rosemary & Thyme Roasted Fingerling Potatoes

Servings: 4
Cooking Time: 25 Minutes
Ingredients:
- 1 small bag baby fingerling potatoes
- 3 tablespoons olive oil
- Salt and pepper to taste
- 2 teaspoons rosemary
- 2 teaspoons thyme

Directions:
1. Start by preheating the toaster oven to 400°F.
2. Toss potatoes in olive oil and place on a baking sheet.
3. Pierce each potato to prevent overexpansion.
4. Sprinkle salt, pepper, rosemary, and thyme over the potatoes.
5. Roast for 25 minutes.

Nutrition Info: Calories: 123, Sodium: 3 mg, Dietary Fiber: 1.2 g, Total Fat: 10.7 g, Total Carbs: 7.5 g, Protein: 0.9 g.

383. Cheddar Cheese Cauliflower Casserole

Servings: 8
Cooking Time: 35 Minutes
Ingredients:
- 4 cups cauliflower florets
- 1 1/2 cups cheddar cheese, shredded
- 1 cup sour cream
- 4 bacon slices, cooked and crumbled
- 3 green onions, chopped

Directions:
1. Fit the oven with the rack in position
2. Boil water in a large pot. Add cauliflower in boiling water and cook for 8-10 minutes or until tender. Drain well.
3. Transfer cauliflower in a large bowl.
4. Add half bacon, half green onion, 1 cup cheese, and sour cream in cauliflower bowl and mix well.
5. Transfer mixture into a greased baking dish and sprinkle with remaining cheese.
6. Set to bake at 350 F for 30 minutes. After 5 minutes place the baking dish in the preheated oven.
7. Garnish with remaining green onion and bacon.
8. Serve and enjoy.

Nutrition Info: Calories 213 Fat 17.1 g Carbohydrates 4.7 g Sugar 1.5 g Protein 10.8 g Cholesterol 45 mg

384. Bbq Chicken Wings

Servings: 4
Cooking Time: 19 Minutes
Ingredients:
- 2 lbs. chicken wings
- 1 teaspoon olive oil
- 1 teaspoon smoked paprika
- 1 teaspoon garlic powder
- Salt and ground black pepper, as required
- ¼ cup BBQ sauce

Directions:
1. In a large bowl combine chicken wings, smoked paprika, garlic powder, oil, salt, and pepper and mix well.
2. Press "Power Button" of Air Fry Oven and turn the dial to select the "Air Fry" mode.
3. Press the Time button and again turn the dial to set the cooking time to 19 minutes.
4. Now push the Temp button and rotate the dial to set the temperature at 360 degrees F.
5. Press "Start/Pause" button to start.
6. When the unit beeps to show that it is preheated, open the lid.
7. Arrange the chicken wings in "Air Fry Basket" and insert in the oven.
8. After 12 minutes of cooking, flip the wings and coat with barbecue sauce evenly.
9. Serve immediately.

Nutrition Info: Calories 468 Total Fat 18.1 g Saturated Fat 4.8 g Cholesterol 202mg Sodium 409 mg Total Carbs 6.5 g Fiber 0.4 g Sugar 4.3 g Protein 65.8 g

385. Healthy Green Beans

Servings: 2
Cooking Time: 10 Minutes
Ingredients:
- 8 oz green beans, trimmed and cut in half
- 1 tbsp tamari
- 1 tsp toasted sesame oil

Directions:
1. Fit the oven with the rack in position 2.
2. Add all ingredients into the large bowl and toss well.
3. Transfer green beans in the air fryer basket then place an air fryer basket in the baking pan.
4. Place a baking pan on the oven rack. Set to air fry at 400 F for 10 minutes.
5. Serve and enjoy.

Nutrition Info: Calories 61 Fat 2.4 g Carbohydrates 8.6 g Sugar 1.7 g Protein 3 g Cholesterol 0 mg

386. Sweet Coconut Shrimp

Servings: 4
Cooking Time: 25 Minutes
Ingredients:
- 1 lb jumbo shrimp, peeled and deveined
- ¾ cup shredded coconut
- 1 tbsp maple syrup
- ½ cup breadcrumbs
- ⅓ cup cornstarch
- ½ cup milk

Directions:
1. Pour the cornstarch in a zipper bag and add in the shrimp. Seal the bag and shake vigorously to coat. In a bowl, mix the syrup with milk. In a separate bowl, combine the breadcrumbs and coconut. Open the zipper bag and remove the shrimp while shaking off excess starch.
2. Dip shrimp in the milk mixture and then in the crumbs, pressing loosely to trap enough crumbs and coconut. Place the coated shrimp in the basket without overcrowding. Select AirFry function, adjust the temperature to 360 F, and press Start. Cook for 12 minutes until crispy.

387. Cabbage Wedges With Parmesan

Servings: 4
Cooking Time: 30 Minutes
Ingredients:
- ½ head of cabbage, cut into 4 wedges
- 4 tbsp butter, melted
- 2 cups Parmesan cheese, grated
- Salt and black pepper to taste
- 1 tsp smoked paprika

Directions:
1. Preheat on Air Fry function to 330 F. Line a baking sheet with parchment paper. Brush the cabbage wedges with the butter. Season with salt and pepper.
2. Coat cabbage with Parmesan cheese and arrange on the baking pan; sprinkle with paprika. Cook for 15 minutes, flip, and cook for an additional 10 minutes. Serve with yogurt dip.

388. Air Fried Green Tomatoes(1)

Servings: 4
Cooking Time: 20 Minutes
Ingredients:
- 2 medium green tomatoes
- ⅓ cup grated Parmesan cheese.
- ¼ cup blanched finely ground almond flour.
- 1 large egg.

Directions:
1. Slice tomatoes into ½-inch-thick slices. Take a medium bowl, whisk the egg. Take a large bowl, mix the almond flour and Parmesan.
2. Dip each tomato slice into the egg, then dredge in the almond flour mixture. Place the slices into the air fryer basket

3. Adjust the temperature to 400 Degrees F and set the timer for 7 minutes. Flip the slices halfway through the cooking time. Serve immediately
Nutrition Info: Calories: 106; Protein: 6.2g; Fiber: 1.4g; Fat: 6.7g; Carbs: 5.9g

389. Cheese Scones With Chives

Servings: 6
Cooking Time: 25 Minutes
Ingredients:
- 1 cup flour
- Salt and black pepper to taste
- 3 tbsp butter
- 1 tsp fresh chives, chopped
- 1 whole egg
- 1 tbsp milk
- 1 cup cheddar cheese, shredded

Directions:
1. Preheat Breville on AirFry function to 340 F. In a bowl, mix butter, flour, cheddar cheese, chives, milk, and egg to get a sticky dough. Dust a flat surface with flour. Roll the dough into small balls. Place the balls in the frying basket and place in the oven. Press Start and cook for 20 minutes.

390. Air Fryer Corn

Servings: 2
Cooking Time: 10 Minutes
Ingredients:
- 2 fresh ears of corn, remove husks, wash, and pat dry
- 1 tbsp fresh lemon juice
- 2 tsp oil
- Pepper
- Salt

Directions:
1. Fit the oven with the rack in position 2.
2. Cut the corn to fit in the air fryer basket.
3. Drizzle oil over the corn. Season with pepper and salt.
4. Place corn in the air fryer basket then places an air fryer basket in the baking pan.
5. Place a baking pan on the oven rack. Set to air fry at 400 F for 10 minutes.
6. Serve and enjoy.
7. Drizzle lemon juice over corn and serve.
Nutrition Info: Calories 122 Fat 5.6 g Carbohydrates 18.2 g Sugar 4.2 g Protein 3.1 g Cholesterol 0 mg

391. Garlic Brussels Sprouts

Servings: 4
Cooking Time: 25 Minutes
Ingredients:
- 1 pound Brussels sprouts
- 1 garlic clove, minced
- 2 tbsp olive oil
- Salt and black pepper to taste

Directions:
1. Wash the Brussels sprouts thoroughly under cold water and trim off the outer leaves, keeping only the head of the sprouts. In a bowl, mix olive oil and garlic. Season with salt and pepper.
2. Add in the prepared sprouts let rest for 5 minutes. Place the coated sprouts in the frying basket. Select AirFry function, adjust the temperature to 380 F, and press Start. Cook for 15 minutes.

392. Creamy Broccoli Casserole

Servings: 6
Cooking Time: 30 Minutes
Ingredients:
- 16 oz frozen broccoli florets, defrosted and drained
- 1/2 tsp onion powder
- 10.5 oz can cream of mushroom soup
- 1 cup cheddar cheese, shredded
- 1/3 cup almond milk
- For topping:
- 1 tbsp butter, melted
- 1/2 cup cracker crumbs

Directions:
1. Fit the oven with the rack in position
2. Add all ingredients except topping ingredients into the 1.5-qt casserole dish.
3. In a small bowl, mix together cracker crumbs and melted butter and sprinkle over the casserole dish mixture.
4. Set to bake at 350 F for 35 minutes. After 5 minutes place the casserole dish in the preheated oven.
5. Serve and enjoy.
Nutrition Info: Calories 203 Fat 13.5 g Carbohydrates 11.9 g Sugar 3.6 g Protein 6.9 g Cholesterol 26 mg

393. Salmon Croquettes

Servings: 8
Cooking Time: 7 Minutes
Ingredients:
- ½ of large can red salmon, drained
- 1 egg, lightly beaten
- 1 tablespoon fresh parsley, chopped
- Salt and freshly ground black pepper, as needed
- 3 tablespoons vegetable oil
- ½ cup breadcrumbs

Directions:
1. In a bowl, add the salmon and with a fork, mash it completely.
2. Add the eggs, parsley, salt, and black pepper and mix until well combined.
3. Make 8 equal-sized croquettes from the mixture.

4. In a shallow dish, mix together the oil, and breadcrumbs.
5. Coat the croquettes with the breadcrumb mixture.
6. Press "Power Button" of Air Fry Oven and turn the dial to select the "Air Fry" mode.
7. Press the Time button and again turn the dial to set the cooking time to 7 minutes.
8. Now push the Temp button and rotate the dial to set the temperature at 390 degrees F.
9. Press "Start/Pause" button to start.
10. When the unit beeps to show that it is preheated, open the lid.
11. Arrange the croquettes in "Air Fry Basket" and insert in the oven.
12. Serve warm.
Nutrition Info: Calories 117 Total Fat 7.8 g Saturated Fat 1.5 g Cholesterol 33 mg Sodium 89 mg Total Carbs 4.9 g Fiber 0.3 g Sugar 0.5 g Protein 7.1 g

394. Savory Parsley Crab Cakes

Servings: 6
Cooking Time: 20 Minutes
Ingredients:
- 1 lb crab meat, shredded
- 2 eggs, beaten
- ½ cup breadcrumbs
- ⅓ cup finely chopped green onion
- ¼ cup parsley, chopped
- 1 tbsp mayonnaise
- 1 tsp sweet chili sauce
- ½ tsp paprika
- Salt and black pepper to taste

Directions:
1. In a bowl, add crab meat, eggs, crumbs, green onion, parsley, mayo, chili sauce, paprika, salt and black pepper; mix well with your hands.
2. Shape into 6 cakes and grease them lightly with oil. Arrange them in the fryer basket without overcrowding. Fit in the baking tray and cook for 8 minutes at 400 F on Air Fry function, turning once halfway through.

395. Sausage Mushroom Caps(1)

Servings: 2
Cooking Time: 20 Minutes
Ingredients:
- ½ lb. Italian sausage
- 6 large Portobello mushroom caps
- ¼ cup grated Parmesan cheese.
- ¼ cup chopped onion
- 2 tbsp. blanched finely ground almond flour
- 1 tsp. minced fresh garlic

Directions:
1. Use a spoon to hollow out each mushroom cap, reserving scrapings.
2. In a medium skillet over medium heat, brown the sausage about 10 minutes or until fully cooked and no pink remains. Drain and then add reserved mushroom scrapings, onion, almond flour, Parmesan and garlic.
3. Gently fold ingredients together and continue cooking an additional minute, then remove from heat
4. Evenly spoon the mixture into mushroom caps and place the caps into a 6-inch round pan. Place pan into the air fryer basket
5. Adjust the temperature to 375 Degrees F and set the timer for 8 minutes. When finished cooking, the tops will be browned and bubbling. Serve warm.
Nutrition Info: Calories: 404; Protein: 23g; Fiber: 5g; Fat: 28g; Carbs: 12g

396. Simple Baked Potatoes

Servings: 6
Cooking Time: 55 Minutes
Ingredients:
- 1 1/2 lbs baby potatoes
- 3 tbsp olive oil
- Pepper
- Salt

Directions:
1. Fit the oven with the rack in position
2. Add baby potatoes, salt, and water to a large pot and bring to boil over medium heat.
3. Cook potatoes until tender. Drain well and transfer to the skillet.
4. Gently smash each potato using the back of a spoon.
5. Drizzle potatoes with oil. Season with pepper and salt. Place potatoes in baking pan.
6. Set to bake at 450 F for 45 minutes. After 5 minutes place the baking pan in the preheated oven.
7. Serve and enjoy.
Nutrition Info: Calories 126 Fat 7.1 g Carbohydrates 14.1 g Sugar 0 g Protein 2.9 g Cholesterol 0 mg

397. Jalapeno Bread

Servings: 10
Cooking Time: 50 Minutes
Ingredients:
- 3 cups all-purpose flour
- 8 oz cheddar cheese, shredded
- 1/2 tsp ground white pepper
- 1 1/2 tbsp baking powder
- 1/4 cup butter, melted
- 1 1/2 cups buttermilk
- 3 jalapeno peppers, chopped
- 2 tbsp sugar
- 1 1/4 tsp salt

Directions:
1. Fit the oven with the rack in position

2. In a mixing bowl, mix flour, baking powder, sugar, white pepper, and salt.
3. Add jalapenos and cheese and stir to combine.
4. Whisk butter and buttermilk together and add to the flour mixture. Stir until just combined.
5. Pour batter into the greased 9*5-inch loaf pan.
6. Set to bake at 375 F for 55 minutes. After 5 minutes place the loaf pan in the preheated oven.
7. Slice and serve.
Nutrition Info: Calories 297 Fat 12.9 g Carbohydrates 34.5 g Sugar 4.5 g Protein 10.9 g Cholesterol 37 mg

398. Cheesy Squash Casserole

Servings: 6
Cooking Time: 30 Minutes
Ingredients:
- 2 lbs yellow summer squash, cut into chunks
- 1/2 cup liquid egg substitute
- 3/4 cup cheddar cheese, shredded
- 1/4 cup mayonnaise
- 1/4 tsp salt

Directions:
1. Fit the oven with the rack in position
2. Add squash in a saucepan then pour enough water in a saucepan to cover the squash. Bring to boil.
3. Turn heat to medium and cook for 10 minutes or until tender. Drain well.
4. In a large mixing bowl, combine together squash, egg substitute, mayonnaise, 1/2 cup cheese, and salt.
5. Transfer squash mixture into a greased baking dish.
6. Set to bake at 375 F for 35 minutes. After 5 minutes place the baking dish in the preheated oven.
7. Sprinkle remaining cheese on top.
8. Serve and enjoy.
Nutrition Info: Calories 130 Fat 8.2 g Carbohydrates 7.7 g Sugar 3.5 g Protein 8 g Cholesterol 18 mg

399. Mixed Nuts With Cinnamon

Servings: 4
Cooking Time: 25 Minutes
Ingredients:
- ½ cup pecans
- ½ cup walnuts
- ½ cup almonds
- A pinch cayenne pepper
- 2 tbsp sugar
- 2 tbsp egg whites
- 2 tsp cinnamon

Directions:
1. Add the pepper, sugar, and cinnamon to a bowl and mix well; set aside. In another bowl, combine the pecans, walnuts, almonds, and egg whites. Add the spice mixture to the nuts and give it a good mix. Lightly grease the baking tray with cooking spray.
2. Pour in the nuts and cook for 10 minutes on Bake function at 350 F. Shake and cook for further for 10 minutes. Pour the nuts in a bowl. Let cool before serving.

400. Avocado, Tomato, And Grape Salad With Crunchy Potato Croutons

Servings: 2
Cooking Time: 10 Minutes
Ingredients:
- Potato croutons:
- 1 medium-small russet potato
- 2 cloves garlic
- 1 tablespoon extra light olive oil
- 1 tablespoon nutritional yeast
- 1/2 teaspoon garlic powder
- 1/2 teaspoon onion powder
- 1/2 teaspoon dried thyme
- 1/2 teaspoon dried rosemary
- 1/2 teaspoon dried oregano
- 1/2 teaspoon chili powder
- 1/4 teaspoon Himalayan sea salt
- 1/3 teaspoon cayenne pepper
- Pinch red pepper flakes
- Black pepper to taste
- Salad:
- 1 cup grape tomatoes
- Small handful dried cranberries
- Small handful green grapes
- 2-3 sprigs cilantro
- 1 avocado
- 2 tablespoons extra-virgin olive oil
- 1 tablespoon nutritional yeast
- 1 tablespoon lemon juice
- 1/2 teaspoon pure maple syrup
- 1/4 teaspoon salt
- Few sprinkles ground pepper
- Small handful toasted pecans

Directions:
1. Peel and cut potatoes into 1-inch cubes.
2. Place potatoes in water with a pinch of salt for 1 hour.
3. When the hour has passed, preheat the toaster oven to 450°F.
4. Drain potatoes and dry them on multiple layers of paper towels, then return to bowl.
5. Peel and mince garlic, then add to bowl.
6. Add rest of crouton ingredients to the bowl and stir together.
7. Lay potatoes mixture across a greased baking sheet in a single layer and bake for 35 minutes, flipping halfway through.
8. Combine oil, yeast, syrup, lemon juice, salt and pepper together to create salad dressing.
9. Slice tomatoes in half and put in a bowl with cranberries and grapes.

10. Chop cilantro and add to bowl. Scoop out avocado and cut it into smaller pieces and add to bowl.
11. Drizzle dressing and mix well. Add potatoes and mix again, top with pecans and serve.
Nutrition Info: Calories: 1032, Sodium: 560 mg, Dietary Fiber: 22.8 g, Total Fat: 84.9 g, Total Carbs: 64.2 g, Protein: 17.0 g.

401. Bok Choy And Butter Sauce(3)

Servings: 4
Cooking Time: 20 Minutes
Ingredients:
- 2 bok choy heads; trimmed and cut into strips
- 1 tbsp. butter; melted
- 2 tbsp. chicken stock
- 1 tsp. lemon juice
- 1 tbsp. olive oil
- A pinch of salt and black pepper

Directions:
1. In a pan that fits your air fryer, mix all the ingredients, toss, introduce the pan in the air fryer and cook at 380°F for 15 minutes.
2. Divide between plates and serve as a side dish

Nutrition Info: Calories: 141; Fat: 3g; Fiber: 2g; Carbs: 4g; Protein: 3g

402. Garlic & Olive Oil Spring Vegetables

Servings: 4
Cooking Time: 20 Minutes
Ingredients:
- 1 pound assorted spring vegetables (such as carrots, asparagus, radishes, spring onions, or sugar snap peas)
- 4 unpeeled garlic cloves
- 2 tablespoons olive oil
- Salt and pepper to taste

Directions:
1. Start by preheating toaster oven to 450°F.
2. Combine vegetables, garlic, oil, salt, and pepper in a bowl and toss.
3. Roast for 20 minutes or until vegetables start to brown.

Nutrition Info: Calories: 105, Sodium: 255 mg, Dietary Fiber: 4.4 g, Total Fat: 7.3 g, Total Carbs: 9.1 g, Protein: 1.8 g.

403. Pancetta & Goat Cheese Bombs With Almonds

Servings: 4
Cooking Time: 25 Minutes
Ingredients:
- 16 oz soft goat cheese
- 2 tbsp fresh rosemary, finely chopped
- 1 cup almonds, chopped into small pieces
- Salt and black pepper
- 15 dried plums, chopped
- 15 pancetta slices

Directions:
1. Line the frying basket with baking paper. In a bowl, add cheese, rosemary, almonds, salt, pepper and plums and stir well. Roll into balls and wrap with pancetta slices. Arrange the bombs on the frying basket. Select AirFry function, adjust the temperature to 400 F, and press Start. Cook for 10 minutes. Check at the 5-minute mark to avoid overcooking. Serve with toothpicks.

404. Grandma's Apple Cinnamon Chips

Servings: 2
Cooking Time: 25 Minutes
Ingredients:
- 1 tsp sugar
- 1 tsp salt
- 1 whole apple, sliced
- ½ tsp cinnamon
- Confectioners' sugar for serving

Directions:
1. Preheat your to 400 F on Bake function. In a bowl, mix cinnamon, salt, and sugar. Add in the apple slices and toss to coat. Place the prepared apple slices in the greased air fryer basket andfit in the cooking tray. Cook for 10 minutes, flipping once. Dust with sugar and serve.

405. Homemade French Fries

Servings: 2
Cooking Time: 25 Minutes
Ingredients:
- 2 russet potatoes, cut into strips
- 2 tbsp olive oil
- Salt and black pepper to taste

Directions:
1. In a bowl, toss the strips with olive oil and season with salt and pepper. Arrange them on the frying basket. Select AirFry function, adjust the temperature to 400 F, and press Start. Cook for 18-22 minutes. Check for crispiness and serve with aioli, ketchup, or crumbled feta cheese.

406. Bacon Croquettes

Servings: 8
Cooking Time: 8 Minutes
Ingredients:
- 1 pound sharp cheddar cheese block
- 1 pound thin bacon slices
- 1 cup all-purpose flour
- 3 eggs

- 1 cup breadcrumbs
- Salt, as required
- ¼ cup olive oil

Directions:
1. Cut the cheese block into 1-inch rectangular pieces.
2. Wrap 2 bacon slices around 1 piece of cheddar cheese, covering completely.
3. Repeat with the remaining bacon and cheese pieces.
4. Arrange the croquettes in a baking dish and freeze for about 5 minutes.
5. In a shallow dish, place the flour.
6. In a second dish, crack the eggs and beat well.
7. In a third dish, mix together the breadcrumbs, salt, and oil.
8. Coat the croquettes with flour, then dip into beaten eggs and finally, coat with the breadcrumbs mixture.
9. Press "Power Button" of Air Fry Oven and turn the dial to select the "Air Fry" mode.
10. Press the Time button and again turn the dial to set the cooking time to 8 minutes.
11. Now push the Temp button and rotate the dial to set the temperature at 390 degrees F.
12. Press "Start/Pause" button to start.
13. When the unit beeps to show that it is preheated, open the lid.
14. Arrange the croquettes in "Air Fry Basket" and insert in the oven.
15. Serve warm.

Nutrition Info: Calories 723 Total Fat 51.3 g Saturated Fat 21.3 g Cholesterol 183 mg Sodium 1880 mg Total Carbs 23.3 g Fiber 1 g Sugar 1.3 g Protein 40.6 g

407. Roasted Brussels Sprouts

Servings: 6
Cooking Time: 30 Minutes

Ingredients:
- 1-1/2 pounds Brussels sprouts, ends trimmed and yellow leaves removed
- 3 tablespoons olive oil
- 1 teaspoon salt
- 1/2 teaspoon black pepper

Directions:
1. Start by preheating toaster oven to 400°F.
2. Toss Brussels sprouts in a large bowl, drizzle with olive oil, sprinkle with salt and pepper, then toss.
3. Roast for 30 minutes.

Nutrition Info: Calories: 109, Sodium: 416 mg, Dietary Fiber: 4.3 g, Total Fat: 7.4 g, Total Carbs: 10.4 g, Protein: 3.9 g.

408. Cheddar & Prosciutto Strips

Servings: 6
Cooking Time: 50 Minutes

Ingredients:
- 1 lb cheddar cheese
- 12 prosciutto slices
- 1 cup flour
- 2 eggs, beaten
- 4 tbsp olive oil
- 1 cup breadcrumbs

Directions:
1. Cut the cheese into 6 equal pieces. Wrap each piece with 2 prosciutto slices. Place them in the freezer just enough to set, about 5 minutes; note that they mustn't be frozen.
2. Preheat Breville on AirFry function to 390 F. Dip the Strips into flour first, then in eggs, and coat with breadcrumbs. Place in the frying basket and drizzle with olive oil. Press Start and cook for 10 minutes or until golden brown. Serve with tomato dip.

MEAT RECIPES

409. Gold Livers

Servings: 4
Cooking Time: 10 Minutes
Ingredients:
- 2 eggs
- 2 tablespoons water
- ¾ cup flour
- 2 cups panko bread crumbs
- 1 teaspoon salt
- ½ teaspoon ground black pepper
- 20 ounces (567 g) chicken livers
- Cooking spray

Directions:
1. Spritz the air fryer basket with cooking spray.
2. Whisk the eggs with water in a large bowl. Pour the flour in a separate bowl. Pour the panko on a shallow dish and sprinkle with salt and pepper.
3. Dredge the chicken livers in the flour. Shake the excess off, then dunk the livers in the whisked eggs, and then roll the livers over the panko to coat well.
4. Arrange the livers in the basket and spritz with cooking spray.
5. Put the air fryer basket on the baking pan and slide into Rack Position 2, select Air Fry, set temperature to 390°F (199°C) and set time to 10 minutes.
6. Flip the livers halfway through.
7. When cooking is complete, the livers should be golden and crispy.
8. Serve immediately.

410. Chicken Breasts In Onion-mushroom Sauce

Servings: 4
Cooking Time: 20 Minutes
Ingredients:
- 4 chicken breasts, cubed
- 1 ½ cup onion soup mix
- 1 cup mushroom soup
- ½ cup heavy cream

Directions:
1. Preheat Breville Air Fryer oven to 400 F on Bake function. Mix mushrooms, onion mix, and heavy cream in a bowl. Pour the mixture over chicken and allow to sit for 25 minutes. Place the marinated chicken in the basket and press Start. Cook for 15 minutes. Serve warm.

411. Minty Chicken-fried Pork Chops

Servings: 6
Cooking Time: 30 Minutes
Ingredients:
- 4 medium-sized pork chops, approximately 3.5 ounces each
- 1 cup of breadcrumbs (Panko brand works well)
- 2 medium-sized eggs
- Pinch of salt and pepper
- ½ tablespoon of mint, either dried and ground; or fresh, rinsed and finely chopped

Directions:
1. Preparing the Ingredients. Cover the basket of the air fryer oven with a lining of tin foil, leaving the edges uncovered to allow air to circulate through the basket. Preheat the air fryer oven to 350 degrees.
2. In a mixing bowl, beat the eggs until fluffy and until the yolks and whites are fully combined, and set aside.
3. In a separate mixing bowl, combine the breadcrumbs, mint, salt, and pepper, and set aside. One by one, dip each raw pork chop into the bowl with dry ingredients, coating all sides; then submerge into the bowl with wet ingredients, then dip again into the dry ingredients. This double coating will ensure an extra crisp air-fry. Lay the coated pork chops on the foil covering the Oven rack/basket, in a single flat layer. Place the Rack on the middle-shelf of the air fryer oven.
4. Air Frying. Set the air fryer oven timer for 15 minutes. After 15 minutes, the air fryer oven will turn off, and the pork should be mid-way cooked and the breaded coating starting to brown. Using tongs, turn each piece of steak over to ensure a full all-over fry. Reset the air fryer oven to 320 degrees for 15 minutes.
5. After 15 minutes, when the air fryer shuts off, remove the fried pork chops using tongs and set on a serving plate. Eat as soon as cool enough to handle – and enjoy!

412. Ranch Chicken Thighs

Servings: 4
Cooking Time: 30 Minutes
Ingredients:
- 2 lbs chicken thighs
- 1 oz ranch seasoning
- 1 cup cheddar cheese, shredded
- 1/2 cup mayonnaise
- 2 tsp garlic, minced

Directions:
1. Fit the oven with the rack in position
2. Place chicken thighs into the baking dish.
3. Mix together mayonnaise, garlic, cheddar cheese, and ranch seasoning and pour over chicken thighs.
4. Set to bake at 400 F for 35 minutes. After 5 minutes place the baking dish in the preheated oven.
5. Serve and enjoy.

Nutrition Info: Calories 684 Fat 36 g Carbohydrates 7.8 g Sugar 2 g Protein 73 g Cholesterol 239 mg

413. Cheesy Pepperoni And Chicken Pizza

Servings: 6
Cooking Time: 15 Minutes
Ingredients:
- 2 cups cooked chicken, cubed
- 1 cup pizza sauce
- 20 slices pepperoni
- ¼ cup grated Parmesan cheese
- 1 cup shredded Mozzarella cheese
- Cooking spray

Directions:
1. Spritz the baking pan with cooking spray.
2. Arrange the chicken cubes in the prepared baking pan, then top the cubes with pizza sauce and pepperoni. Stir to coat the cubes and pepperoni with sauce. Scatter the cheeses on top.
3. Put the air fryer basket on the baking pan and slide into Rack Position 2, select Air Fry, set temperature to 375ºF (190ºC) and set time to 15 minutes.
4. When cooking is complete, the pizza should be frothy and the cheeses should be melted.
5. Serve immediately.

414. Easy Creamy Chicken

Servings: 4
Cooking Time: 55 Minutes
Ingredients:
- 4 chicken breasts
- 1 tsp garlic powder
- 1 tsp dried basil
- 1 tsp dried oregano
- 3/4 cup parmesan cheese, grated
- 1 cup sour cream
- 1 cup mozzarella cheese, shredded
- 1/2 tsp pepper
- 1/2 tsp salt

Directions:
1. Fit the oven with the rack in position
2. Season chicken with pepper and salt and place into the greased baking dish.
3. Mix together sour cream, mozzarella cheese, parmesan cheese, oregano, basil, garlic powder, and salt and pour over chicken.
4. Set to bake at 375 F for 60 minutes. After 5 minutes place the baking dish in the preheated oven.
5. Serve and enjoy.

Nutrition Info: Calories 479 Fat 27.8 g Carbohydrates 4.2 g Sugar 0.3 g Protein 51.7 g Cholesterol 171 mg

415. Pork Wellington

Servings: 6
Cooking Time: 30 Minutes
Ingredients:
- 1 ½ lb. pork tenderloin
- ½ tsp salt
- ½ tsp pepper
- 1 tsp thyme
- 1 sheet puff pastry
- 4 oz. prosciutto, sliced thin
- 1 tbsp. Dijon mustard
- 1 tbsp. olive oil
- 1 tbsp. butter
- 8 oz. mushrooms, chopped
- 1 shallot, chopped
- 1 egg, beaten

Directions:
1. Season tenderloin with salt, pepper, and thyme on all sides.
2. On parchment covered work surface, roll out pastry as long as the tenderloin and wide enough to cover it completely.
3. Lay the prosciutto across the pastry to cover it and spread with mustard.
4. Melt butter and oil in a large skillet over high heat. Add mushrooms and shallot and cook 5-10 minutes, until golden brown. Remove from pan.
5. Add tenderloin to the skillet and brown on all sides.
6. Spread mushrooms over mustard and add pork. Roll up to completely cover tenderloin. Use beaten egg to seal the edge.
7. Set oven to bake on 425°F for 35 minutes.
8. Line baking pan with parchment paper and place pork on it, seam side down. Brush top with remaining egg. After oven preheats 5 minutes, place pan in position 1 and cook 30 or until puffed and golden brown.
9. Remove from oven and let rest 5 minutes before slicing and serving.

Nutrition Info: Calories 457, Total Fat 25g, Saturated Fat 7g, Total Carbs 20g, Net Carbs 19g, Protein 38g, Sugar 1g, Fiber 1g, Sodium 627mg, Potassium 706mg, Phosphorus 409mg

416. Chicken Pizza

Ingredients:
- One pizza base
- Grated pizza cheese (mozzarella cheese preferably) for topping
- Some pizza topping sauce
- Use cooking oil for brushing and topping purposes
- ingredients for topping:
- 2 onions chopped
- ½ lb. chicken (Cut the chicken into tiny pieces)
- 2 capsicums chopped
- 2 tomatoes that have been deseeded and chopped
- 1 tbsp. (optional) mushrooms/corns

- 2 tsp. pizza seasoning
- Some cottage cheese that has been cut into small cubes (optional)

Directions:
1. Put the pizza base in a pre-heated oven for around 5 minutes. (Pre heated to 340 Fahrenheit).
2. Take out the base. Pour some pizza sauce on top of the base at the center. Using a spoon spread the sauce over the base making sure that you leave some gap around the circumference. Grate some mozzarella cheese and sprinkle it over the sauce layer.
3. Take all the vegetables and the chicken mentioned in the ingredient list above and mix them in a bowl. Add some oil and seasoning. Also add some salt and pepper according to taste. Mix them properly. Put this topping over the layer of cheese on the pizza. Now sprinkle some more grated cheese and pizza seasoning on top of this layer.
4. Pre heat the oven at 250 Fahrenheit for around 5 minutes. Open the fry basket and place the pizza inside. Close the basket and keep the fryer at 170 degrees for another 10 minutes. If you feel that it is undercooked you may put it at the same temperature for another 2 minutes or so.

417. Chicken Pasta Broccoli Casserole

Servings: 8
Cooking Time: 35 Minutes
Ingredients:
- 2 lbs chicken breasts, cut into large chunks
- 16 oz pasta, cooked and drained
- 12 oz frozen broccoli, thawed
- 1/2 cup cheddar cheese, shredded
- 1 can cream of chicken condensed soup
- 1 tbsp olive oil
- Pepper
- Salt

Directions:
1. Fit the oven with the rack in position
2. Heat oil in a pan over medium heat.
3. Season chicken with pepper and salt and place into the pan. Cook chicken until lightly browned, about 3-4 minutes on each side.
4. Remove pan from heat and set aside.
5. Add chicken and remaining ingredients into the mixing bowl and mix well.
6. Pour chicken mixture into the 9*13-inch greased casserole dish.
7. Set to bake at 400 F for 40 minutes. After 5 minutes place the casserole dish in the preheated oven.
8. Serve and enjoy.

Nutrition Info: Calories 446 Fat 14.2 g Carbohydrates 35.2 g Sugar 0.9 g Protein 42.4 g Cholesterol 151 mg

418. Mustard & Thyme Chicken

Servings: 4
Cooking Time: 20 Minutes
Ingredients:
- 1 tsp garlic powder
- 1 lb chicken breasts, sliced
- 1 tsp dried thyme
- ½ cup dry wine
- ½ cup Dijon mustard
- 1 cup breadcrumbs
- 1 tbsp lemon zest
- 2 tbsp olive oil

Directions:
1. In a bowl, mix breadcrumbs with garlic powder, lemon zest, salt, and pepper. In another bowl, mix mustard, olive oil, and wine. Dip chicken slices in the wine mixture and then in the crumb mixture. Place the chicken in the basket and cook for 15 minutes at 350 F on AirFry function.

419. Meatballs(10)

Servings: 6
Cooking Time: 20 Minutes
Ingredients:
- 2 lbs ground chicken
- 1/2 cup parmesan cheese, grated
- 1 cup breadcrumbs
- 1 egg, lightly beaten
- 1 tbsp fresh parsley, chopped
- 1 tsp Italian seasoning
- 1 tsp garlic, minced
- 2 tbsp olive oil
- Pepper
- Salt

Directions:
1. Fit the oven with the rack in position
2. Add all ingredients into the bowl and mix until well combined.
3. Make small balls from meat mixture and place in baking pan.
4. Set to bake at 400 F for 25 minutes. After 5 minutes place the baking pan in the preheated oven.
5. Serve and enjoy.

Nutrition Info: Calories 436 Fat 19.4 g Carbohydrates 13.6 g Sugar 1.3 g Protein 49.5 g Cholesterol 168 mg

420. Sweet & Spicy Chicken

Servings: 6
Cooking Time: 30 Minutes
Ingredients:
- 6 chicken breasts, skinless, boneless, cut in 1-inch pieces
- 1 cup corn starch
- 2 cups water

- 1 cup ketchup
- ½ cup brown sugar
- 1 tbsp. sesame oil
- 3 tbsp. soy sauce
- 2 tbsp. black sesame seeds
- 2 tbsp. white sesame seeds
- ½ tsp red pepper flakes
- ½ tsp garlic powder
- 2 tbsp. green onion, chopped

Directions:
1. Place baking pan in position 2. Lightly spray fryer basket with cooking spray.
2. Place the cornstarch in a large bowl. Add chicken and toss to coat chicken thoroughly.
3. Working in batches, place chicken in a single layer in the basket and place on baking pan. Set oven to air fryer on 350°F for 10 minutes. Stir the chicken halfway through cooking time. Transfer chicken to baking sheet.
4. In a large skillet over medium heat, whisk together remaining ingredients, except green onion. Bring to a boil, stirring occasionally. Cook until sauce has thickened, about 3-5 minutes.
5. Add chicken and stir to coat. Cook another 3-5 minutes, stirring frequently. Serve garnished with green onions.

Nutrition Info: Calories 556, Total Fat 12g, Saturated Fat 3g, Total Carbs 50g, Net Carbs 49g, Protein 62g, Sugar 26g, Fiber 1g, Sodium 730mg, Potassium 957mg, Phosphorus 569mg

421. Caraway Crusted Beef Steaks

Servings: 4
Cooking Time: 10 Minutes
Ingredients:
- 4 beef steaks
- 2 teaspoons caraway seeds
- 2 teaspoons garlic powder
- Sea salt and cayenne pepper, to taste
- 1 tablespoon melted butter
- 1/3 cup almond flour
- 2 eggs, beaten

Directions:
1. Add the beef steaks to a large bowl and toss with the caraway seeds, garlic powder, salt and pepper until well coated.
2. Stir together the melted butter and almond flour in a bowl. Whisk the eggs in a different bowl.
3. Dredge the seasoned steaks in the eggs, then dip in the almond and butter mixture.
4. Arrange the coated steaks in the basket.
5. Put the air fryer basket on the baking pan and slide into Rack Position 2, select Air Fry, set temperature to 355ºF (179ºC) and set time to 10 minutes.
6. Flip the steaks once halfway through to ensure even cooking.
7. When cooking is complete, the internal temperature of the beef steaks should reach at least 145ºF (63ºC) on a meat thermometer.
8. Transfer the steaks to plates. Let cool for 5 minutes and serve hot.

422. Ham Muffins With Swiss Cheese

Servings: 6
Cooking Time: 25 Minutes
Ingredients:
- 5 whole eggs, beaten
- 2 ¼ oz ham, sliced
- 1 cup milk
- ¼ tsp pepper
- 1 ½ cups Swiss cheese, grated
- ¼ tsp salt
- ¼ cup green onion, chopped
- ½ tsp thyme

Directions:
1. Preheat Breville oven to 350 F on AirFry function. In a bowl, mix beaten eggs, thyme, onion, salt, Swiss cheese, pepper, and milk. Line baking forms with ham slices. Pour in the egg mixture. Transfer the muffins to the cooking basket and cook for 15 minutes. Serve chilled.

423. Balsamic Chicken With Mozzarella Cheese

Servings: 4
Cooking Time: 25 Minutes
Ingredients:
- 4 chicken breasts, cubed
- 4 fresh basil leaves
- ¼ cup balsamic vinegar
- 2 tomatoes, chopped
- 1 tbsp butter, melted
- 4 mozzarella cheese, grated

Directions:
1. In a bowl, mix butter and balsamic vinegar. Add in the chicken and toss to coat. Transfer to a baking tray and press Start. Cook for 20 minutes at 400 F on AirFry function. Top with mozzarella cheese and Bake until the cheese melts. Top with basil and tomatoes and serve.

424. Pineapple & Ginger Chicken Kabobs

Servings: 2
Cooking Time: 20 Minutes
Ingredients:
- 2 chicken breasts, cut into 2-inch pieces
- ½ cup soy sauce
- ½ cup pineapple juice
- ¼ cup sesame oil
- 4 cloves garlic, chopped

- 1 tbsp fresh ginger, grated
- 4 scallions, chopped
- 2 tbsp toasted sesame seeds
- A pinch of black pepper

Directions:
1. In a bowl, toss to coat all the ingredients except the chicken. Let sit for 10 minutes.
2. Preheat your oven on Air Fry function to 390 F. Remove the chicken pieces and pat them dry using paper towels. Thread the chicken pieces onto skewers and trim any fat. Place in the AirFryer basket and fit in the baking tray. Cook for 7-10 minutes, flipping once. Serve.

425. Mexican Salsa Chicken

Servings: 6
Cooking Time: 30 Minutes
Ingredients:
- 4 chicken breasts, skinless & boneless
- 1/4 tsp cumin
- 1/4 tsp garlic powder
- 1 3/4 cups Mexican shredded cheese
- 12 oz salsa
- 1/4 tsp pepper
- 1/4 tsp salt

Directions:
1. Fit the oven with the rack in position
2. Place chicken breasts into the baking dish and season with cumin, garlic powder, pepper, and salt.
3. Pour salsa over chicken breasts.
4. Sprinkle shredded cheese on top of chicken.
5. Set to bake at 375 F for 35 minutes. After 5 minutes place the baking dish in the preheated oven.
6. Serve and enjoy.

Nutrition Info: Calories 330 Fat 17.8 g Carbohydrates 6.1 g Sugar 1.8 g Protein 36.1 g Cholesterol 116 mg

426. Cayenne Turkey Breasts

Servings: 4
Cooking Time: 25 Minutes
Ingredients:
- 1 lb turkey breast, boneless and skinless
- 2 cups panko breadcrumbs
- Cayenne pepper and salt to taste
- 1 stick butter, melted

Directions:
1. Preheat Breville on AirFry function to 350 F. In a bowl, mix breadcrumbs, cayenne pepper, and salt. Brush the butter onto the turkey and coat with the breadcrumbs. Cook for 15 minutes.

427. Simple Herbed Hens

Servings: 8
Cooking Time: 30 Minutes

Ingredients:
- 4 (1¼-pound / 567-g) Cornish hens, giblets removed, split lengthwise
- 2 cups white wine, divided
- 2 garlic cloves, minced
- 1 small onion, minced
- ½ teaspoon celery seeds
- ½ teaspoon poultry seasoning
- ½ teaspoon paprika
- ½ teaspoon dried oregano
- ¼ teaspoon freshly ground black pepper

Directions:
1. Place the hens, cavity side up, in the baking pan. Pour 1½ cups of the wine over the hens. Set aside.
2. In a shallow bowl, combine the garlic, onion, celery seeds, poultry seasoning, paprika, oregano, and pepper. Sprinkle half of the combined seasonings over the cavity of each split half. Cover and refrigerate. Allow the hens to marinate for 2 hours.
3. Transfer the hens to the pan. Slide the baking pan into Rack Position 1, select Convection Bake, set temperature to 350ºF (180ºC) and set time to 90 minutes.
4. Flip the breast halfway through and remove the skin. Pour the remaining ½ cup of wine over the top, and sprinkle with the remaining seasonings.
5. When cooking is complete, the inner temperature of the hens should be at least 165ºF (74ºC). Transfer the hens to a serving platter and serve hot.

428. Sweet & Spicy Chicken Wings

Servings: 4
Cooking Time: 30 Minutes
Ingredients:
- 12 chicken wings
- 1/2 cup hot sauce
- 1/2 cup honey
- Pepper
- Salt

Directions:
1. Fit the oven with the rack in position 2.
2. Season chicken wings with pepper and salt.
3. Arrange chicken wings in the air fryer basket then place an air fryer basket in the baking pan.
4. Place a baking pan on the oven rack. Set to air fry at 400 F for 25 minutes.
5. Meanwhile, add honey and hot sauce in a saucepan and heat over medium heat for 5 minutes.
6. Add chicken wings in a bowl. Pour
7. sauce over chicken wings and toss well.
8. Serve and enjoy.

Nutrition Info: Calories 698 Fat 22.2 g Carbohydrates 35.4 g Sugar 35.2 g Protein 89.4 g Cholesterol 256 mg

429. Italian Sausage Jambalaya

Ingredients:
- 2 cups water
- 3 spicy Italian sausages
- 2 Tbsp extra-virgin olive oil
- 2 cups frozen mirepoix
- 1 cup canned crushed tomatoes
- 1½ tsp Cajun seasoning
- 2 (8.8-oz) packages precooked rice
- Salt and freshly ground black pepper, to taste

Directions:
1. Remove the casings from the sausage and discard, then crumble the meat.
2. In oven over medium heat, heat the olive oil.
3. Brown the sausage, stirring occasionally, for about 3 minutes.
4. Add the mirepoix and cook until tender, about 4 minutes.
5. Stir in the tomatoes, Cajun seasoning, and rice. Season with salt and pepper.
6. Simmer for about 5 minutes, and serve.

430. Chicken Oregano Fingers

Ingredients:
- 1 lb. boneless chicken breast cut into Oregano Fingers
- 2 cup dry breadcrumbs
- 2 tsp. oregano
- 1 ½ tbsp. ginger-garlic paste
- 4 tbsp. lemon juice
- 2 tsp. salt
- 1 tsp. pepper powder
- 1 tsp. red chili powder
- 6 tbsp. corn flour
- 4 eggs

Directions:
1. Mix all the ingredients for the marinade and put the chicken Oregano Fingers inside and let it rest overnight.
2. Mix the breadcrumbs, oregano and red chili flakes well and place the marinated Oregano Fingers on this mixture. Cover it with plastic wrap and leave it till right before you serve to cook.
3. Pre heat the oven at 160 degrees Fahrenheit for 5 minutes. Place the Oregano Fingers in the fry basket and close it. Let them cook at the same temperature for another 15 minutes or so. Toss the Oregano Fingers well so that they are cooked uniformly.

431. Veal Patti With Boiled Peas

Ingredients:
- ½ lb. minced veal
- ½ cup breadcrumbs
- A pinch of salt to taste
- ½ cup of boiled peas
- ¼ tsp. ginger finely chopped
- 1 green chili finely chopped
- 1 tsp. lemon juice
- 1 tbsp. fresh coriander leaves. Chop them finely
- ¼ tsp. red chili powder
- ¼ tsp. cumin powder
- ¼ tsp. dried mango powder

Directions:
1. Take a container and into it pour all the masalas, onions, green chilies, peas, coriander leaves, lemon juice, and ginger and 1-2 tbsp. breadcrumbs. Add the minced veal as well. Mix all the ingredients well. Mold the mixture into round patties. Press them gently. Now roll them out carefully.
2. Pre heat the oven at 250 Fahrenheit for 5 minutes. Open the basket of the Fryer and arrange the patties in the basket. Close it carefully. Keep the fryer at 150 degrees for around 10 or 12 minutes. In between the cooking process, turn the patties over to get a uniform cook. Serve hot with mint sauce.

432. Beef And Spinach Meatloaves

Servings: 2
Cooking Time: 45 Minutes

Ingredients:
- 1 large egg, beaten
- 1 cup frozen spinach
- $^1/_3$ cup almond meal
- ¼ cup chopped onion
- ¼ cup plain Greek milk
- ¼ teaspoon salt
- ¼ teaspoon dried sage
- 2 teaspoons olive oil, divided
- Freshly ground black pepper, to taste
- ½ pound (227 g) extra-lean ground beef
- ¼ cup tomato paste
- 1 tablespoon granulated stevia
- ¼ teaspoon Worcestershire sauce
- Cooking spray

Directions:
1. Coat a shallow baking pan with cooking spray.
2. In a large bowl, combine the beaten egg, spinach, almond meal, onion, milk, salt, sage, 1 teaspoon of olive oil, and pepper.
3. Crumble the beef over the spinach mixture. Mix well to combine. Divide the meat mixture in half. Shape each half into a loaf. Place the loaves in the prepared pan.
4. In a small bowl, whisk together the tomato paste, stevia, Worcestershire sauce, and remaining 1 teaspoon of olive oil. Spoon half of the sauce over each meatloaf.
5. Slide the baking pan into Rack Position 1, select Convection Bake, set the temperature to 350ºF (180ºC) and set the time to 40 minutes.

6. When cooking is complete, an instant-read thermometer inserted in the center of the meatloaves should read at least 165ºF (74ºC).
7. Serve immediately.

433. Parmesan Chicken Fingers With Plum Sauce

Servings: 2
Cooking Time: 20 Minutes
Ingredients:
- 2 chicken breasts, cut in strips
- 3 tbsp Parmesan cheese, grated
- ¼ tbsp fresh chives, chopped
- ⅓ cup breadcrumbs
- 1 egg white
- 2 tbsp plum sauce, optional
- ½ tbsp fresh thyme, chopped
- ½ tbsp black pepper
- 1 tbsp water

Directions:
1. Preheat on Air Fry function to 360 F. Mix the chives, Parmesan cheese, thyme, pepper and breadcrumbs. In another bowl, whisk the egg white and mix with the water. Dip the chicken strips into the egg mixture and then in the breadcrumb mixture. Place the strips in the greased basket and fit in the baking tray. Cook for 10 minutes, flipping once. Serve with plum sauce.

434. Baked Chicken Fritters

Servings: 4
Cooking Time: 25 Minutes
Ingredients:
- 1 lb ground chicken
- 1 cup breadcrumbs
- 1 egg, lightly beaten
- 1 garlic clove, minced
- 1 1/2 cup mozzarella cheese, shredded
- 1/2 cup shallots, chopped
- 2 cups broccoli, chopped
- Pepper
- Salt

Directions:
1. Fit the oven with the rack in position
2. Add all ingredients into the bowl and mix until well combined.
3. Make small patties and place them in a parchment-lined baking pan.
4. Set to bake at 390 F for 30 minutes. After 5 minutes place the baking pan in the preheated oven.
5. Serve and enjoy.

Nutrition Info: Calories 399 Fat 13 g Carbohydrates 26.5 g Sugar 2.5 g Protein 42.6 g Cholesterol 147 mg

435. Rosemary Turkey Scotch Eggs

Servings: 4
Cooking Time: 12 Minutes
Ingredients:
- 1 egg
- 1 cup panko bread crumbs
- ½ teaspoon rosemary
- 1 pound (454 g) ground turkey
- 4 hard-boiled eggs, peeled
- Salt and ground black pepper, to taste
- Cooking spray

Directions:
1. Spritz the air fryer basket with cooking spray.
2. Whisk the egg with salt in a bowl. Combine the bread crumbs with rosemary in a shallow dish.
3. Stir the ground turkey with salt and ground black pepper in a separate large bowl, then divide the ground turkey into four portions.
4. Wrap each hard-boiled egg with a portion of ground turkey. Dredge in the whisked egg, then roll over the breadcrumb mixture.
5. Place the wrapped eggs in the basket and spritz with cooking spray.
6. Put the air fryer basket on the baking pan and slide into Rack Position 2, select Air Fry, set temperature to 400ºF (205ºC) and set time to 12 minutes.
7. Flip the eggs halfway through.
8. When cooking is complete, the scotch eggs should be golden brown and crunchy.
9. Serve immediately.

436. Mayo Chicken Breasts With Basil & Cheese

Servings: 4
Cooking Time: 20 Minutes
Ingredients:
- 4 chicken breasts, cubed
- 1 tsp garlic powder
- 1 cup mayonnaise
- Salt and black pepper to taste
- ½ cup cream cheese, softened
- Chopped basil for garnish

Directions:
1. In a bowl, mix cream cheese, mayonnaise, garlic powder, and salt. Add in the chicken and toss to coat. Place the chicken in the basket and Press Start. Cook for 15 minutes at 380 F on AirFry function. Serve garnished with roughly chopped fresh basil.

437. Barbecue Flavored Pork Ribs

Servings: 6
Cooking Time: 15 Minutes
Ingredients:
- ¼ cup honey, divided
- ¾ cup BBQ sauce

- 2 tablespoons tomato ketchup
- 1 tablespoon Worcestershire sauce
- 1 tablespoon soy sauce
- ½ teaspoon garlic powder
- Freshly ground white pepper, to taste
- 1¾ pound pork ribs

Directions:
1. Preparing the Ingredients. In a large bowl, mix together 3 tablespoons of honey and remaining ingredients except pork ribs.
2. Refrigerate to marinate for about 20 minutes.
3. Preheat the air fryer oven to 355 degrees F.
4. Place the ribs in an Air fryer rack/basket.
5. Air Frying. Cook for about 13 minutes.
6. Remove the ribs from the air fryer oven and coat with remaining honey.
7. Serve hot.

438. Baked Beef & Broccoli

Servings: 2
Cooking Time: 25 Minutes
Ingredients:
- 1/2 lb beef meat, cut into pieces
- 1 tbsp vinegar
- 1 garlic clove, minced
- 1 tbsp olive oil
- 1/2 tsp Italian seasoning
- 1/2 cup broccoli florets
- 1 onion, sliced
- Pepper
- Salt

Directions:
1. Fit the oven with the rack in position
2. Add meat and remaining ingredients into the large bowl and toss well and spread in baking pan.
3. Set to bake at 390 F for 30 minutes. After 5 minutes place the baking pan in the preheated oven.
4. Serve and enjoy.

Nutrition Info: Calories 316 Fat 16.1 g Carbohydrates 7.4 g Sugar 2.9 g Protein 34.4 g Cholesterol 102 mg

439. Meatballs(15)

Servings: 4
Cooking Time: 20 Minutes
Ingredients:
- 1 lb ground beef
- 2 tbsp parmesan cheese, grated
- 2 tsp Italian seasoning
- 1/4 cup rolled oats
- 1 egg, lightly beaten
- 1/2 cup spinach, chopped
- 1 tsp garlic, minced
- 1/2 onion, minced
- 4 oz mushrooms, chopped
- 3/4 cup cooked quinoa

Directions:
1. Fit the oven with the rack in position
2. Add all ingredients into the mixing bowl and mix until well combined.
3. Make small balls from the meat mixture and place it into the parchment-lined baking pan.
4. Set to bake at 400 F for 25 minutes. After 5 minutes place the baking pan in the preheated oven.
5. Serve and enjoy.

Nutrition Info: Calories 395 Fat 12 g Carbohydrates 27 g Sugar 1.4 g Protein 43.3 g Cholesterol 146 mg

440. Spiced Pork Chops

Servings: 4
Cooking Time: 16 Minutes
Ingredients:
- 4 pork chops, boneless
- 1/2 tsp granulated onion
- 1/2 tsp granulated garlic
- 1/4 tsp sugar
- 2 tsp olive oil
- 1/2 tsp celery seed
- 1/2 tsp parsley
- 1/2 tsp salt

Directions:
1. Fit the oven with the rack in position 2.
2. Brush pork chops with olive oil.
3. Mix celery seed, parsley, granulated onion, garlic, sugar, and salt and sprinkle over pork chops.
4. Place pork chops in the air fryer basket then place an air fryer basket in the baking pan.
5. Place a baking pan on the oven rack. Set to air fry at 350 F for 16 minutes.
6. Serve and enjoy.

Nutrition Info: Calories 279 Fat 22.3 g Carbohydrates 0.6 g Sugar 0.3 g Protein 18.1 g Cholesterol 69 mg

441. Air Fried Chicken Wings With Buffalo Sauce

Servings: 6
Cooking Time: 20 Minutes
Ingredients:
- 16 chicken drumettes (party wings)
- Chicken seasoning or rub, to taste
- 1 teaspoon garlic powder
- Ground black pepper, to taste
- ¼ cup buffalo wings sauce
- Cooking spray

Directions:
1. Spritz the air fryer basket with cooking spray.
2. Rub the chicken wings with chicken seasoning, garlic powder, and ground black pepper on a clean work surface.
3. Arrange the chicken wings in the basket. Spritz with cooking spray.

4. Put the air fryer basket on the baking pan and slide into Rack Position 2, select Air Fry, set temperature to 400°F (205°C) and set time to 10 minutes.
5. Flip the chicken wings halfway through.
6. When cooking is complete, the chicken wings should be lightly browned.
7. Transfer the chicken wings in a large bowl, then pour in the buffalo wings sauce and toss to coat well.
8. Put the wings back to the oven and set time to 7 minutes. Flip the wings halfway through.
9. When cooking is complete, the wings should be heated through. Serve immediately.

442. Korean-style Chicken Wings

Servings: 4
Cooking Time: 20 Minutes
Ingredients:
- 1 pound chicken wings
- 8 oz flour
- 8 oz breadcrumbs
- 3 beaten eggs
- 4 tbsp canola oil
- Salt and black pepper to taste
- 2 tbsp sesame seeds
- 2 tbsp Korean red pepper paste
- 1 tbsp apple cider vinegar
- 2 tbsp honey
- 1 tbsp soy sauce
- Sesame seeds, to serve

Directions:
1. Separate the chicken wings into winglets and drumettes. In a bowl, mix salt, olive oil, and pepper. Coat the chicken with flour followed by eggs and breadcrumbs. Place in the basket and fit in the baking tray. Oil with cooking spray and cook for 15 minutes on Air Fry mode at 350 F.
2. Mix red pepper paste, apple cider vinegar, soy sauce, honey, and ¼ cup of water in a saucepan and bring to a boil over medium heat. Simmer until the sauce thickens, about 3-4 minutes. Pour the sauce over the chicken pieces. Garnish with sesame seeds and serve.

443. Guacamole Stuffed Chicken

Servings: 4
Cooking Time: 10 Minutes
Ingredients:
- Nonstick cooking spray
- 2 chicken breasts, boneless & skinless
- ½ cup guacamole
- 2/3 cup cheddar cheese, grated
- 1 cup panko bread crumbs
- ½ tsp Adobo seasoning

Directions:
1. Place baking pan in position 2. Spray the fryer basket with cooking spray.
2. Cut the chicken breasts in half, similar to butterflying them but cut all the way through. Place the chicken between two sheets of plastic wrap and pound really thin.
3. Spread 2 tablespoons guacamole over each piece of chicken. Sprinkle with the cheese. Fold the chicken pieces in half covering the filling.
4. In a shallow dish, combine bread crumbs and seasoning. Coat each side of chicken with mixture and place in the fryer basket.
5. Place the basket in the oven and set to air fry on 375°F for 10 minutes. Turn chicken over halfway through cooking time. Serve immediately.
Nutrition Info: Calories 363, Total Fat 15g, Saturated Fat 5g, Total Carbs 22g, Net Carbs 19g, Protein 35g, Sugar 2g, Fiber 3g, Sodium 441mg, Potassium 604mg, Phosphorus 400mg

444. Easy Baked Chicken Drumsticks

Servings: 6
Cooking Time: 45 Minutes
Ingredients:
- 6 chicken legs
- 1/4 cup Worcestershire sauce
- 2 tbsp olive oil
- 1/2 tsp paprika
- 1/2 tsp oregano
- 1 1/2 tsp onion powder
- 1 1/2 tsp garlic powder
- 1/2 tsp pepper
- 1/2 tsp salt

Directions:
1. Fit the oven with the rack in position
2. Add chicken legs and remaining ingredients into the zip-lock bag, seal bag shake well and place in the fridge for 2 hours.
3. Place marinated chicken legs in a baking pan.
4. Set to bake at 375 F for 50 minutes. After 5 minutes place the baking pan in the preheated oven.
5. Serve and enjoy.
Nutrition Info: Calories 182 Fat 9.7 g Carbohydrates 3.3 g Sugar 2.4 g Protein 19.5 g Cholesterol 59 mg

445. Tonkatsu

Servings: 4
Cooking Time: 10 Minutes
Ingredients:
- $2/3$ cup all-purpose flour
- 2 large egg whites
- 1 cup panko bread crumbs
- 4 (4-ounce / 113-g) center-cut boneless pork loin chops (about ½ inch thick)
- Cooking spray

Directions:

1. Pour the flour in a bowl. Whisk the egg whites in a separate bowl. Spread the bread crumbs on a large plate.
2. Dredge the pork loin chops in the flour first, press to coat well, then shake the excess off and dunk the chops in the eggs whites, and then roll the chops over the bread crumbs. Shake the excess off.
3. Arrange the pork chops in the basket and spritz with cooking spray.
4. Put the air fryer basket on the baking pan and slide into Rack Position 2, select Air Fry, set temperature to 375ºF (190ºC) and set time to 10 minutes.
5. After 5 minutes, remove from the oven. Flip the pork chops. Return to the oven and continue cooking.
6. When cooking is complete, the pork chops should be crunchy and lightly browned.
7. Serve immediately.

446. Spiced Pork Roast

Servings: 8
Cooking Time: 50 Minutes
Ingredients:
- Nonstick cooking spray
- 3 1/3 tbsp. brown sugar
- 2/3 tbsp. sugar
- 1 ½ tsp pepper
- 1 tsp salt
- 1 tsp ginger
- ¾ tsp garlic powder
- ¾ tsp onion salt
- ½ tbsp. dry mustard
- ¼ tsp cayenne pepper
- ¼ tsp crushed red pepper flakes
- ¼ tsp cumin
- ¼ tsp paprika
- ¾ tsp thyme
- 2 ½ lb. pork loin roast, boneless

Directions:
1. Place baking pan in position 1 of the oven. Spray the fryer basket with cooking spray.
2. In a small bowl, combine sugars and spices, mix well.
3. Rub spice mixture into all sides of the pork roast. Place roast in the basket.
4. Set oven to convection bake on 300°F for 60 minutes. After 5 minutes, place the basket on the pan and cook 45-50 minutes.
5. Remove from oven and let rest 10 minutes before slicing and serving.

Nutrition Info: Calories 224, Total Fat 6g, Saturated Fat 2g, Total Carbs 8g, Net Carbs 8g, Protein 32g, Sugar 8g, Fiber 0g, Sodium 362mg, Potassium 549mg, Phosphorus 321mg

447. Tamarind Pork Chops With Green Beans

Servings: 4
Cooking Time: 30 Minutes + Marinating Time
Ingredients:
- 2 tbsp tamarind paste
- ½ lb green beans, trimmed
- 1 tbsp garlic, minced
- ½ cup green mole sauce
- 3 tbsp corn syrup
- 1 tbsp olive oil
- 2 tbsp molasses
- 4 tbsp southwest seasoning
- 2 tbsp ketchup
- 4 pork chops

Directions:
1. In a bowl, mix all the ingredients, except for potatoes, pork chops, and mole sauce. Add in 2 tbsp of water. Let the pork chops marinate in the mixture for 30 minutes.
2. Place pork chops in the basket and fit in the baking tray; cook for 25 minutes on Air Fry function at 350 F. Blanch the green beans in salted water in a pot over medium heat for 2-3 minutes until tender. Drain and season with salt and pepper. Serve the pork with green beans and mole sauce.

448. Cayenne Chicken Drumsticks

Servings: 4
Cooking Time: 50 Minutes
Ingredients:
- 8 chicken drumsticks
- 2 tbsp oregano
- 2 tbsp thyme
- 2 oz oats
- ¼ cup milk
- ¼ steamed cauliflower florets
- 1 egg
- 1 tbsp ground cayenne pepper
- Salt and black pepper to taste

Directions:
1. Preheat on Air Fry function to 350 F. Season the drumsticks with salt and pepper; rub them with the milk. Place all the other ingredients except the egg in a food processor. Process until smooth. Dip drumsticks in the egg first and then in the oat mixture. Arrange on the greased AitjrFryer basket and fit in the baking tray. Cook for 20 minutes until golden brown.

449. Cajun Burger Patties

Servings: 2
Cooking Time: 10 Minutes
Ingredients:
- 1 egg, lightly beaten

- 1/2 lb ground pork
- 1/2 cup breadcrumbs
- 1 tbsp Cajun seasoning
- Pepper
- Salt

Directions:
1. Fit the oven with the rack in position 2.
2. Line the air fryer basket with parchment paper.
3. Add all ingredients into the large bowl and mix until well combined.
4. Make two equal shapes of patties from meat mixture and place in the air fryer basket then place an air fryer basket in the baking pan.
5. Place a baking pan on the oven rack. Set to air fry at 360 F for 10 minutes.
6. Serve and enjoy.

Nutrition Info: Calories 300 Fat 7.6 g Carbohydrates 19.6 g Sugar 1.8 g Protein 36.1 g Cholesterol 165 mg

450. Parmesan Herb Meatballs

Servings: 6
Cooking Time: 20 Minutes
Ingredients:
- 1 lb ground beef
- 1/2 small onion, minced
- 2 garlic cloves, minced
- 1 egg, lightly beaten
- 1 1/2 tbsp fresh basil, chopped
- 1 tbsp fresh parsley, chopped
- 1/2 tbsp fresh rosemary, chopped
- 1/4 cup parmesan cheese, grated
- 1/2 cup breadcrumbs
- Pepper
- Salt

Directions:
1. Fit the oven with the rack in position
2. Add all ingredients into the mixing bowl and mix until well combined.
3. Make small balls from the meat mixture and place them into the baking pan.
4. Set to bake at 375 F for 25 minutes. After 5 minutes place the baking pan in the preheated oven.
5. Serve and enjoy.

Nutrition Info: Calories 204 Fat 6.8 g Carbohydrates 7.8 g Sugar 0.9 g Protein 26.5 g Cholesterol 98 mg

451. Perfect Chicken Parmesan

Servings: 2
Cooking Time: 25 Minutes
Ingredients:
- 2 large white meat chicken breasts, approximately 5-6 ounces
- 1 cup of breadcrumbs (Panko brand works well)
- 2 medium-sized eggs
- Pinch of salt and pepper
- 1 tablespoon of dried oregano
- 1 cup of marinara sauce (store-bought or homemade will do equally well)
- 2 slices of provolone cheese
- 1 tablespoon of parmesan cheese

Directions:
1. Preparing the Ingredients. Cover the basket of the air fryer oven with a lining of tin foil, leaving the edges uncovered to allow air to circulate through the basket.
2. Preheat the air fryer oven to 350 degrees.
3. In a mixing bowl, beat the eggs until fluffy and until the yolks and whites are fully combined, and set aside.
4. In a separate mixing bowl, combine the breadcrumbs, oregano, salt and pepper, and set aside.
5. One by one, dip the raw chicken breasts into the bowl with dry ingredients, coating both sides; then submerge into the bowl with wet ingredients, then dip again into the dry ingredients. This double coating will ensure an extra crisp-and-delicious air-fry!
6. Lay the coated chicken breasts on the foil covering the Oven rack/basket, in a single flat layer. Place the Rack on the middle-shelf of the air fryer oven.
7. Air Frying. Set the air fryer oven timer for 10 minutes.
8. After 10 minutes, the air fryer will turn off and the chicken should be mid-way cooked and the breaded coating starting to brown.
9. Using tongs, turn each piece of chicken over to ensure a full all-over fry.
10. Reset the air fryer oven to 320 degrees for another 10 minutes.
11. While the chicken is cooking, pour half the marinara sauce into a 7-inch heat-safe pan.
12. After 15 minutes, when the air fryer shuts off, remove the fried chicken breasts using tongs and set in the marinara-covered pan. Drizzle the rest of the marinara sauce over the fried chicken, then place the slices of provolone cheese atop both of them and sprinkle the parmesan cheese over the entire pan.
13. Reset the air fryer oven to 350 degrees for 5 minutes.
14. After 5 minutes, when the air fryer shuts off, remove the dish from the air fryer using tongs or oven mitts. The chicken will be perfectly crisped and the cheese melted and lightly toasted. Serve while hot!

452. Turkey Burger Cutlets

Ingredients:
- ½ lb. minced turkey
- ½ cup breadcrumbs
- A pinch of salt to taste
- ¼ tsp. ginger finely chopped
- 1 green chili finely chopped
- 1 tsp. lemon juice

- 1 tbsp. fresh coriander leaves. Chop them finely
- ¼ tsp. red chili powder
- ½ cup of boiled peas
- ¼ tsp. cumin powder
- ¼ tsp. dried mango powder

Directions:
1. Take a container and into it pour all the masalas, onions, green chilies, peas, coriander leaves, lemon juice, ginger and 1-2 tbsp. breadcrumbs. Add the minced turkey as well. Mix all the ingredients well. Mold the mixture into round Cutlets. Press them gently. Now roll them out carefully. Pre heat the oven at 250 Fahrenheit for 5 minutes.
2. Open the basket of the Fryer and arrange the Cutlets in the basket. Close it carefully.
3. Keep the fryer at 150 degrees for around 10 or 12 minutes. In between the cooking process, turn the Cutlets over to get a uniform cook. Serve hot with mint sauce.

453. Air Fried Beef And Mushroom Stroganoff

Servings: 4
Cooking Time: 14 Minutes
Ingredients:
- 1 pound (454 g) beef steak, thinly sliced
- 8 ounces (227 g) mushrooms, sliced
- 1 whole onion, chopped
- 2 cups beef broth
- 1 cup sour cream
- 4 tablespoons butter, melted
- 2 cups cooked egg noodles

Directions:
1. Combine the mushrooms, onion, beef broth, sour cream and butter in a bowl until well blended. Add the beef steak to another bowl.
2. Spread the mushroom mixture over the steak and let marinate for 10 minutes.
3. Pour the marinated steak in the baking pan.
4. Slide the baking pan into Rack Position 1, select Convection Bake, set temperature to 400ºF (205ºC) and set time to 14 minutes.
5. Flip the steak halfway through the cooking time.
6. When cooking is complete, the steak should be browned and the vegetables should be tender.
7. Serve hot with the cooked egg noodles.

454. Chicken Thighs In Waffles

Servings: 4
Cooking Time: 20 Minutes
Ingredients:
- For the chicken:
- 4 chicken thighs, skin on
- 1 cup low-fat buttermilk
- ½ cup all-purpose flour
- ½ teaspoon garlic powder
- ½ teaspoon mustard powder
- 1 teaspoon kosher salt
- ½ teaspoon freshly ground black pepper
- ¼ cup honey, for serving
- Cooking spray
- For the waffles:
- ½ cup all-purpose flour
- ½ cup whole wheat pastry flour
- 1 large egg, beaten
- 1 cup low-fat buttermilk
- 1 teaspoon baking powder
- 2 tablespoons canola oil
- ½ teaspoon kosher salt
- 1 tablespoon granulated sugar

Directions:
1. Combine the chicken thighs with buttermilk in a large bowl. Wrap the bowl in plastic and refrigerate to marinate for at least an hour.
2. Spritz the air fryer basket with cooking spray.
3. Combine the flour, mustard powder, garlic powder, salt, and black pepper in a shallow dish. Stir to mix well.
4. Remove the thighs from the buttermilk and pat dry with paper towels. Sit the bowl of buttermilk aside.
5. Dip the thighs in the flour mixture first, then into the buttermilk, and then into the flour mixture. Shake the excess off.
6. Arrange the thighs in the basket and spritz with cooking spray.
7. Put the air fryer basket on the baking pan and slide into Rack Position 2, select Air Fry, set temperature to 360ºF (182ºC) and set time to 20 minutes.
8. Flip the thighs halfway through.
9. When cooking is complete, an instant-read thermometer inserted in the thickest part of the chicken thighs should register at least 165ºF (74ºC).
10. Meanwhile, make the waffles: combine the ingredients for the waffles in a large bowl. Stir to mix well, then arrange the mixture in a waffle iron and cook until a golden and fragrant waffle forms.
11. Remove the waffles from the waffle iron and slice into 4 pieces. Remove the chicken thighs from the oven and allow to cool for 5 minutes.
12. Arrange each chicken thigh on each waffle piece and drizzle with 1 tablespoon of honey. Serve warm.

455. Juicy & Tender Pork Chops

Servings: 4
Cooking Time: 15 Minutes
Ingredients:
- 4 pork chops, boneless
- 1 tsp onion powder
- 1 tsp smoked paprika
- 1/4 cup olive oil
- 1 tsp pepper

- 2 tsp salt

Directions:
1. Fit the oven with the rack in position
2. Brush pork chops with oil and season with onion powder, paprika, pepper, and salt.
3. Place pork chops in a baking pan.
4. Set to bake at 400 F for 20 minutes. After 5 minutes place the baking pan in the preheated oven.
5. Serve and enjoy.

Nutrition Info: Calories 369 Fat 32.6 g Carbohydrates 1.1 g Sugar 0.3 g Protein 18.2 g Cholesterol 69 mg

456. Italian Chicken Breasts With Tomatoes

Servings: 8
Cooking Time: 35 Minutes
Ingredients:
- 3 pounds (1.4 kg) chicken breasts, bone-in
- 1 teaspoon minced fresh basil
- 1 teaspoon minced fresh rosemary
- 2 tablespoons minced fresh parsley
- 1 teaspoon cayenne pepper
- ½ teaspoon salt
- ½ teaspoon freshly ground black pepper
- 4 medium Roma tomatoes, halved
- Cooking spray

Directions:
1. Spritz the air fryer basket with cooking spray.
2. Combine all the ingredients, except for the chicken breasts and tomatoes, in a large bowl. Stir to mix well.
3. Dunk the chicken breasts in the mixture and press to coat well.
4. Transfer the chicken breasts in the basket.
5. Put the air fryer basket on the baking pan and slide into Rack Position 2, select Air Fry, set temperature to 370ºF (188ºC) and set time to 20 minutes.
6. Flip the breasts halfway through the cooking time.
7. When cooking is complete, the internal temperature of the thickest part of the breasts should reach at least 165ºF (74ºC).
8. Remove the cooked chicken breasts from the oven and adjust the temperature to 350ºF (180ºC).
9. Place the tomatoes in the basket and spritz with cooking spray. Sprinkle with a touch of salt.
10. Set time to 10 minutes. Stir the tomatoes halfway through the cooking time.
11. When cooking is complete, the tomatoes should be tender.
12. Serve the tomatoes with chicken breasts on a large serving plate.

457. Juicy Baked Chicken Breast

Servings: 4
Cooking Time: 25 Minutes
Ingredients:
- 4 chicken breasts
- 1 tbsp fresh parsley, chopped
- 1/4 tsp red pepper flakes
- 1/2 tsp black pepper
- 1 tsp Italian seasoning
- 2 tbsp olive oil
- 1/4 cup balsamic vinegar
- 1 tsp kosher salt

Directions:
1. Fit the oven with the rack in position
2. Place chicken breasts into the mixing bowl.
3. Mix together remaining ingredients and pour over chicken breasts and coat well and let marinate for 30 minutes.
4. Arrange marinated chicken breasts into a greased baking dish.
5. Set to bake at 425 F for 30 minutes. After 5 minutes place the baking dish in the preheated oven.
6. Slice and serve.

Nutrition Info: Calories 345 Fat 18.2 g Carbohydrates 0.6 g Sugar 0.2 g Protein 42.3 g Cholesterol 131 mg

458. Seafood Grandma's Easy To Cook Wontons

Ingredients:
- 1 ½ cup all-purpose flour
- ½ tsp. salt
- 5 tbsp. water
- For filling:
- 2 cups minced seafood (prawns, shrimp, oysters, scallops)
- 2 tbsp. oil
- 2 tsp. ginger-garlic paste
- 2 tsp. soya sauce
- 2 tsp. vinegar

Directions:
1. Squeeze the dough and cover it with plastic wrap and set aside. Next, cook the ingredients for the filling and try to ensure that the seafood is covered well with the sauce. Roll the dough and place the filling in the center. Now, wrap the dough to cover the filling and pinch the edges together. Pre heat the oven at 200° F for 5 minutes.
2. Place the wontons in the fry basket and close it. Let them cook at the same temperature for another 20 minutes. Recommended sides are chili sauce or ketchup.

459. Pork Schnitzel

Servings: 10

Cooking Time: 30 Minutes
Ingredients:
- 10 pork cutlets
- 1 tsp salt
- 1 tsp pepper
- 1 cup flour
- 2 eggs
- 1 cup Panko bread crumbs
- Nonstick cooking spray

Directions:
1. Place each cutlet between plastic wrap and pound to ¼-inch thick. Sprinkle both sides with salt and pepper.
2. Place the flour in a shallow dish.
3. In a separate shallow dish, beat the eggs.
4. Place the bread crumbs in another shallow dish.
5. Place the baking pan in position 2 of the oven. Spray the fryer basket with cooking spray.
6. Dip each cutlet first in flour, then egg, then coat with bread crumbs. Place in basket in a single layer, these will need to be cooked in batches.
7. Place basket on the pan and set oven to air fry on 375°F for 10 minutes. Cook each cutlet 3-4 minutes per side, or until nicely browned. Repeat with remaining cutlets. Serve immediately.

Nutrition Info: Calories 320, Total Fat 8g, Saturated Fat 3g, Total Carbs 17g, Net Carbs 16g, Protein 45g, Sugar 1g, Fiber 1g, Sodium 417mg, Potassium 768mg, Phosphorus 484mg

460. Tasty Steak Tips

Servings: 4
Cooking Time: 5 Minutes
Ingredients:
- 1 lb steak, cut into cubes
- 1 tsp olive oil
- 1/4 tsp garlic powder
- 1 tsp Montreal steak seasoning
- Pepper
- Salt

Directions:
1. Fit the oven with the rack in position 2.
2. In a bowl, add steak cubes and remaining ingredients and toss well.
3. Add marinated steak cubes to the air fryer basket then place an air fryer basket in the baking pan.
4. Place a baking pan on the oven rack. Set to air fry at 400 F for 5 minutes.
5. Serve and enjoy.

Nutrition Info: Calories 236 Fat 6.8 g Carbohydrates 0.2 g Sugar 0 g Protein 41 g Cholesterol 102 mg

461. Copycat Chicken Sandwich

Servings: 4
Cooking Time: 15 Minutes
Ingredients:
- 2 chicken breasts, boneless & skinless
- 1 cup buttermilk
- 1 tbsp. + 2 tsp paprika, divided
- 1 tbsp. + 1 ½ tsp garlic powder, divided
- 2 tsp salt, divided
- 2 tsp pepper, divided
- 4 brioche buns
- 1 cup flour
- ½ cup corn starch
- 1 tbsp. onion powder
- 1 tbsp. cayenne pepper
- ½ cup mayonnaise
- 1 tsp hot sauce
- Sliced pickles

Directions:
1. Place chicken between two sheets of plastic wrap and pound to ½-inch thick. Cut crosswise to get 4 cutlets.
2. In a large bowl, whisk together buttermilk and one teaspoon each paprika, garlic powder, salt, and pepper. Add chicken, cover, and refrigerate overnight.
3. Place the buns on the baking pan and place in position 2 of the oven. Set to toast for about 2-5 minutes depending how toasted you want them. Set aside.
4. In a medium shallow dish, combine flour, cornstarch, onion powder, cayenne pepper, and remaining paprika, garlic powder, salt, and pepper.
5. Whisk in 2-3 tablespoons of the buttermilk batter chicken was marinating in until smooth.
6. Lightly spray fryer basket with cooking spray.
7. Dredge chicken in the flour mixture forming a thick coating of the batter. Place in fryer basket.
8. Place basket in the oven. Set oven to air fryer on 375°F for 10 minutes. Cook until crispy and golden brown, turning chicken over halfway through cooking time.
9. In a small bowl, whisk together mayonnaise, hot sauce, 1 teaspoon paprika, and ½ teaspoon garlic powder.
10. To serve, spread top of buns with mayonnaise mixture. Place chicken on bottom buns and top with pickles then top bun.

Nutrition Info: Calories 689, Total Fat 27g, Saturated Fat 5g, Total Carbs 71g, Net Carbs 67g, Protein 38g, Sugar 7g, Fiber 4g, Sodium 1734mg, Potassium 779mg, Phosphorus 435mg

462. Cheesy Bacon Chicken

Servings: 4
Cooking Time: 30 Minutes
Ingredients:
- 4 chicken breasts, sliced in half
- 1 cup cheddar cheese, shredded
- 8 bacon slices, cooked & chopped
- 6 oz cream cheese
- Pepper

- Salt

Directions:
1. Fit the oven with the rack in position
2. Place season chicken with pepper and salt and place it into the greased baking dish.
3. Add cream cheese and bacon on top of chicken.
4. Sprinkle shredded cheddar cheese on top of chicken.
5. Set to bake at 400 F for 35 minutes. After 5 minutes place the baking dish in the preheated oven.
6. Serve and enjoy.

Nutrition Info: Calories 745 Fat 50.9 g Carbohydrates 2.1 g Sugar 0.2 g Protein 66.6 g Cholesterol 248 mg

463. Crispy Crusted Pork Chops

Servings: 2
Cooking Time: 15 Minutes
Ingredients:
- 2 pork chops, bone-in
- 1 cup pork rinds, crushed
- 1/2 tsp parsley
- 1 tbsp olive oil
- 1/2 tsp garlic powder
- 1/2 tsp onion powder
- 1/2 tsp paprika

Directions:
1. Fit the oven with the rack in position 2.
2. In a large bowl, mix pork rinds, garlic powder, onion powder, parsley, and paprika.
3. Brush pork chops with oil and coat with pork rind mixture.
4. place coated pork chops in air fryer basket then place air fryer basket in baking pan.
5. Place a baking pan on the oven rack. Set to air fry at 400 F for 15 minutes.
6. Serve and enjoy.

Nutrition Info: Calories 413 Fat 32.7 g Carbohydrates 1.3 g Sugar 0.4 g Protein 28.5 g Cholesterol 92 mg

464. Chicken Momo's Recipe

Ingredients:
- 1 ½ cup all-purpose flour
- ½ tsp. salt
- 5 tbsp. water
- 2 cups minced chicken
- 2 tbsp. oil
- 2 tsp. ginger-garlic paste
- 2 tsp. soya sauce
- 2 tsp. vinegar

Directions:
1. Squeeze the dough and cover it with plastic wrap and set aside. Next, cook the ingredients for the filling and try to ensure that the beef is covered well with the sauce.
2. Roll the dough and cut it into a square. Place the filling in the center. Now, wrap the dough to cover the filling and pinch the edges together. Pre heat the oven at 200° F for 5 minutes. Place the wontons in the fry basket and close it. Let them cook at the same temperature for another 20 minutes. Recommended sides are chili sauce or ketchup.

465. Tender Baked Pork Chops

Servings: 4
Cooking Time: 15 Minutes
Ingredients:
- 4 pork chops, boneless
- 1/4 tsp onion powder
- 1/2 tsp garlic powder
- 2 tbsp olive oil
- 2 tbsp brown sugar
- 1/2 tsp chili powder
- Pepper
- Salt

Directions:
1. Fit the oven with the rack in position
2. Brush pork chops with oil.
3. In a small bowl, mix brown sugar, chili powder, onion powder, garlic powder, pepper, and salt and rub all over pork chops.
4. Place pork chops in a baking pan.
5. Set to bake at 400 F for 20 minutes. After 5 minutes place the baking pan in the preheated oven.
6. Serve and enjoy.

Nutrition Info: Calories 336 Fat 26.9 g Carbohydrates 5 g Sugar 4.5 g Protein 18.1 g Cholesterol 69 mg

466. Chicken Wings With Honey & Cashew Cream

Servings: 4
Cooking Time: 25 Minutes
Ingredients:
- 2 lb chicken wings
- 1 tbsp fresh cilantro, chopped
- Salt and black pepper to taste
- 1 tbsp cashews cream
- 1 garlic clove, minced
- 1 tbsp plain yogurt
- 2 tbsp honey
- ½ tbsp white wine vinegar
- ½ tbsp ginger, minced
- ½ tbsp garlic chili sauce

Directions:
1. Preheat Breville on AirFry function to 360 F. Season the wings with salt and black pepper, place them in a baking dish. Press Start and cook for 15 minutes. In a bowl, mix the remaining ingredients. Top the chicken with sauce and cook for 5 more minutes. Serve warm.

467. Ham & Cheese Stuffed Chicken Breasts

Servings: 4
Cooking Time: 40 Minutes
Ingredients:
- 4 skinless and boneless chicken breasts
- 4 slices ham
- 4 slices Swiss cheese
- 3 tbsp all-purpose flour
- 4 tbsp butter
- 1 tbsp paprika
- 1 tbsp chicken bouillon granules
- ½ cup dry white wine
- 1 cup heavy whipping cream

Directions:
1. Preheat on Air Fry function to 380 F. Pound the chicken breasts and top with a slice of ham and Swiss cheese. Fold the edges of the chicken over the filling and secure the borders with toothpicks. In a medium bowl, combine the paprika and flour and coat in the chicken rolls. Fry the chicken in your for 20 minutes, turning once.
2. In a large skillet over low heat, melt the butter and add the heavy cream, bouillon granules, and wine; bring to a boil. Add in the chicken and let simmer for around 5-10 minutes. Serve.

468. Italian Veggie Chicken

Servings: 4
Cooking Time: 30 Minutes
Ingredients:
- 4 chicken breasts
- 1 cup mozzarella cheese, shredded
- 6 bacon slices, cooked & chopped
- 8 oz can artichoke hearts, sliced
- 1 cup cherry tomatoes, cut in half
- 1 zucchini, sliced
- 1 tbsp dried basil
- 1/4 tsp salt

Directions:
1. Fit the oven with the rack in position
2. Place chicken breasts into the casserole dish and sprinkle with basil and salt.
3. Spread artichoke hearts, cherry tomatoes, and zucchini on top of chicken.
4. Sprinkle shredded cheese and bacon on top of vegetables.
5. Set to bake at 375 F for 35 minutes. After 5 minutes place the casserole dish in the preheated oven.
6. Serve and enjoy.

Nutrition Info: Calories 484 Fat 24.2 g Carbohydrates 6.9 g Sugar 2.5 g Protein 56.8 g Cholesterol 165 mg

469. White Wine Chicken Wings

Servings: 2
Cooking Time: 30 Minutes
Ingredients:
- 8 chicken wings
- ½ tbsp sugar
- 2 tbsp cornflour
- ½ tbsp white wine
- 1 tbsp fresh ginger, grated
- ½ tbsp olive oil

Directions:
1. In a bowl, mix olive oil, ginger, white wine, and sugar. Add in the chicken wings and toss to coat. Roll up in the flour. Place the chicken in the frying basket and press Start. Cook for 20 minutes until crispy on the outside at 320 F on AirFry function. Serve warm.

470. Easy Pesto Chicken

Servings: 4
Cooking Time: 35 Minutes
Ingredients:
- 4 chicken breasts, sliced into 8 pieces
- 8 oz mozzarella cheese, shredded
- 1/4 cup pesto
- 1/4 tsp pepper
- 1/2 tsp salt

Directions:
1. Fit the oven with the rack in position
2. Season chicken with pepper and salt and place in a greased baking dish.
3. Spread pesto and cheese on top of chicken.
4. Set to bake at 350 F for 40 minutes. After 5 minutes place the baking dish in the preheated oven.
5. Serve and enjoy.

Nutrition Info: Calories 505 Fat 27.3 g Carbohydrates 3.1 g Sugar 1 g Protein 59.8 g Cholesterol 164 mg

471. Baked Spinach Cheese Chicken

Servings: 2
Cooking Time: 20 Minutes
Ingredients:
- 2 chicken breasts, boneless & skinless
- 1/2 tsp garlic powder
- 1/4 cup sun-dried tomatoes, chopped
- 1/4 cup cheddar cheese, shredded
- 3 oz cream cheese
- 2 cups fresh spinach, chopped
- 3/4 tsp pepper
- 3/4 tsp salt

Directions:
1. Fit the oven with the rack in position

2. Slice the chicken breasts into the half and place them into the baking dish. Season with pepper and salt.
3. Cook spinach in the pan until wilted.
4. In a bowl, mix spinach, garlic powder, tomatoes, cheddar cheese, and cream cheese.
5. Spread spinach mixture on top of chicken breasts.
6. Set to bake at 425 F for 25 minutes. After 5 minutes place the baking dish in the preheated oven.
7. Serve and enjoy.
Nutrition Info: Calories 498 Fat 30.5 g Carbohydrates 4.3 g Sugar 1.1 g Protein 50.2 g Cholesterol 192 mg

472. Teriyaki Pork Rolls

Servings: 6
Cooking Time: 8 Minutes
Ingredients:
- 1 tsp. almond flour
- 4 tbsp. low-sodium soy sauce
- 4 tbsp. mirin
- 4 tbsp. brown sugar
- Thumb-sized amount of ginger, chopped
- Pork belly slices
- Enoki mushrooms

Directions:
1. Preparing the Ingredients. Mix brown sugar, mirin, soy sauce, almond flour, and ginger together until brown sugar dissolves.
2. Take pork belly slices and wrap around a bundle of mushrooms. Brush each roll with teriyaki sauce. Chill half an hour.
3. Preheat your air fryer oven to 350 degrees and add marinated pork rolls.
4. Air Frying. Set temperature to 350°F, and set time to 8 minutes.
Nutrition Info: CALORIES: 412; FAT: 9G; PROTEIN:19G; SUGAR:4G

473. Spicy Thai Beef Stir-fry

Servings: 4
Cooking Time: 9 Minutes
Ingredients:
- 1 pound sirloin steaks, thinly sliced
- 2 tablespoons lime juice, divided
- ⅓ cup crunchy peanut butter
- ½ cup beef broth
- 1 tablespoon olive oil
- 1½ cups broccoli florets
- 2 cloves garlic, sliced
- 1 to 2 red chile peppers, sliced

Directions:
1. Preparing the Ingredients. In a medium bowl, combine the steak with 1 tablespoon of the lime juice. Set aside.
2. Combine the peanut butter and beef broth in a small bowl and mix well. Drain the beef and add the juice from the bowl into the peanut butter mixture.
3. In a 6-inch metal bowl, combine the olive oil, steak, and broccoli.
4. Air Frying. Cook for 3 to 4 minutes or until the steak is almost cooked and the broccoli is crisp and tender, shaking the basket once during cooking time.
5. Add the garlic, chile peppers, and the peanut butter mixture and stir.
6. Cook for 3 to 5 minutes or until the sauce is bubbling and the broccoli is tender.
7. Serve over hot rice.
Nutrition Info: CALORIES: 387; FAT: 22G; PROTEIN:42G; FIBER:2G

474. Duck Poppers

Ingredients:
- ½ cup hung curd
- 1 tsp. lemon juice
- 1 tsp. red chili flakes
- 1 cup cubed duck
- 1 ½ tsp. garlic paste
- Salt and pepper to taste
- 1 tsp. dry oregano
- 1 tsp. dry basil

Directions:
1. Add the ingredients into a separate bowl and mix them well to get a consistent mixture.
2. Dip the duck pieces in the above mixture and leave them aside for some time.
3. Pre heat the oven at 180° C for around 5 minutes. Place the coated duck pieces in the fry basket and close it properly. Let them cook at the same temperature for 20 more minutes. Keep turning them over in the basket so that they are cooked properly. Serve with tomato ketchup.

475. Chicken And Eggs

Ingredients:
- Bread slices (brown or white)
- ½ lb. sliced chicken
- 1 egg white for every 2 slices
- 1 tsp sugar for every 2 slices

Directions:
1. Put two slices together and cut them along the diagonal. In a bowl, whisk the egg whites and add some sugar.
2. Dip the bread triangles into this mixture. Cook the chicken now.
3. Pre heat the oven at 180° C for 4 minutes. Place the coated bread triangles in the fry basket and close it. Let them cook at the same temperature for another 20 minutes at least. Halfway through the process, turn the triangles over so that you get a uniform cook. Top with chicken and serve.

476. Beer Corned Beef With Carrots

Servings: 4
Cooking Time: 35 Minutes
Ingredients:
- 1 tbsp beef spice
- 1 white onion, chopped
- 2 carrots, chopped
- 12 oz bottle beer
- 1 ½ cups chicken broth
- 4 pounds corned beef

Directions:
1. Cover beef with beer and let sit in the fridge for 30 minutes. Transfer to a pot over medium heat and add in chicken broth, carrots, and onion. Bring to a boil and simmer for 10 minutes. Drain boiled meat and veggies and place them in a baking dish. Sprinkle with beef spice. Select Bake function, adjust the temperature to 400 F, and press Start. Cook for 30 minutes.

SNACKS AND DESSERTS RECIPES

477. Chocolate Donuts

Servings: 8-10
Cooking Time: 20 Minutes
Ingredients:
- (8-ounce) can jumbo biscuits
- Cooking oil
- Chocolate sauce, such as Hershey's

Directions:
1. Preparing the Ingredients. Separate the biscuit dough into 8 biscuits and place them on a flat work surface. Use a small circle cookie cutter or a biscuit cutter to cut a hole in the center of each biscuit. You can also cut the holes using a knife.
2. Spray the Oven rack/basket with cooking oil. Place the Rack on the middle-shelf of the air fryer oven.
3. Air Frying. Place 4 donuts in the air fryer oven. Do not stack. Spray with cooking oil. Cook for 4 minutes.
4. Open the air fryer oven and flip the donuts. Cook for an additional 4 minutes.
5. Remove the cooked donuts from the air fryer, then repeat steps 3 and 4 for the remaining 4 donuts.
6. Drizzle chocolate sauce over the donuts and enjoy while warm.

Nutrition Info: CALORIES: 181; FAT:98G; PROTEIN:3G; FIBER:1G

478. Strawberry Muffins

Servings: 12
Cooking Time: 20 Minutes
Ingredients:
- 4 eggs
- 1/4 cup water
- 1/2 cup butter, melted
- 2 tsp baking powder
- 2 cups almond flour
- 2/3 cup strawberries, chopped
- 2 tsp vanilla
- 1/4 cup erythritol
- Pinch of salt

Directions:
1. Fit the oven with the rack in position
2. Line 12-cups muffin tin with cupcake liners and set aside.
3. In a medium bowl, mix together almond flour, baking powder, and salt.
4. In a separate bowl, whisk eggs, sweetener, vanilla, water, and butter.
5. Add almond flour mixture into the egg mixture and mix until well combined.
6. Add strawberries and stir well.
7. Pour batter into the prepared muffin tin.
8. Set to bake at 350 F for 25 minutes. After 5 minutes place muffin tin in the preheated oven.
9. Serve and enjoy.

Nutrition Info: Calories 201 Fat 18.5 g Carbohydrates 5.2 g Sugar 1.3 g Protein 6 g Cholesterol 75 mg

479. Garlicky-lemon Zucchini

Ingredients:
- Coarse salt and black pepper, to taste
- ½ tsp thyme, minced
- ½ lemon
- 4 small green zucchinis, any color, sliced about ¼-inch thick
- 1½ Tbsp extra virgin olive oil
- 1 Tbsp garlic, minced

Directions:
1. Heat oven over medium-low heat. Add oil and let heat for 1 minute.
2. Sprinkle zucchini with salt and pepper.
3. Add to the pan in a single layer. When zucchini is nicely browned, flip
4. and brown on other side.
5. Add garlic and saute for 1 minute.
6. Sprinkle thyme and additional salt if necessary.
7. Remove from pan and squeeze lemon juice on zucchini.

480. Toasted Coco Flakes

Servings: 4
Cooking Time: 15 Minutes
Ingredients:
- 1 cup unsweetened coconut flakes
- ¼ cup granular erythritol.
- 2 tsp. coconut oil
- ⅛ tsp. salt

Directions:
1. Toss coconut flakes and oil in a large bowl until coated. Sprinkle with erythritol and salt. Place coconut flakes into the air fryer basket.
2. Adjust the temperature to 300 Degrees F and set the timer for 3 minutes.
3. Toss the flakes when 1 minute remains. Add an extra minute if you would like a more golden coconut flake. Store in an airtight container up to 3 days.

Nutrition Info: Calories: 165; Protein: 1.3g; Fiber: 2.7g; Fat: 15.5g; Carbs: 20.3g

481. Nutella Brownies

Ingredients:
- ½ stick unsalted butter
- ¼ cup half-and-half
- 4 oz chocolate chips
- ½ cup Nutella spread
- 1 cup sugar

- 3 large eggs
- 1 cup all-purpose flour
- ½ cup Dutch cocoa powder
- ½ tsp salt
- ½ tsp vanilla extract

Directions:
1. Preheat oven to 350°F.
2. Whisk together sugar and eggs in one bowl.
3. Whisk together flour, cocoa and salt in another bowl.
4. In oven, simmer butter and half-and-half together over low heat.
5. Add chocolate chips and stir until melted, about 2 minutes.
6. Add in Nutella and continue stirring until incorporated. Remove from heat.
7. Pour sugar mixture into chocolate mixture in oven.
8. Carefully add flour mixture and fold until just incorporated.
9. Bake for 25 minutes, but start checking at 20 minutes. At about 20-22 minutes, you will have a brownie with a fudge-like consistency.

482. Choco Cookies

Servings: 8
Cooking Time: 8 Minutes
Ingredients:
- 3 egg whites
- 3/4 cup cocoa powder, unsweetened
- 1 3/4 cup confectioner sugar
- 1 1/2 tsp vanilla

Directions:
1. Fit the oven with the rack in position
2. In a mixing bowl, whip egg whites until fluffy soft peaks. Slowly add in cocoa, sugar, and vanilla.
3. Drop teaspoonful onto parchment-lined baking pan into 32 small cookies.
4. Set to bake at 350 F for 8 minutes. After 5 minutes place the baking pan in the preheated oven.
5. Serve and enjoy.

Nutrition Info: Calories 132 Fat 1.1 g Carbohydrates 31 g Sugar 0.3 g Protein 2 g Cholesterol 0 mg

483. Apple Dumplings

Servings: 4
Cooking Time: 25 Minutes
Ingredients:
- 2 tbsp. melted coconut oil
- 2 puff pastry sheets
- 1 tbsp. brown sugar
- 2 tbsp. raisins
- 2 small apples of choice

Directions:
1. Preparing the Ingredients. Ensure your air fryer oven is preheated to 356 degrees.
2. Core and peel apples and mix with raisins and sugar.
3. Place a bit of apple mixture into puff pastry sheets and brush sides with melted coconut oil.
4. Air Frying. Place into the air fryer oven. Cook 25 minutes, turning halfway through. Will be golden when done.

Nutrition Info: CALORIES: 367; FAT:7G; PROTEIN:2G; SUGAR:5G

484. Three Berry Crumble

Ingredients:
- ¾ cup brown sugar
- ¾ cup old fashioned oats
- ½ cup chopped almonds
- 1 tsp cinnamon
- 6 cups of fresh mixed berries (blueberries, raspberries), washed and dried
- ¼ cup sugar
- ¼ cup flour
- 1 Tbsp lemon juice
- ¾ cup flour
- 1 stick cold butter, cut into cubes

Directions:
1. Preheat oven to 375°F.
2. Lightly toss the berries, sugar, flour and lemon juice inside your oven.
3. In a bowl, mix the flour, brown sugar, oats, almonds and cinnamon.
4. Incorporate cold butter with your fingertips into the oat mixture until small clumps form.
5. Pour topping onto fruit and bake for 45 minutes to 1 hour, until bubbles form and top appears browned and crispy.
6. Serve with vanilla ice cream right out of oven.

485. Mozzarella And Tomato Salad

Servings: 6
Cooking Time: 15 Minutes
Ingredients:
- 1 lb. tomatoes; sliced
- 1 cup mozzarella; shredded
- 1 tbsp. ginger; grated
- 1 tbsp. balsamic vinegar
- 1 tsp. sweet paprika
- 1 tsp. chili powder
- ½ tsp. coriander, ground

Directions:
1. In a pan that fits your air fryer, mix all the ingredients except the mozzarella, toss, introduce the pan in the air fryer and cook at 360°F for 12 minutes
2. Divide into bowls and serve cold as an appetizer with the mozzarella sprinkled all over.

Nutrition Info: Calories: 185; Fat: 8g; Fiber: 2g; Carbs: 4g; Protein: 8g

486. Sausage And Mushroom Empanadas

Servings: 4
Cooking Time: 12 Minutes
Ingredients:
- ½ pound (227 g) Kielbasa smoked sausage, chopped
- 4 chopped canned mushrooms
- 2 tablespoons chopped onion
- ½ teaspoon ground cumin
- ¼ teaspoon paprika
- Salt and black pepper, to taste
- ½ package puff pastry dough, at room temperature
- 1 egg, beaten
- Cooking spray

Directions:
1. Combine the sausage, mushrooms, onion, cumin, paprika, salt, and pepper in a bowl and stir to mix well.
2. Make the empanadas: Place the puff pastry dough on a lightly floured surface. Cut circles into the dough with a glass. Place 1 tablespoon of the sausage mixture into the center of each pastry circle. Fold each in half and pinch the edges to seal. Using a fork, crimp the edges. Brush them with the beaten egg and mist with cooking spray.
3. Spritz the air fryer basket with cooking spray. Place the empanadas in the basket.
4. Put the air fryer basket on the baking pan and slide into Rack Position 2, select Air Fry, set temperature to 360ºF (182ºC), and set time to 12 minutes.
5. Flip the empanadas halfway through the cooking time.
6. When cooking is complete, the empanadas should be golden brown. Remove from the oven. Allow them to cool for 5 minutes and serve hot.

487. Currant Cookies

Servings: 6
Cooking Time: 15 Minutes
Ingredients:
- ½ cup currants
- ½ cup swerve
- 2 cups almond flour
- ½ cup ghee; melted
- 1 tsp. vanilla extract
- 2 tsp. baking soda

Directions:
1. Take a bowl and mix all the ingredients and whisk well.
2. Spread this on a baking sheet lined with parchment paper, put the pan in the air fryer and cook at 350°F for 30 minutes.
3. Cool down; cut into rectangles and serve.

Nutrition Info: Calories: 172; Fat: 5g; Fiber: 2g; Carbs: 3g; Protein: 5g

488. Cheese And Ham Stuffed Baby Bella

Servings: 8
Cooking Time: 12 Minutes
Ingredients:
- 4 ounces (113 g) Mozzarella cheese, cut into pieces
- ½ cup diced ham
- 2 green onions, chopped
- 2 tablespoons bread crumbs
- ½ teaspoon garlic powder
- ¼ teaspoon ground oregano
- ¼ teaspoon ground black pepper
- 1 to 2 teaspoons olive oil
- 16 fresh Baby Bella mushrooms, stemmed removed

Directions:
1. Process the cheese, ham, green onions, bread crumbs, garlic powder, oregano, and pepper in a food processor until finely chopped.
2. With the food processor running, slowly drizzle in 1 to 2 teaspoons olive oil until a thick paste has formed. Transfer the mixture to a bowl.
3. Evenly divide the mixture into the mushroom caps and lightly press down the mixture.
4. Lay the mushrooms in the air fryer basket in a single layer.
5. Put the air fryer basket on the baking pan and slide into Rack Position 2, select Roast, set temperature to 390ºF (199ºC), and set time to 12 minutes.
6. When cooking is complete, the mushrooms should be lightly browned and tender. Remove from the oven to a plate. Let the mushrooms cool for 5 minutes and serve warm.

489. Lemon Blackberries Cake(2)

Servings: 4
Cooking Time: 15 Minutes
Ingredients:
- 2 eggs, whisked
- ¼ cup almond milk
- 1 ½ cups almond flour
- 1 cup blackberries; chopped.
- 2 tbsp. ghee; melted
- 4 tbsp. swerve
- 1 tsp. lemon zest, grated
- 1 tsp. lemon juice
- ½ tsp. baking powder

Directions:
1. Take a bowl and mix all the ingredients and whisk well.
2. Pour this into a cake pan that fits the air fryer lined with parchment paper, put the pan in your air fryer and cook at 340°F for 25 minutes. Cool the cake down, slice and serve

Nutrition Info: Calories: 193; Fat: 5g; Fiber: 1g; Carbs: 4g; Protein: 4g

490. Crispy Cod Fingers

Servings: 4
Cooking Time: 12 Minutes
Ingredients:
- 2 eggs
- 2 tablespoons milk
- 2 cups flour
- 1 cup cornmeal
- 1 teaspoon seafood seasoning
- Salt and black pepper, to taste
- 1 cup bread crumbs
- 1 pound (454 g) cod fillets, cut into 1-inch strips

Directions:
1. Beat the eggs with the milk in a shallow bowl. In another shallow bowl, combine the flour, cornmeal, seafood seasoning, salt, and pepper. On a plate, place the bread crumbs.
2. Dredge the cod strips, one at a time, in the flour mixture, then in the egg mixture, finally roll in the bread crumb to coat evenly.
3. Transfer the cod strips to the air fryer basket.
4. Put the air fryer basket on the baking pan and slide into Rack Position 2, select Air Fry, set temperature to 400°F (205°C), and set time to 12 minutes.
5. When cooking is complete, the cod strips should be crispy. Remove from the oven to a paper towel-lined plate and serve warm.

491. Rosemary Russet Potato Chips

Servings: 4
Cooking Time: 1 Hour
Ingredients:
- 4 russet potatoes
- ½ tsp. salt
- 1 tbsp. olive oil
- 2 tsps. chopped rosemary

Directions:
1. Rinse the potatoes and scrub to clean. Peel and cut them in a lengthwise manner similar to thin chips.
2. Put them in a bowl and soak in water for 30 minutes.
3. Pat the potato chips with paper towels to dry.
4. Toss the chips in a bowl with olive oil. Transfer them to the cooking basket.
5. Cook for 30 minutes at 330F. Shake several times during the cooking process.
6. Toss the cooked chips in a bowl with salt and rosemary while warm.

Nutrition Info: Calories: 322 Fat: 3.69g Carbs: 66g Protein: 7.5g

492. Apple-peach Crumble With Honey

Servings: 4
Cooking Time: 11 Minutes
Ingredients:
- 1 apple, peeled and chopped
- 2 peaches, peeled, pitted, and chopped
- 2 tablespoons honey
- ½ cup quick-cooking oatmeal
- $1/3$ cup whole-wheat pastry flour
- 2 tablespoons unsalted butter, at room temperature
- 3 tablespoons packed brown sugar
- ½ teaspoon ground cinnamon

Directions:
1. Mix together the apple, peaches, and honey in the baking pan until well incorporated.
2. In a bowl, combine the oatmeal, pastry flour, butter, brown sugar, and cinnamon and stir to mix well. Spread this mixture evenly over the fruit.
3. Slide the baking pan into Rack Position 1, select Convection Bake, set temperature to 380°F (193°C), and set time to 11 minutes.
4. When cooking is complete, the fruit should be bubbling around the edges and the topping should be golden brown.
5. Remove from the oven and serve warm.

493. Gooey Chocolate Fudge Cake

Ingredients:
- 3 Tbsp cocoa powder
- ½ cup water
- ¼ cup whole milk
- 1 egg
- 1 tsp vanilla extract
- 1 cup flour
- ½ tsp baking soda
- 1 cup sugar
- Pinch of salt
- ½ cup vegetable oil

Directions:
1. Preheat the oven to 350°F.
2. In a large bowl, whisk flour, baking soda, sugar and salt.
3. Combine oil, cocoa powder and water in another bowl.
4. Whisk in flour mixture and pour into oven.
5. Incorporate milk, egg and vanilla into the batter.
6. Bake for 25 minutes, or until edges are set and center is only slightly jiggly.

494. Crispy Eggplant Bites

Servings: 4
Cooking Time: 20 Minutes
Ingredients:
- 1 eggplant, cut into 1-inch pieces

- 1 tsp garlic powder
- 2 tbsp olive oil
- 1/2 tsp Italian seasoning
- 1 tsp paprika
- 1/2 tsp red pepper

Directions:
1. Fit the oven with the rack in position 2.
2. Add all ingredients into the large mixing bowl and toss well.
3. Transfer eggplant mixture in air fryer basket then places air fryer basket in baking pan.
4. Place a baking pan on the oven rack. Set to air fry at 375 F for 20 minutes.
5. Serve and enjoy.

Nutrition Info: Calories 99 Fat 7.5 g Carbohydrates 8.7 g Sugar 4.5 g Protein 1.5 g Cholesterol 0 mg

495. Rocky Road Squares

Servings: 16
Cooking Time: 15 Minutes
Ingredients:
- 3 oz. dark chocolate, chopped
- 1/2 cup butter
- 2 cups graham cracker crumbs
- 1 cup walnuts, chopped, divided
- 1 cup coconut, divided
- ½ cup mini semi-sweet chocolate chips
- 1 ½ cups mini marshmallows
- ½ can sweetened condensed milk

Directions:
1. Place rack in position Line an 8-inch square pan with parchment paper.
2. In a microwave safe bowl, place the chocolate and butter and microwave on high in 30 second intervals until melted and smooth, stirring after each interval.
3. Stir in crumbs, ½ cup nuts, and ½ cup coconut and mix well. Press evenly on the bottom of prepared pan.
4. Sprinkle the following over crust, in this order, marshmallows, coconut, remaining nuts, and chocolate chips. Drizzle milk evenly over the top.
5. Set oven to bake on 350°F for 25 minutes. After 5 minutes, add the pan to the oven and bake 15-20 minutes or until marshmallows are golden brown.
6. Remove from oven and let cool completely. Cover and refrigerate at least 1 hour before cutting and serving.

Nutrition Info: Calories 323, Total Fat 17g, Saturated Fat 7g, Total Carbs 36g, Net Carbs 34g, Protein 4g, Sugar 21g, Fiber 2g, Sodium 139mg, Potassium 203mg, Phosphorus 106mg

496. Moist Baked Donuts

Servings: 12
Cooking Time: 15 Minutes

Ingredients:
- 2 eggs
- 3/4 cup sugar
- 1/2 cup buttermilk
- 1/4 cup vegetable oil
- 1 cup all-purpose flour
- 1/2 tsp vanilla
- 1 tsp baking powder
- 1/2 tsp salt

Directions:
1. Fit the oven with the rack in position
2. Spray donut pan with cooking spray and set aside.
3. In a bowl, mix together oil, vanilla, baking powder, sugar, eggs, buttermilk, and salt until well combined.
4. Stir in flour and mix until smooth.
5. Pour batter into the prepared donut pan.
6. Set to bake at 350 F for 20 minutes. After 5 minutes place the donut pan in the preheated oven.
7. Serve and enjoy.

Nutrition Info: Calories 140 Fat 5.5 g Carbohydrates 21.2 g Sugar 13.1 g Protein 2.3 g Cholesterol 28 mg

497. Keto Mixed Berry Crumble Pots

Servings: 6
Cooking Time: 15 Minutes
Ingredients:
- 2 ounces unsweetened mixed berries
- 1/2 cup granulated swerve
- 2 tablespoons golden flaxseed meal
- 1/4 teaspoon ground star anise
- 1/2 teaspoon ground cinnamon
- 1 teaspoon xanthan gum
- 2/3 cup almond flour
- 1 cup powdered swerve
- 1/2 teaspoon baking powder
- 1/3 cup unsweetened coconut, finely shredded
- 1/2 stick butter, cut into small pieces

Directions:
1. Toss the mixed berries with the granulated swerve, golden flaxseed meal, star anise, cinnamon, and xanthan gum. Divide between six custard cups coated with cooking spray.
2. In a mixing dish, thoroughly combine the remaining ingredients. Sprinkle over the berry mixture.
3. Bake in the preheated Air Fryer at 330 degrees F for 35 minutes. Work in batches if needed.

Nutrition Info: 155 Calories; 13g Fat; 1g Carbs; 1g Protein; 8g Sugars; 6g Fiber

498. Corn And Black Bean Salsa

Servings: 4
Cooking Time: 10 Minutes
Ingredients:

- ½ (15-ounce / 425-g) can corn, drained and rinsed
- ½ (15-ounce / 425-g) can black beans, drained and rinsed
- ¼ cup chunky salsa
- 2 ounces (57 g) reduced-fat cream cheese, softened
- ¼ cup shredded reduced-fat Cheddar cheese
- ½ teaspoon paprika
- ½ teaspoon ground cumin
- Salt and freshly ground black pepper, to taste

Directions:
1. Combine the corn, black beans, salsa, cream cheese, Cheddar cheese, paprika, and cumin in a medium bowl. Sprinkle with salt and pepper and stir until well blended.
2. Pour the mixture into the baking pan.
3. Slide the baking pan into Rack Position 2, select Air Fry, set temperature to 325ºF (163ºC), and set time to 10 minutes.
4. When cooking is complete, the mixture should be heated through. Rest for 5 minutes and serve warm.

499. Delicious Banana Cake

Servings: 8
Cooking Time: 40 Minutes
Ingredients:
- 2 large eggs, beaten
- 1 tsp baking powder
- 1 1/2 cup sugar, granulated
- 1 tsp vanilla extract
- 1/2 cup butter
- 1 cup milk
- 2 cups all-purpose flour
- 2 bananas, mashed
- 1 tsp baking soda

Directions:
1. Fit the oven with the rack in position
2. In a mixing bowl, beat together sugar and butter until creamy. Add beaten eggs and mix well.
3. Add milk, vanilla extract, baking soda, baking powder, flour, and mashed bananas into the mixture and beat for 2 minutes. Mix well.
4. Pour batter into the greased baking dish.
5. Set to bake at 350 F for 45 minutes. After 5 minutes place the baking dish in the preheated oven.
6. Slices and serve.

Nutrition Info: Calories 418 Fat 13.8 g Carbohydrates 80 g Sugar 42.7 g Protein 6.2 g Cholesterol 80 mg

500. Nutella Banana Muffins

Servings: 12
Cooking Time: 25 Minutes
Ingredients:
- 1 2/3 cups plain flour
- 1 teaspoon baking soda
- 1 teaspoon baking powder
- 1 teaspoon ground cinnamon
- ¼ teaspoon salt
- 4 ripe bananas, peeled and mashed
- 2 eggs
- ½ cup brown sugar
- 1 teaspoon vanilla essence
- 3 tablespoons milk
- 1 tablespoon Nutella
- ¼ cup walnuts

Directions:
1. Grease 12 muffin molds. Set aside.
2. In a large bowl, sift together the flour, baking soda, baking powder, cinnamon, and salt.
3. In another bowl, mix together the remaining ingredients except walnuts.
4. Add the banana mixture into flour mixture and mix until just combined.
5. Fold in the walnuts.
6. Place the mixture into the prepared muffin molds.
7. Press "Power Button" of Air Fry Oven and turn the dial to select the "Air Fry" mode.
8. Press the Time button and again turn the dial to set the cooking time to 25 minutes.
9. Now push the Temp button and rotate the dial to set the temperature at 250 degrees F.
10. Press "Start/Pause" button to start.
11. When the unit beeps to show that it is preheated, open the lid.
12. Arrange the muffin molds in "Air Fry Basket" and insert in the oven.
13. Place the muffin molds onto a wire rack to cool for about 10 minutes.
14. Carefully, invert the muffins onto the wire rack to completely cool before serving.

Nutrition Info: Calories 227 Total Fat 6.6 g Saturated Fat 1.5 g Cholesterol 45 mg Sodium 221 mg Total Carbs 38.1 g Fiber 2.4 g Sugar 15.8 g Protein 5.2 g

501. Healthy Carrot Fries

Servings: 4
Cooking Time: 25 Minutes
Ingredients:
- 4 medium carrots, peel and cut into fries shape
- 1/2 tbsp paprika
- 1 1/2 tbsp olive oil
- 1/2 tsp salt

Directions:
1. Fit the oven with the rack in position
2. Add carrots, paprika, oil, and salt into the mixing bowl and toss well.
3. Transfer carrot fries in baking pan.
4. Set to bake at 450 F for 30 minutes. After 5 minutes place the baking pan in the preheated oven.

5. Serve and enjoy.
Nutrition Info: Calories 73 Fat 5.4 g Carbohydrates 6.5 g Sugar 3.1 g Protein 0.6 g Cholesterol 0 mg

502. Pumpkin Bread

Servings: 10
Cooking Time: 40 Minutes
Ingredients:
- 1 1/3 cups all-purpose flour
- 1 cup sugar
- ¾ teaspoon baking soda
- 1 teaspoon pumpkin pie spice
- 1/3 teaspoon ground cinnamon
- ¼ teaspoon salt
- 2 eggs
- ½ cup pumpkin puree
- 1/3 cup vegetable oil
- ¼ cup water

Directions:
1. In a bowl, mix together the flour, sugar, baking soda, spices and salt
2. In another large bowl, add the eggs, pumpkin, oil and water and beat until well combined.
3. In a large mixing bowl or stand mixer.
4. Add the flour mixture and mix until just combined.
5. Place the mixture into a lightly greased loaf pan.
6. With a piece of foil, cover the pan loosely.
7. Press "Power Button" of Air Fry Oven and turn the dial to select the "Air Bake" mode.
8. Press the Time button and again turn the dial to set the cooking time to 40 minutes.
9. Now push the Temp button and rotate the dial to set the temperature at 325 degrees F.
10. Press "Start/Pause" button to start.
11. When the unit beeps to show that it is preheated, open the lid.
12. Arrange the pan in "Air Fry Basket" and insert in the oven.
13. After 25 minutes of cooking, remove the foil.
14. Place the pan onto a wire rack to cool for about 10 minutes.
15. Carefully, invert the bread onto wire rack to cool completely before slicing.
16. Cut the bread into desired-sized slices and serve.
Nutrition Info: Calories 217 Total Fat 8.4 g Saturated Fat 1.4 g Cholesterol 33 mg Sodium 167 mg Total Carbs 34 g Fiber 0.9 g Sugar 20.5g Protein 3 g

503. Apricot Crumble With Blackberries

Servings: 4
Cooking Time: 30 Minutes
Ingredients:
- 2 ½ cups fresh apricots, de-stoned and cubed
- 1 cup fresh blackberries
- ½ cup sugar
- 2 tbsp lemon Juice
- 1 cup flour
- 5 tbsp butter

Directions:
1. Preheat Breville on Bake function to 360 F. Add the apricot cubes to a bowl and mix with lemon juice, 2 tbsp sugar, and blackberries. Scoop the mixture into a greased dish and spread it evenly.
2. In another bowl, mix flour and remaining sugar. Add 1 tbsp of cold water and butter and keep mixing until you have a crumbly mixture. Pour over the fruit mixture and cook for 20 minutes.

504. Chocolate Chip Waffles

Ingredients:
- Salt and Pepper to taste
- 3 tbsp. Butter
- 1 cup chocolate chips
- 3 cups cocoa powder
- 3 eggs
- 2 tsp. dried basil
- 2 tsp. dried parsley

Directions:
1. Preheat the air fryer to 250 Fahrenheit.
2. In a small bowl, mix the ingredients, except for the chocolate chips, together. Ensure that the mixture is smooth and well balanced. Take a waffle mold and grease it with butter. Add the batter to the mold and place it in the air fryer basket. Cook till both the sides have browned. Garnish with chips and serve.

505. Maple Pecan Pie

Servings: 4
Cooking Time: 1 Hr 10 Minutes
Ingredients:
- ¾ cup maple syrup
- 2 eggs
- ½ tsp salt
- ¼ tsp nutmeg
- ½ tsp cinnamon
- 2 tbsp almond butter
- 2 tbsp brown sugar
- ½ cup chopped pecans
- 1 tbsp butter, melted
- 1 8-inch pie dough
- ¾ tsp vanilla extract

Directions:
1. Preheat Breville on Toast function to 350 F. Coat the pecans with the melted butter. Toast them for 5 minutes. Place the pie crust into the baking pan and scatter the pecans over.
2. Whisk together all remaining ingredients in a bowl. Pour the maple mixture over the pecans. Set Breville to 320 F and press Start. Bake the pie for 25 minutes on Bake function.

506. Tasty Gingersnap Cookies

Servings: 8
Cooking Time: 10 Minutes
Ingredients:
- 1 egg
- 1/2 tsp ground cinnamon
- 1/2 tsp ground ginger
- 1 tsp baking powder
- 3/4 cup erythritol
- 1/2 tsp vanilla
- 1/8 tsp ground cloves
- 1/4 tsp ground nutmeg
- 2/4 cup butter, melted
- 1 1/2 cups almond flour
- Pinch of salt

Directions:
1. Fit the oven with the rack in position
2. In a mixing bowl, mix together all dry ingredients.
3. In another bowl, mix together all wet ingredients.
4. Add dry ingredients to the wet ingredients and mix until a dough-like mixture is formed.
5. Cover and place in the refrigerator for 30 minutes.
6. Make cookies from dough and place onto a parchment-lined baking pan.
7. Set to bake at 350 F for 15 minutes. After 5 minutes place the baking pan in the preheated oven.
8. Serve and enjoy.

Nutrition Info: Calories 142 Fat 14.7 g Carbohydrates 1.8 g Sugar 0.3 g Protein 2 g Cholesterol 51 mg

507. Sweet Cream Cheese Wontons

Servings: 16
Cooking Time: 5 Minutes
Ingredients:
- 1 egg mixed with a bit of water
- Wonton wrappers
- ½ C. powdered erythritol
- 8 ounces softened cream cheese
- Olive oil

Directions:
1. Preparing the Ingredients. Mix sweetener and cream cheese together.
2. Lay out 4 wontons at a time and cover with a dish towel to prevent drying out.
3. Place ½ of a teaspoon of cream cheese mixture into each wrapper.
4. Dip finger into egg/water mixture and fold diagonally to form a triangle. Seal edges well.
5. Repeat with remaining ingredients.
6. Air Frying. Place filled wontons into the air fryer oven and cook 5 minutes at 400 degrees, shaking halfway through cooking.

Nutrition Info: CALORIES: 303; FAT:3G; PROTEIN:0.5G; SUGAR:4G

508. Delicious Jalapeno Poppers

Servings: 10
Cooking Time: 7 Minutes
Ingredients:
- 10 jalapeno peppers, cut in half, remove seeds & membranes
- 1/2 cup cheddar cheese, shredded
- 4 oz cream cheese
- 1/4 tsp paprika
- 1 tsp ground cumin
- 1 tsp salt

Directions:
1. Fit the oven with the rack in position 2.
2. In a small bowl, mix together cream cheese, cheddar cheese, cumin, paprika, and salt.
3. Stuff cream cheese mixture into each jalapeno half.
4. Place stuffed jalapeno peppers in air fryer basket then place air fryer basket in baking pan.
5. Place a baking pan on the oven rack. Set to air fry at 350 F for 7 minutes.
6. Serve and enjoy.

Nutrition Info: Calories 69 Fat 6.1 g Carbohydrates 1.5 g Sugar 0.5 g Protein 2.5 g Cholesterol 18 mg

509. Yogurt Pumpkin Bread

Servings: 4
Cooking Time: 15 Minutes
Ingredients:
- 2 large eggs
- 8 tablespoons pumpkin puree
- 6 tablespoons banana flour
- 4 tablespoons honey
- 4 tablespoons plain Greek yogurt
- 2 tablespoons vanilla essence
- Pinch of ground nutmeg 6 tablespoons oats

Directions:
1. In a bowl, add in all the ingredients except oats and with a hand mixer, mix until smooth.
2. Add the oats and with a fork, mix well.
3. Grease and flour a loaf pan.
4. Place the mixture into the prepared loaf pan.
5. Press "Power Button" of Air Fry Oven and turn the dial to select the "Air Crisp" mode.
6. Press the Time button and again turn the dial to set the cooking time to 15 minutes.
7. Now push the Temp button and rotate the dial to set the temperature at 360 degrees F.
8. Press "Start/Pause" button to start.

9. When the unit beeps to show that it is preheated, open the lid.
10. Arrange the pan in "Air Fry Basket" and insert in the oven.
11. Carefully, invert the bread onto wire rack to cool completely before slicing.
12. Cut the bread into desired-sized slices and serve.
Nutrition Info: Calories 232 Total Fat 8.33 g Saturated Fat 1.5 g Cholesterol 94 mg Sodium 53 mg Total Carbs 29.3 g Fiber 2.8 g Sugar 20.5 g Protein 7.7 g

510. Garlic Edamame

Servings: 4
Cooking Time: 9 Minutes
Ingredients:
- 1 (16-ounce / 454-g) bag frozen edamame in pods
- 2 tablespoon olive oil, divided
- ½ teaspoon garlic salt
- ½ teaspoon salt
- ¼ teaspoon freshly ground black pepper
- ½ teaspoon red pepper flakes (optional)

Directions:
1. Place the edamame in a medium bowl and drizzle with 1 tablespoon of olive oil. Toss to coat well.
2. Stir together the garlic salt, salt, pepper, and red pepper flakes (if desired) in a small bowl. Pour the mixture into the bowl of edamame and toss until the edamame is fully coated.
3. Grease the air fryer basket with the remaining 1 tablespoon of olive oil.
4. Place the edamame in the greased basket.
5. Put the air fryer basket on the baking pan and slide into Rack Position 2, select Air Fry, set temperature to 375ºF (190ºC), and set time to 9 minutes.
6. Stir the edamame once halfway through the cooking time.
7. When cooking is complete, the edamame should be crisp. Remove from the oven to a plate and serve warm.

511. Pan-fried Bananas

Servings: 6
Cooking Time: 15 Minutes
Ingredients:
- 8 bananas
- 3 tbsp vegetable oil
- 3 tbsp cornflour
- 1 egg white
- ¾ cup breadcrumbs

Directions:
1. Preheat Breville on Toast function to 350 F. Combine oil and breadcrumbs in a bowl. Coat the bananas with the cornflour, brush with egg white, and dip in the breadcrumb mixture. Arrange on a lined baking sheet and press Start. Cook for 8-12 minutes.

512. Apple Cake

Servings: 12
Cooking Time: 45 Minutes
Ingredients:
- 2 cups apples, peeled and chopped
- 1/4 cup sugar
- 1/4 cup butter, melted
- 12 oz apple juice
- 3 cups all-purpose flour
- 3 tsp baking powder
- 1 1/2 tbsp ground cinnamon
- 1 tsp Salt

Directions:
1. Fit the oven with the rack in position
2. In a large bowl, mix together flour, salt, sugar, cinnamon, and baking powder.
3. Add melted butter and apple juice and mix until well combined.
4. Add apples and fold well.
5. Pour batter into the greased baking dish.
6. Set to bake at 350 F for 45 minutes. After 5 minutes place the baking dish in the preheated oven.
7. Serve and enjoy.
Nutrition Info: Calories 200 Fat 4 g Carbohydrates 38 g Sugar 11 g Protein 3 g Cholesterol 10 mg

513. Artichoke Cashews Spinach Dip

Servings: 10
Cooking Time: 20 Minutes
Ingredients:
- 28 oz can artichokes, drained and rinsed
- 1 small onion, diced
- 4 garlic cloves
- 1 1/2 cups cashews
- 1 tsp olive oil
- 4 cups fresh spinach
- 2 tbsp fresh lemon juice
- 1/4 cup nutritional yeast
- 1 1/2 cups milk
- 1 1/2 tsp salt

Directions:
1. Fit the oven with the rack in position 2.
2. Soak cashews in boiling water for 5 minutes. Drain well.
3. Heat oil in a pan over medium heat. Add onion and garlic and sauté for 2-3 minutes.
4. Remove pan from heat and set aside.
5. Add soaked cashews, milk, nutritional yeast, lemon juice, and salt into the blender and blend until smooth.

6. Add sautéed garlic onion, artichokes, and spinach and blend for few minutes until getting chunky texture.
7. Transfer blended mixture into the baking dish.
8. Set to bake at 425 F for 25 minutes. After 5 minutes place the baking dish in the preheated oven.
9. Serve and enjoy.

Nutrition Info: Calories 205 Fat 11.3 g Carbohydrates 21.4 g Sugar 3.9 g Protein 9 g Cholesterol 3 mg

514. Cheese And Leeks Dip

Servings: 6
Cooking Time: 15 Minutes
Ingredients:
- 2 spring onions; minced
- 4 leeks; sliced
- ¼ cup coconut cream
- 3 tbsp. coconut milk
- 2 tbsp. butter; melted
- Salt and white pepper to the taste

Directions:
1. In a pan that fits your air fryer, mix all the ingredients and whisk them well.
2. Introduce the pan in the fryer and cook at 390°F for 12 minutes. Divide into bowls and serve

Nutrition Info: Calories: 204; Fat: 12g; Fiber: 2g; Carbs: 4g; Protein: 14g

515. Tuna Melts With Scallions

Servings: 6
Cooking Time: 6 Minutes
Ingredients:
- 2 (5- to 6-ounce / 142- to 170-g) cans oil-packed tuna, drained
- 1 large scallion, chopped
- 1 small stalk celery, chopped
- ⅓ cup mayonnaise
- 1 tablespoon chopped fresh dill
- 1 tablespoon capers, drained
- ¼ teaspoon celery salt
- 12 slices cocktail rye bread
- 2 tablespoons butter, melted
- 6 slices sharp Cheddar cheese

Directions:
1. In a medium bowl, stir together the tuna, scallion, celery, mayonnaise, dill, capers and celery salt.
2. Brush one side of the bread slices with the butter. Arrange the bread slices in the baking pan, buttered-side down. Scoop a heaping tablespoon of the tuna mixture on each slice of bread, spreading it out evenly to the edges.
3. Cut the cheese slices to fit the dimensions of the bread and place a cheese slice on each piece.
4. Slide the baking pan into Rack Position 2, select Roast, set temperature to 375ºF (190ºC) and set time to 6 minutes.
5. After 4 minutes, remove from the oven and check the tuna melts. The tuna melts are done when the cheese has melted and the tuna is heated through. If needed, continue cooking.
6. When cooking is complete, remove from the oven. Use a spatula to transfer the tuna melts to a clean work surface and slice each one in half diagonally. Serve warm.

516. Vegetables Balls

Servings: 6
Cooking Time: 10 Minutes
Ingredients:
- 2 cups cauliflower florets
- 1 tsp paprika
- 1 tsp chives
- 2 tsp garlic
- 1 medium Parsnip
- 1 medium carrot
- 1 cup breadcrumbs
- 1/2 cup desiccated coconut
- 2 tsp oregano
- 1 tsp mixed spice
- 1/2 cup sweet potato
- Pepper
- Salt

Directions:
1. Fit the oven with the rack in position
2. Add all vegetables into the food processor and process until resemble breadcrumbs.
3. Add process vegetables into the mixing bowl.
4. Add all remaining ingredients into the bowl and mix well until combine.
5. Make small balls from the mixture and place in the air fryer basket then place an air fryer basket in the baking pan.
6. Place a baking pan on the oven rack. Set to air fry at 400 F for 10 minutes.
7. Serve and enjoy.

Nutrition Info: Calories 131 Fat 2.7 g Carbohydrates 23.6 g Sugar 4.5 g Protein 4 g Cholesterol 0 mg

517. Vanilla Lemon Cupcakes

Servings: 6
Cooking Time: 15 Minutes
Ingredients:
- 1 egg
- 1/2 cup milk
- 2 tbsp canola oil
- 1/4 tsp baking soda
- 3/4 tsp baking powder
- 1 tsp lemon zest, grated
- 1/2 cup sugar

- 1 cup flour
- 1/2 tsp vanilla
- 1/2 tsp salt

Directions:
1. Fit the oven with the rack in position
2. Line 12-cups muffin tin with cupcake liners and set aside.
3. In a bowl, whisk egg, vanilla, milk, oil, and sugar until creamy.
4. Add remaining ingredients and stir until just combined.
5. Pour batter into the prepared muffin tin.
6. Set to bake at 350 F for 20 minutes. After 5 minutes place muffin tin in the preheated oven.
7. Serve and enjoy.

Nutrition Info: Calories 200 Fat 6 g Carbohydrates 35 g Sugar 17 g Protein 3 g Cholesterol 30 mg

518. Almond Cookies With Dark Chocolate

Servings: 4
Cooking Time: 45 Minutes
Ingredients:
- 8 egg whites
- ½ tsp almond extract
- 1 ⅓ cups sugar
- ¼ tsp salt
- 2 tsp lemon juice
- 1 ½ tsp vanilla extract
- Melted dark chocolate to drizzle

Directions:
1. In a mixing bowl, add egg whites, salt, and lemon juice. Beat using an electric mixer until foamy.
2. Slowly add the sugar and continue beating until completely combined; add the almond and vanilla extracts. Beat until stiff and glossy peaks form.
3. Line a baking sheet with parchment paper. Fill a piping bag with the meringue mixture and pipe as many mounds on the baking sheet as you can leaving 2-inch spaces between each mound.
4. Place the baking sheet in the preheated Breville oven and press Start. Bake at 250 F for 5 minutes on Bake function. Reduce the temperature to 220 F and bake for 15 more minutes.
5. Then, reduce the temperature to 190 F and cook for 15 minutes. Remove the baking sheet and let the meringues cool for 2 hours. Drizzle with dark chocolate and serve.

519. Butter Cookies

Servings: 24
Cooking Time: 15 Minutes
Ingredients:
- 1 egg, lightly beaten
- 1 tsp vanilla
- 3/4 cup Swerve
- 1 1/4 cups almond flour

- 1 tsp baking powder
- 1 stick butter
- Pinch of salt

Directions:
1. Fit the oven with the rack in position
2. In a bowl, beat butter and sweetener until creamy.
3. In a separate bowl, mix together almond flour and baking powder.
4. Add egg and vanilla in butter mixture and beat until smooth.
5. Add dry ingredients to the wet ingredients and mix until well combined.
6. Wrap dough in plastic wrap and place in the fridge for 1 hour.
7. Make cookies from dough and place onto a parchment-lined baking pan.
8. Set to bake at 325 F for 20 minutes. After 5 minutes place the baking pan in the preheated oven.
9. Serve and enjoy.

Nutrition Info: Calories 46 Fat 4.7 g Carbohydrates 0.5 g Sugar 0.1 g Protein 0.6 g Cholesterol 17 mg

520. Buttermilk Biscuits

Ingredients:
- 4 tsp baking powder
- ¼ tsp baking soda
- ¼ tsp salt
- 4 Tbsp softened butter
- 1 cup all-purpose flour
- 1 cup whole wheat flour
- 2 Tbsp sugar
- 1¼ cups cold buttermilk

Directions:
1. Preheat oven to 400°F.
2. In a bowl, combine flours, sugar, baking powder, baking soda and salt.
3. Add softened butter and use your Oregano Fingers to work the butter into the flour until the mixture resembles coarse crumbs.
4. Stir in the buttermilk, forming a soft dough.
5. Turn the dough onto a floured surface and pat into a ¾ inch thick circle.
6. With a 2-inch biscuit cutter, cut out biscuits, gathering dough as needed to shape more biscuits.
7. Arrange biscuits in oven and bake until golden brown, about 12 minutes.

521. Crab Stuffed Mushrooms

Servings: 16
Cooking Time: 8 Minutes
Ingredients:
- 16 mushrooms, clean and chop stems
- 2 oz crab meat, chopped
- 8 oz cream cheese, softened
- 1/4 tsp chili powder

- 1/4 cup mozzarella cheese, shredded

Directions:
1. Fit the oven with the rack in position 2.
2. In a bowl, mix chopped stems, chili powder, cheese, crabmeat, and cream cheese.
3. Stuff cheese mixture in mushrooms and place in air fryer basket then place air fryer basket in baking pan.
4. Place a baking pan on the oven rack. Set to air fry at 370 F for 8 minutes.
5. Serve and enjoy.

Nutrition Info: Calories 59 Fat 5.1 g Carbohydrates 1.2 g Sugar 0.4 g Protein 2.2 g Cholesterol 18 mg

522. Peanut Butter Fudge Cake

Servings: 10
Cooking Time: 15 Minutes
Ingredients:
- 1 cup peanut butter
- 1 ¼ cups monk fruit
- 3 eggs
- 1 cup almond flour
- 1 teaspoon baking powder
- 1/4 teaspoon kosher salt
- 1 cup unsweetened bakers' chocolate, broken into chunks

Directions:
1. Start by preheating your Air Fryer to 350 degrees F. Now, spritz the sides and bottom of a baking pan with cooking spray.
2. In a mixing dish, thoroughly combine the peanut butter with the monk fruit until creamy. Next, fold in the egg and beat until fluffy.
3. After that, stir in the almond flour, baking powder, salt, and bakers'chocolate. Mix until everything is well combined.
4. Bake in the preheated Air Fryer for 20 to 22 minutes. Transfer to a wire rack to cool before slicing and serving.

Nutrition Info: 207 Calories; 11g Fat; 4g Carbs; 4g Protein; 1g Sugars; 4g Fiber

523. Mixed Berry Compote With Coconut Chips

Servings: 6
Cooking Time: 15 Minutes
Ingredients:
- 1 tablespoon butter
- 12 ounces mixed berries
- 1/3 cup granulated swerve
- 1/4 teaspoon grated nutmeg
- 1/4 teaspoon ground cloves
- 1/2 teaspoon ground cinnamon
- 1 teaspoon pure vanilla extract
- 1/2 cup coconut chips

Directions:
1. Start by preheating your Air Fryer to 330 degrees F. Grease a baking pan with butter.
2. Place all ingredients, except for the coconut chips, in a baking pan. Bake in the preheated Air Fryer for 20 minutes.
3. Serve in individual bowls, garnished with coconut chips.

Nutrition Info: 76 Calories; 3g Fat; 5g Carbs; 6g Protein; 1g Sugars; 1g Fiber

524. Chocolate Chip Pan Cookie

Servings: 4
Cooking Time: 15 Minutes
Ingredients:
- ½ cup blanched finely ground almond flour.
- 1 large egg.
- ¼ cup powdered erythritol
- 2 tbsp. unsalted butter; softened.
- 2 tbsp. low-carb, sugar-free chocolate chips
- ½ tsp. unflavored gelatin
- ½ tsp. baking powder.
- ½ tsp. vanilla extract.

Directions:
1. Take a large bowl, mix almond flour and erythritol. Stir in butter, egg and gelatin until combined.
2. Stir in baking powder and vanilla and then fold in chocolate chips
3. Pour batter into 6-inch round baking pan. Place pan into the air fryer basket.
4. Adjust the temperature to 300 Degrees F and set the timer for 7 minutes.
5. When fully cooked, the top will be golden brown and a toothpick inserted in center will come out clean. Let cool at least 10 minutes.

Nutrition Info: Calories: 188; Protein: 5.6g; Fiber: 2.0g; Fat: 15.7g; Carbs: 16.8g

525. Blueberry Pudding

Ingredients:
- 2 tbsp. custard powder
- 3 tbsp. powdered sugar
- 3 tbsp. unsalted butter
- 1 cup blueberry juice
- 2 cups milk

Directions:
1. Boil the milk and the sugar in a pan and add the custard powder followed by the blueberry juice and stir till you get a thick mixture.
2. Preheat the fryer to 300 Fahrenheit for five minutes. Place the dish in the basket and reduce the temperature to 250 Fahrenheit. Cook for ten minutes and set aside to cool.

526. Strawberry Tart

Ingredients:
- 2 cups sliced strawberries
- 1 cup fresh cream
- 3 tbsp. butter
- 1 ½ cup plain flour
- 3 tbsp. unsalted butter
- 2 tbsp. powdered sugar
- 2 cups cold water

Directions:
1. In a large bowl, mix the flour, cocoa powder, butter and sugar with your Oregano Fingers. The mixture should resemble breadcrumbs. Squeeze the dough using the cold milk and wrap it and leave it to cool for ten minutes. Roll the dough out into the pie and prick the sides of the pie.
2. Mix the ingredients for the filling in a bowl. Make sure that it is a little
3. thick. Preheat the fryer to 300 Fahrenheit for five minutes. You will need to place the tin in the basket and cover it. When the pastry has turned golden brown, you will need to remove the tin and let it cool. Cut into slices and serve with a dollop of cream.

527. Choco Lava Cakes

Servings: 4
Cooking Time: 20 Minutes
Ingredients:
- 3 ½ oz butter, melted
- 3 ½ tbsp sugar
- 1 ½ tbsp self-rising flour
- 3 ½ oz dark chocolate, melted
- 2 eggs

Directions:
1. Preheat Breville on Bake function to 375 F. Beat eggs and sugar until frothy. Stir in butter and chocolate; gently fold in the flour.
2. Divide the mixture between 4 buttered ramekins and press Start. Bake in the fryer for 10 minutes. Let cool for 2 minutes before turning the cakes upside down onto serving plates.

528. Chocolate Paradise Cake

Servings: 6
Cooking Time: 15 Minutes
Ingredients:
- 2 eggs, beaten
- 2/3 cup sour cream
- 1 cup almond flour
- 2/3 cup swerve
- 1/3 cup coconut oil, softened
- 1/4 cup cocoa powder
- 2 tablespoons chocolate chips, unsweetened
- 1 ½ teaspoons baking powder
- 1 teaspoon vanilla extract
- 1/2 teaspoon pure rum extract
- Chocolate Frosting:
- 1/2 cup butter, softened
- 1/4 cup cocoa powder
- 1 cup powdered swerve
- 2 tablespoons milk

Directions:
1. Mix all ingredients for the chocolate cake with a hand mixer on low speed. Scrape the batter into a cake pan.
2. Bake at 330 degrees F for 25 to 30 minutes. Transfer the cake to a wire rack
3. Meanwhile, whip the butter and cocoa until smooth. Stir in the powdered swerve. Slowly and gradually, pour in the milk until your frosting reaches desired consistency.
4. Whip until smooth and fluffy; then, frost the cooled cake. Place in your refrigerator for a couple of hours. Serve well chilled.

Nutrition Info: 433 Calories; 44g Fat; 8g Carbs; 5g Protein; 9g Sugars; 9g Fiber

529. Sweet Potato Croquettes

Servings: 6
Cooking Time: 55 Minutes
Ingredients:
- 2 cups cooked quinoa
- 1/4 cup parsley, chopped
- 1/4 cup flour
- 2 cups sweet potatoes, mashed
- 2 tsp Italian seasoning
- 1 garlic clove, minced
- 1/4 cup celery, diced
- 1/4 cup scallions, chopped
- Pepper
- Salt

Directions:
1. Fit the oven with the rack in position
2. Add all ingredients into the mixing bowl and mix until well combined.
3. Make 1-inch round croquettes from mixture and place in baking pan.
4. Set to bake at 375 F for 60 minutes. After 5 minutes place the baking pan in the preheated oven.
5. Serve and enjoy.

Nutrition Info: Calories 295 Fat 4.1 g Carbohydrates 55.2 g Sugar 0.6 g Protein 9.5 g Cholesterol 1 mg

530. Crispy Shrimps

Servings: 2
Cooking Time: 8 Minutes
Ingredients:
- 1 egg
- ¼ pound nacho chips, crushed
- 10 shrimps, peeled and deveined

- 1 tablespoon olive oil
- Salt and black pepper, to taste

Directions:
1. Preheat the Air fryer to 36F and grease an Air fryer basket.
2. Crack egg in a shallow dish and beat well.
3. Place the nacho chips in another shallow dish.
4. Season the shrimps with salt and black pepper, coat into egg and then roll into nacho chips.
5. Place the coated shrimps into the Air fryer basket and cook for about 8 minutes.
6. Dish out and serve warm.

Nutrition Info: Calories: 514, Fat: 25.8g, Carbohydrates: 36.9g, Sugar: 2.3g, Protein: 32.5g, Sodium: 648mg

531. Air Fryer Pepperoni Chips

Servings: 6
Cooking Time: 8 Minutes
Ingredients:
- 6 oz pepperoni slices

Directions:
1. Fit the oven with the rack in position 2.
2. Place pepperoni slices in an air fryer basket then place an air fryer basket in baking pan.
3. Place a baking pan on the rack. Set to air fry at 360 F for 8 minutes.
4. Serve and enjoy.

Nutrition Info: Calories 51 Fat 1 g Carbohydrates 2 g Sugar 0 g Protein 9.1 g Cholesterol 0 mg

532. Bread Pudding

Ingredients:
- 2 tbsp. custard powder
- 3 tbsp. powdered sugar
- 3 tbsp. unsalted butter
- 6 slices bread
- 2 cups milk

Directions:
1. Spread butter and jam on the slices of bread and cut them into the shapes you would like. Place them in a greased dish.
2. Boil the milk and the sugar in a pan and add the custard powder and stir till you get a thick mixture.
3. Preheat the fryer to 300 Fahrenheit for five minutes. Place the dish in the basket and reduce the temperature to 250 Fahrenheit. Cook for ten minutes and set aside to cool.

533. Coffee Chocolate Cake

Servings: 8
Cooking Time: 30 Minutes
Ingredients:
- Dry Ingredients:
- 1½ cups almond flour
- ½ cup coconut meal
- $^2/_3$ cup Swerve
- 1 teaspoon baking powder
- ¼ teaspoon salt
- Wet Ingredients:
- 1 egg
- 1 stick butter, melted
- ½ cup hot strongly brewed coffee
- Topping:
- ½ cup confectioner's Swerve
- ¼ cup coconut flour
- 3 tablespoons coconut oil
- 1 teaspoon ground cinnamon
- ½ teaspoon ground cardamom

Directions:
1. In a medium bowl, combine the almond flour, coconut meal, Swerve, baking powder, and salt.
2. In a large bowl, whisk the egg, melted butter, and coffee until smooth.
3. Add the dry mixture to the wet and stir until well incorporated. Transfer the batter to a greased baking pan.
4. Stir together all the ingredients for the topping in a small bowl. Spread the topping over the batter and smooth the top with a spatula.
5. Slide the baking pan into Rack Position 1, select Convection Bake, set temperature to 330ºF (166ºC), and set time to 30 minutes.
6. When cooking is complete, the cake should spring back when gently pressed with your fingers.
7. Rest for 10 minutes before serving.

534. Sweet Cinnamon Peaches

Servings: 4
Cooking Time: 10 Minutes
Ingredients:
- 2 tablespoons sugar
- ¼ teaspoon ground cinnamon
- 4 peaches, cut into wedges
- Cooking spray

Directions:
1. Spritz the air fryer basket with cooking spray.
2. In a large bowl, stir together the sugar and cinnamon. Add the peaches to the bowl and toss to coat evenly.
3. Spread the coated peaches in a single layer on the basket.
4. Put the air fryer basket on the baking pan and slide into Rack Position 2, select Air Fry, set temperature to 350ºF (180ºC) and set time to 10 minutes.
5. After 5 minutes, remove from the oven. Turn the peaches over. Lightly mist them with cooking spray. Return to the oven to continue cooking.

6. When cooking is complete, the peaches will be lightly browned and caramelized. Remove from the oven and let rest for 5 minutes before serving.

535. Lemon-raspberry Muffins

Servings: 6
Cooking Time: 15 Minutes
Ingredients:
- 2 cups almond flour
- ¾ cup Swerve
- 1¼ teaspoons baking powder
- 1/3 teaspoon ground allspice
- 1/3 teaspoon ground anise star
- ½ teaspoon grated lemon zest
- ¼ teaspoon salt
- 2 eggs
- 1 cup sour cream
- ½ cup coconut oil
- ½ cup raspberries

Directions:
1. Line a muffin pan with 6 paper liners.
2. In a mixing bowl, mix the almond flour, Swerve, baking powder, allspice, anise, lemon zest, and salt.
3. In another mixing bowl, beat the eggs, sour cream, and coconut oil until well mixed. Add the egg mixture to the flour mixture and stir to combine. Mix in the raspberries.
4. Scrape the batter into the prepared muffin cups, filling each about three-quarters full.
5. Put the muffin pan into Rack Position 1, select Convection Bake, set temperature to 345ºF (174ºC), and set time to 15 minutes.
6. When cooking is complete, the tops should be golden and a toothpick inserted in the middle should come out clean.
7. Allow the muffins to cool for 10 minutes in the muffin pan before removing and serving.

536. Coconut Broccoli Pop-corn

Servings: 4
Cooking Time: 6 Minutes
Ingredients:
- 2 cups broccoli florets
- 4 eggs yolks
- 2 cups coconut flour
- 1/4 cup butter, melted
- Pepper
- Salt

Directions:
1. Fit the oven with the rack in position 2.
2. In a bowl whisk egg yolks with melted butter, pepper, and salt. Add coconut flour and stir to combine.
3. Coat each broccoli floret with egg mixture and place in the air fryer basket then place an air fryer basket in the baking pan.
4. Place a baking pan on the oven rack. Set to air fry at 400 F for 6 minutes.
5. Serve and enjoy.
Nutrition Info: Calories 201 Fat 17.2 g Carbohydrates 7.7 g Sugar 1.4 g Protein 5.1 g Cholesterol 240 mg

537. Crumble With Blackberries & Apricots

Servings: 4
Cooking Time: 30 Minutes
Ingredients:
- 2 ½ cups fresh apricots, cubed
- 1 cup fresh blackberries
- ½ cup sugar
- 2 tbsp lemon Juice
- 1 cup flour
- 5 tbsp butter

Directions:
1. Preheat on Bake function to 390 F. Add apricots to a bowl and mix with lemon juice, 2 tbsp sugar, and blackberries. Spread the mixture onto the greased Air Fryer baking pan. In another bowl, mix flour and remaining sugar. Add 1 tbsp of cold water and butter and keep mixing until you have a crumbly mixture; top with crumb mixture. Cook for 20 minutes.

538. Raspberry-coco Desert

Servings: 12
Cooking Time: 20 Minutes
Ingredients:
- Vanilla bean, 1 tsp.
- Pulsed raspberries, 1 cup
- Coconut milk, 1 cup
- Desiccated coconut, 3 cup
- Coconut oil, ¼ cup
- Erythritol powder, 1/3 cup

Directions:
1. Preheat the air fryer for 5 minutes.
2. Combine all ingredients in a mixing bowl.
3. Pour into a greased baking dish.
4. Bake in the air fryer for 20 minutes at 37F.
Nutrition Info: Calories: 132 Carbs: 9.7g Fat: 9.7g Protein: 1.5g

539. Mozzarella Pepperoni Pizza Bites

Servings: 8
Cooking Time: 12 Minutes
Ingredients:

- 1 cup finely shredded Mozzarella cheese
- ½ cup chopped pepperoni
- ¼ cup Marinara sauce
- 1 (8-ounce / 227-g) can crescent roll dough
- All-purpose flour, for dusting

Directions:
1. In a small bowl, stir together the cheese, pepperoni and Marinara sauce.
2. Lay the dough on a lightly floured work surface. Separate it into 4 rectangles. Firmly pinch the perforations together and pat the dough pieces flat.
3. Divide the cheese mixture evenly between the rectangles and spread it out over the dough, leaving a ¼-inch border. Roll a rectangle up tightly, starting with the short end. Pinch the edge down to seal the roll. Repeat with the remaining rolls.
4. Slice the rolls into 4 or 5 even slices. Place the slices in the baking pan, leaving a few inches between each slice.
5. Slide the baking pan into Rack Position 2, select Roast, set temperature to 350ºF (180ºC) and set time to 12 minutes.
6. When cooking is complete, the rolls will be golden brown with crisp edges. Remove from the oven and serve hot.

540. Caramelized Fruit Kebabs

Servings: 4
Cooking Time: 4 Minutes
Ingredients:
- 2 peaches, peeled, pitted, and thickly sliced
- 3 plums, halved and pitted
- 3 nectarines, halved and pitted
- 1 tablespoon honey
- ½ teaspoon ground cinnamon
- ¼ teaspoon ground allspice
- Pinch cayenne pepper
- Special Equipment:
- 8 metal skewers

Directions:
1. Thread, alternating peaches, plums, and nectarines onto the metal skewers.
2. Thoroughly combine the honey, cinnamon, allspice, and cayenne in a small bowl. Brush generously the glaze over the fruit skewers.
3. Transfer the fruit skewers to the air fryer basket.
4. Put the air fryer basket on the baking pan and slide into Rack Position 2, select Air Fry, set temperature to 400ºF (205ºC), and set time to 4 minutes.
5. When cooking is complete, the fruit should be caramelized.
6. Remove the fruit skewers from the oven and let rest for 5 minutes before serving.

541. Ruderal Swiss Fondue

Ingredients:
- 1 cup dry white wine
- 1 Tbsp Kirshwasser
- 2 cups grated Emmen haler cheese
- 2 cups grated Gruyere cheese
- 2 Tbsp cornstarch
- Sliced apples and cubed bread, for serving

Directions:
1. In a bowl, mix the two cheeses and the cornstarch with a wooden spoon.
2. Pour the wine and kirshwasser into a 2-quart oven and bring to a gentle simmer over medium-low heat.
3. Add the cheese mixture to the liquid, a handful at a time, and stir until all the cheese is melted.
4. Serve fondue in a bowl over the fire. With a fondue fork, stab a slice of apple or a cube of bread and dip into the melted cheese.

542. Margherita Pizza

Servings: 4
Cooking Time: 18 Minutes
Ingredients:
- 1 whole-wheat pizza crust
- 1/2 cup mozzarella cheese, grated
- 1/2 cup can tomatoes
- 2 tbsp olive oil
- 3 Roma tomatoes, sliced
- 10 basil leaves

Directions:
1. Fit the oven with the rack in position
2. Roll out whole wheat pizza crust using a rolling pin. Make sure the crust is ½-inch thick.
3. Sprinkle olive oil on top of pizza crust.
4. Spread can tomatoes over pizza crust.
5. Arrange sliced tomatoes and basil on pizza crust. Sprinkle grated cheese on top.
6. Place pizza on top of the oven rack and set to bake at 425 F for 23 minutes.
7. Slice and serve.

Nutrition Info: Calories 126 Fat 7.9 g Carbohydrates 11.3 g Sugar 4.2 g Protein 3.6 g Cholesterol 2 mg

543. Cinnamon Fried Bananas

Servings: 2-3
Cooking Time: 10 Minutes
Ingredients:
- 1 C. panko breadcrumbs
- 3 tbsp. cinnamon
- ½ C. almond flour
- 3 egg whites
- 8 ripe bananas

- 3 tbsp. vegan coconut oil

Directions:
1. Preparing the Ingredients. Heat coconut oil and add breadcrumbs. Mix around 2-3 minutes until golden. Pour into bowl.
2. Peel and cut bananas in half. Roll each bananas half into flour, eggs, and crumb mixture.
3. Air Frying. Place into the air fryer oven. Cook 10 minutes at 280 degrees.
4. A great addition to a healthy banana split!

Nutrition Info: CALORIES: 219; FAT:10G; PROTEIN:3G; SUGAR:5G

OTHER FAVORITE RECIPES

544. Spinach And Chickpea Casserole

Servings: 4
Cooking Time: 21 To 22 Minutes
Ingredients:
- 2 tablespoons olive oil
- 2 garlic cloves, minced
- 1 tablespoon ginger, minced
- 1 onion, chopped
- 1 chili pepper, minced
- Salt and ground black pepper, to taste
- 1 pound (454 g) spinach
- 1 can coconut milk
- ½ cup dried tomatoes, chopped
- 1 (14-ounce / 397-g) can chickpeas, drained

Directions:
1. Heat the olive oil in a saucepan over medium heat. Sauté the garlic and ginger in the olive oil for 1 minute, or until fragrant.
2. Add the onion, chili pepper, salt and pepper to the saucepan. Sauté for 3 minutes.
3. Mix in the spinach and sauté for 3 to 4 minutes or until the vegetables become soft. Remove from heat.
4. Pour the vegetable mixture into the baking pan. Stir in coconut milk, dried tomatoes and chickpeas until well blended.
5. Slide the baking pan into Rack Position 1, select Convection Bake, set temperature to 370ºF (188ºC) and set time to 15 minutes.
6. When cooking is complete, transfer the casserole to a serving dish. Let cool for 5 minutes before serving.

545. Fast Cinnamon Toast

Servings: 6
Cooking Time: 5 Minutes
Ingredients:
- 1½ teaspoons cinnamon
- 1½ teaspoons vanilla extract
- ½ cup sugar
- 2 teaspoons ground black pepper
- 2 tablespoons melted coconut oil
- 12 slices whole wheat bread

Directions:
1. Combine all the ingredients, except for the bread, in a large bowl. Stir to mix well.
2. Dunk the bread in the bowl of mixture gently to coat and infuse well. Shake the excess off. Arrange the bread slices in the air fryer basket.
3. Put the air fryer basket on the baking pan and slide into Rack Position 2, select Air Fry, set temperature to 400ºF (205ºC) and set time to 5 minutes.
4. Flip the bread halfway through.
5. When cooking is complete, the bread should be golden brown.
6. Remove the bread slices from the oven and slice to serve.

546. Crispy Cheese Wafer

Servings: 2
Cooking Time: 5 Minutes
Ingredients:
- 1 cup shredded aged Manchego cheese
- 1 teaspoon all-purpose flour
- ½ teaspoon cumin seeds
- ¼ teaspoon cracked black pepper

Directions:
1. Line the air fryer basket with parchment paper.
2. Combine the cheese and flour in a bowl. Stir to mix well. Spread the mixture in the pan into a 4-inch round.
3. Combine the cumin and black pepper in a small bowl. Stir to mix well. Sprinkle the cumin mixture over the cheese round.
4. Put the air fryer basket on the baking pan and slide into Rack Position 2, select Air Fry, set temperature to 375ºF (190ºC) and set time to 5 minutes.
5. When cooked, the cheese will be lightly browned and frothy.
6. Use tongs to transfer the cheese wafer onto a plate and slice to serve.

547. Spicy Air Fried Old Bay Shrimp

Servings: 2 Cups
Cooking Time: 10 Minutes
Ingredients:
- ½ teaspoon Old Bay Seasoning
- 1 teaspoon ground cayenne pepper
- ½ teaspoon paprika
- 1 tablespoon olive oil
- ⅛ teaspoon salt
- ½ pound (227 g) shrimps, peeled and deveined
- Juice of half a lemon

Directions:
1. Combine the Old Bay Seasoning, cayenne pepper, paprika, olive oil, and salt in a large bowl, then add the shrimps and toss to coat well.
2. Put the shrimps in the air fryer basket.
3. Put the air fryer basket on the baking pan and slide into Rack Position 2, select Air Fry, set temperature to 390ºF (199ºC) and set time to 10 minutes.
4. Flip the shrimps halfway through the cooking time.
5. When cooking is complete, the shrimps should be opaque. Serve the shrimps with lemon juice on top.

548. Jewish Blintzes

Servings: 8 Blintzes
Cooking Time: 10 Minutes
Ingredients:
- 2 (7½-ounce / 213-g) packages farmer cheese, mashed
- ¼ cup cream cheese
- ¼ teaspoon vanilla extract
- ¼ cup granulated white sugar
- 8 egg roll wrappers
- 4 tablespoons butter, melted

Directions:
1. Combine the farmer cheese, cream cheese, vanilla extract, and sugar in a bowl. Stir to mix well.
2. Unfold the egg roll wrappers on a clean work surface, spread ¼ cup of the filling at the edge of each wrapper and leave a ½-inch edge uncovering.
3. Wet the edges of the wrappers with water and fold the uncovered edge over the filling. Fold the left and right sides in the center, then tuck the edge under the filling and fold to wrap the filling.
4. Brush the wrappers with melted butter, then arrange the wrappers in a single layer in the air fryer basket, seam side down. Leave a little space between each two wrappers.
5. Put the air fryer basket on the baking pan and slide into Rack Position 2, select Air Fry, set temperature to 375°F (190°C) and set time to 10 minutes.
6. When cooking is complete, the wrappers will be golden brown.
7. Serve immediately.

549. Crunchy And Beery Onion Rings

Servings: 2 To 4
Cooking Time: 16 Minutes
Ingredients:
- ⅔ cup all-purpose flour
- 1 teaspoon paprika
- ½ teaspoon baking soda
- 1 teaspoon salt
- ½ teaspoon freshly ground black pepper
- 1 egg, beaten
- ¾ cup beer
- 1½ cups bread crumbs
- 1 tablespoons olive oil
- 1 large Vidalia onion, peeled and sliced into ½-inch rings
- Cooking spray

Directions:
1. Spritz the air fryer basket with cooking spray.
2. Combine the flour, paprika, baking soda, salt, and ground black pepper in a bowl. Stir to mix well.
3. Combine the egg and beer in a separate bowl. Stir to mix well.
4. Make a well in the center of the flour mixture, then pour the egg mixture in the well. Stir to mix everything well.
5. Pour the bread crumbs and olive oil in a shallow plate. Stir to mix well.
6. Dredge the onion rings gently into the flour and egg mixture, then shake the excess off and put into the plate of bread crumbs. Flip to coat the both sides well. Arrange the onion rings in the basket.
7. Put the air fryer basket on the baking pan and slide into Rack Position 2, select Air Fry, set temperature to 360°F (182°C) and set time to 16 minutes.
8. Flip the rings and put the bottom rings to the top halfway through.
9. When cooked, the rings will be golden brown and crunchy. Remove from the oven and serve immediately.

550. Garlicky Spiralized Zucchini And Squash

Servings: 4
Cooking Time: 10 Minutes
Ingredients:
- 2 large zucchini, peeled and spiralized
- 2 large yellow summer squash, peeled and spiralized
- 1 tablespoon olive oil, divided
- ½ teaspoon kosher salt
- 1 garlic clove, whole
- 2 tablespoons fresh basil, chopped
- Cooking spray

Directions:
1. Spritz the air fryer basket with cooking spray.
2. Combine the zucchini and summer squash with 1 teaspoon of the olive oil and salt in a large bowl. Toss to coat well.
3. Transfer the zucchini and summer squash to the basket and add the garlic.
4. Put the air fryer basket on the baking pan and slide into Rack Position 2, select Air Fry, set temperature to 360°F (182°C) and set time to 10 minutes.
5. Stir the zucchini and summer squash halfway through the cooking time.
6. When cooked, the zucchini and summer squash will be tender and fragrant. Transfer the cooked zucchini and summer squash onto a plate and set aside.
7. Remove the garlic from the oven and allow to cool for 5 minutes. Mince the garlic and combine with remaining olive oil in a small bowl. Stir to mix well.
8. Drizzle the spiralized zucchini and summer squash with garlic oil and sprinkle with basil. Toss to serve.

551. Pastrami Casserole

Servings: 2
Cooking Time: 8 Minutes
Ingredients:
- 1 cup pastrami, sliced
- 1 bell pepper, chopped
- ¼ cup Greek yogurt
- 2 spring onions, chopped
- ½ cup Cheddar cheese, grated
- 4 eggs
- ¼ teaspoon ground black pepper
- Sea salt, to taste
- Cooking spray

Directions:
1. Spritz the baking pan with cooking spray.
2. Whisk together all the ingredients in a large bowl. Stir to mix well. Pour the mixture into the baking pan.
3. Slide the baking pan into Rack Position 1, select Convection Bake, set temperature to 330ºF (166ºC) and set time to 8 minutes.
4. When cooking is complete, the eggs should be set and the casserole edges should be lightly browned.
5. Remove from the oven and allow to cool for 10 minutes before serving.

552. Simple Air Fried Okra Chips

Servings: 6
Cooking Time: 16 Minutes
Ingredients:
- 2 pounds (907 g) fresh okra pods, cut into 1-inch pieces
- 2 tablespoons canola oil
- 1 teaspoon coarse sea salt

Directions:
1. Stir the oil and salt in a bowl to mix well. Add the okra and toss to coat well. Place the okra in the air fryer basket.
2. Put the air fryer basket on the baking pan and slide into Rack Position 2, select Air Fry, set temperature to 400ºF (205ºC) and set time to 16 minutes.
3. Flip the okra at least three times during cooking.
4. When cooked, the okra should be lightly browned. Remove from the oven and serve immediately.

553. Chocolate And Coconut Macaroons

Servings: 24 Macaroons
Cooking Time: 8 Minutes
Ingredients:
- 3 large egg whites, at room temperature
- ¼ teaspoon salt
- ¾ cup granulated white sugar
- 4½ tablespoons unsweetened cocoa powder
- 2¼ cups unsweetened shredded coconut

Directions:
1. Line the air fryer basket with parchment paper.
2. Whisk the egg whites with salt in a large bowl with a hand mixer on high speed until stiff peaks form.
3. Whisk in the sugar with the hand mixer on high speed until the mixture is thick. Mix in the cocoa powder and coconut.
4. Scoop 2 tablespoons of the mixture and shape the mixture in a ball. Repeat with remaining mixture to make 24 balls in total.
5. Arrange the balls in a single layer in the basket and leave a little space between each two balls.
6. Put the air fryer basket on the baking pan and slide into Rack Position 2, select Air Fry, set temperature to 375ºF (190ºC) and set time to 8 minutes.
7. When cooking is complete, the balls should be golden brown.
8. Serve immediately.

554. Taco Beef And Chile Casserole

Servings: 4
Cooking Time: 15 Minutes
Ingredients:
- 1 pound (454 g) 85% lean ground beef
- 1 tablespoon taco seasoning
- 1 (7-ounce / 198-g) can diced mild green chiles
- ½ cup milk
- 2 large eggs
- 1 cup shredded Mexican cheese blend
- 2 tablespoons all-purpose flour
- ½ teaspoon kosher salt
- Cooking spray

Directions:
1. Spritz the baking pan with cooking spray.
2. Toss the ground beef with taco seasoning in a large bowl to mix well. Pour the seasoned ground beef in the prepared baking pan.
3. Combing the remaining ingredients in a medium bowl. Whisk to mix well, then pour the mixture over the ground beef.
4. Slide the baking pan into Rack Position 1, select Convection Bake, set temperature to 350ºF (180ºC) and set time to 15 minutes.
5. When cooking is complete, a toothpick inserted in the center should come out clean.
6. Remove the casserole from the oven and allow to cool for 5 minutes, then slice to serve.

555. Pão De Queijo

Servings: 12 Balls
Cooking Time: 12 Minutes
Ingredients:
- 2 tablespoons butter, plus more for greasing

- ½ cup milk
- 1½ cups tapioca flour
- ½ teaspoon salt
- 1 large egg
- 2/3 cup finely grated aged Asiago cheese

Directions:
1. Put the butter in a saucepan and pour in the milk, heat over medium heat until the liquid boils. Keep stirring.
2. Turn off the heat and mix in the tapioca flour and salt to form a soft dough. Transfer the dough in a large bowl, then wrap the bowl in plastic and let sit for 15 minutes.
3. Break the egg in the bowl of dough and whisk with a hand mixer for 2 minutes or until a sanity dough forms. Fold the cheese in the dough. Cover the bowl in plastic again and let sit for 10 more minutes.
4. Grease the baking pan with butter.
5. Scoop 2 tablespoons of the dough into the baking pan. Repeat with the remaining dough to make dough 12 balls. Keep a little distance between each two balls.
6. Slide the baking pan into Rack Position 1, select Convection Bake, set temperature to 375ºF (190ºC) and set time to 12 minutes.
7. Flip the balls halfway through the cooking time.
8. When cooking is complete, the balls should be golden brown and fluffy.
9. Remove the balls from the oven and allow to cool for 5 minutes before serving.

556. Corn On The Cob With Mayonnaise

Servings: 4
Cooking Time: 10 Minutes
Ingredients:
- 2 tablespoons mayonnaise
- 2 teaspoons minced garlic
- ½ teaspoon sea salt
- 1 cup panko bread crumbs
- 4 (4-inch length) ears corn on the cob, husk and silk removed
- Cooking spray

Directions:
1. Spritz the air fryer basket with cooking spray.
2. Combine the mayonnaise, garlic, and salt in a bowl. Stir to mix well. Pour the panko on a plate.
3. Brush the corn on the cob with mayonnaise mixture, then roll the cob in the bread crumbs and press to coat well.
4. Transfer the corn on the cob in the basket and spritz with cooking spray.
5. Put the air fryer basket on the baking pan and slide into Rack Position 2, select Air Fry, set temperature to 400ºF (205ºC) and set time to 10 minutes.
6. Flip the corn on the cob at least three times during the cooking.
7. When cooked, the corn kernels on the cob should be almost browned. Remove from the oven and serve immediately.

557. Goat Cheese And Asparagus Frittata

Servings: 2 To 4
Cooking Time: 25 Minutes
Ingredients:
- 1 cup asparagus spears, cut into 1-inch pieces
- 1 teaspoon vegetable oil
- 1 tablespoon milk
- 6 eggs, beaten
- 2 ounces (57 g) goat cheese, crumbled
- 1 tablespoon minced chives, optional
- Kosher salt and pepper, to taste
- Add the asparagus spears to a small bowl and drizzle with the vegetable oil. Toss until well coated and transfer to the air fryer basket.

Directions:
1. Put the air fryer basket on the baking pan and slide into Rack Position 2, select Air Fry, set temperature to 400ºF (205ºC) and set time to 5 minutes.
2. Flip the asparagus halfway through.
3. When cooking is complete, the asparagus should be tender and slightly wilted.
4. Remove from the oven to the baking pan.
5. Stir together the milk and eggs in a medium bowl. Pour the mixture over the asparagus in the pan. Sprinkle with the goat cheese and the chives (if using) over the eggs. Season with salt and pepper.
6. Slide the baking pan into Rack Position 1, select Convection Bake, set temperature to 320ºF (160ºC) and set time to 20 minutes.
7. When cooking is complete, the top should be golden and the eggs should be set.
8. Transfer to a serving dish. Slice and serve.

558. Roasted Mushrooms

Servings: About 1½ Cups
Cooking Time: 30 Minutes
Ingredients:
- 1 pound (454 g) button or cremini mushrooms, washed, stems trimmed, and cut into quarters or thick slices
- ¼ cup water
- 1 teaspoon kosher salt or ½ teaspoon fine salt
- 3 tablespoons unsalted butter, cut into pieces, or extra-virgin olive oil

Directions:
1. Place a large piece of aluminum foil on the sheet pan. Place the mushroom pieces in the middle of the foil. Spread them out into an even layer. Pour the water over them, season with the salt, and add the butter. Wrap the mushrooms in the foil.

2. Select Roast, set the temperature to 325ºF (163ºC), and set the time for 15 minutes. Select Start to begin preheating.
3. Once the unit has preheated, place the pan in the oven.
4. After 15 minutes, remove the pan from the oven. Transfer the foil packet to a cutting board and carefully unwrap it. Pour the mushrooms and cooking liquid from the foil onto the sheet pan.
5. Select Roast, set the temperature to 350ºF (180ºC), and set the time for 15 minutes. Return the pan to the oven. Select Start to begin.
6. After about 10 minutes, remove the pan from the oven and stir the mushrooms. Return the pan to the oven and continue cooking for anywhere from 5 to 15 more minutes, or until the liquid is mostly gone and the mushrooms start to brown.
7. Serve immediately.

559. Easy Corn And Bell Pepper Casserole

Servings: 4
Cooking Time: 20 Minutes
Ingredients:
- 1 cup corn kernels
- ¼ cup bell pepper, finely chopped
- ½ cup low-fat milk
- 1 large egg, beaten
- ½ cup yellow cornmeal
- ½ cup all-purpose flour
- ½ teaspoon baking powder
- 2 tablespoons melted unsalted butter
- 1 tablespoon granulated sugar
- Pinch of cayenne pepper
- ¼ teaspoon kosher salt
- Cooking spray

Directions:
1. Spritz the baking pan with cooking spray.
2. Combine all the ingredients in a large bowl. Stir to mix well. Pour the mixture into the baking pan.
3. Slide the baking pan into Rack Position 1, select Convection Bake, set temperature to 330ºF (166ºC) and set time to 20 minutes.
4. When cooking is complete, the casserole should be lightly browned and set.
5. Remove from the oven and serve immediately.

560. Simple Cheesy Shrimps

Servings: 4 To 6
Cooking Time: 8 Minutes
Ingredients:
- ²⁄₃ cup grated Parmesan cheese
- 4 minced garlic cloves
- 1 teaspoon onion powder
- ½ teaspoon oregano
- 1 teaspoon basil
- 1 teaspoon ground black pepper
- 2 tablespoons olive oil
- 2 pounds (907 g) cooked large shrimps, peeled and deveined
- Lemon wedges, for topping
- Cooking spray

Directions:
1. Spritz the air fryer basket with cooking spray.
2. Combine all the ingredients, except for the shrimps, in a large bowl. Stir to mix well.
3. Dunk the shrimps in the mixture and toss to coat well. Shake the excess off. Arrange the shrimps in the basket.
4. Put the air fryer basket on the baking pan and slide into Rack Position 2, select Air Fry, set temperature to 350ºF (180ºC) and set time to 8 minutes.
5. Flip the shrimps halfway through the cooking time.
6. When cooking is complete, the shrimps should be opaque. Transfer the cooked shrimps onto a large plate and squeeze the lemon wedges over before serving.

561. Chicken Divan

Servings: 4
Cooking Time: 24 Minutes
Ingredients:
- 4 chicken breasts
- Salt and ground black pepper, to taste
- 1 head broccoli, cut into florets
- ½ cup cream of mushroom soup
- 1 cup shredded Cheddar cheese
- ½ cup croutons
- Cooking spray

Directions:
1. Spritz the air fryer basket with cooking spray.
2. Put the chicken breasts in the basket and sprinkle with salt and ground black pepper.
3. Put the air fryer basket on the baking pan and slide into Rack Position 2, select Air Fry, set temperature to 390ºF (199ºC) and set time to 14 minutes.
4. Flip the breasts halfway through the cooking time.
5. When cooking is complete, the breasts should be well browned and tender.
6. Remove the breasts from the oven and allow to cool for a few minutes on a plate, then cut the breasts into bite-size pieces.
7. Combine the chicken, broccoli, mushroom soup, and Cheddar cheese in a large bowl. Stir to mix well.
8. Spritz the baking pan with cooking spray. Pour the chicken mixture into the pan. Spread the croutons over the mixture.
9. Slide the baking pan into Rack Position 1, select Convection Bake, set time to 10 minutes.
10. When cooking is complete, the croutons should be lightly browned and the mixture should be set.

11. Remove from the oven and serve immediately.

562. Cheddar Jalapeño Cornbread

Servings: 8
Cooking Time: 20 Minutes
Ingredients:
- ²/₃ cup cornmeal
- ¹/₃ cup all-purpose flour
- ¾ teaspoon baking powder
- 2 tablespoons buttery spread, melted
- ½ teaspoon kosher salt
- 1 tablespoon granulated sugar
- ¾ cup whole milk
- 1 large egg, beaten
- 1 jalapeño pepper, thinly sliced
- ¹/₃ cup shredded sharp Cheddar cheese
- Cooking spray

Directions:
1. Spritz the baking pan with cooking spray.
2. Combine all the ingredients in a large bowl. Stir to mix well. Pour the mixture in the baking pan.
3. Slide the baking pan into Rack Position 1, select Convection Bake, set temperature to 300ºF (150ºC) and set time to 20 minutes.
4. When the cooking is complete, a toothpick inserted in the center of the bread should come out clean.
5. Remove the baking pan from the oven and allow the bread to cool for 5 minutes before slicing to serve.

563. Ritzy Chicken And Vegetable Casserole

Servings: 4
Cooking Time: 15 Minutes
Ingredients:
- 4 boneless and skinless chicken breasts, cut into cubes
- 2 carrots, sliced
- 1 yellow bell pepper, cut into strips
- 1 red bell pepper, cut into strips
- 15 ounces (425 g) broccoli florets
- 1 cup snow peas
- 1 scallion, sliced
- Cooking spray
- Sauce:
- 1 teaspoon Sriracha
- 3 tablespoons soy sauce
- 2 tablespoons oyster sauce
- 1 tablespoon rice wine vinegar
- 1 teaspoon cornstarch
- 1 tablespoon grated ginger
- 2 garlic cloves, minced
- 1 teaspoon sesame oil
- 1 tablespoon brown sugar

Directions:
1. Spritz the baking pan with cooking spray.
2. Combine the chicken, carrot, and bell peppers in a large bowl. Stir to mix well.
3. Combine the ingredients for the sauce in a separate bowl. Stir to mix well.
4. Pour the chicken mixture into the baking pan, then pour the sauce over. Stir to coat well.
5. Slide the baking pan into Rack Position 1, select Convection Bake, set temperature to 370ºF (188ºC) and set time to 13 minutes.
6. Add the broccoli and snow peas to the pan halfway through.
7. When cooking is complete, the vegetables should be tender.
8. Remove from the oven and sprinkle with sliced scallion before serving.

564. Shrimp With Sriracha And Worcestershire Sauce

Servings: 4
Cooking Time: 10 Minutes
Ingredients:
- 1 tablespoon Sriracha sauce
- 1 teaspoon Worcestershire sauce
- 2 tablespoons sweet chili sauce
- ¾ cup mayonnaise
- 1 egg, beaten
- 1 cup panko bread crumbs
- 1 pound (454 g) raw shrimp, shelled and deveined, rinsed and drained
- Lime wedges, for serving
- Cooking spray

Directions:
1. Spritz the air fryer basket with cooking spray.
2. Combine the Sriracha sauce, Worcestershire sauce, chili sauce, and mayo in a bowl. Stir to mix well. Reserve ¹/₃ cup of the mixture as the dipping sauce.
3. Combine the remaining sauce mixture with the beaten egg. Stir to mix well. Put the panko in a separate bowl.
4. Dredge the shrimp in the sauce mixture first, then into the panko. Roll the shrimp to coat well. Shake the excess off.
5. Place the shrimp in the basket, then spritz with cooking spray.
6. Put the air fryer basket on the baking pan and slide into Rack Position 2, select Air Fry, set temperature to 360ºF (182ºC) and set time to 10 minutes.
7. Flip the shrimp halfway through the cooking time.
8. When cooking is complete, the shrimp should be opaque.
9. Remove the shrimp from the oven and serve with reserve sauce mixture and squeeze the lime wedges over.

565. Asian Dipping Sauce

Servings: About 1 Cup
Cooking Time: 0 Minutes
Ingredients:
- ¼ cup rice vinegar
- ¼ cup hoisin sauce
- ¼ cup low-sodium chicken or vegetable stock
- 3 tablespoons soy sauce
- 1 tablespoon minced or grated ginger
- 1 tablespoon minced or pressed garlic
- 1 teaspoon chili-garlic sauce or sriracha (or more to taste)

Directions:
1. Stir together all the ingredients in a small bowl, or place in a jar with a tight-fitting lid and shake until well mixed.
2. Use immediately.

566. Golden Nuggets

Servings: 20 Nuggets
Cooking Time: 4 Minutes
Ingredients:
- 1 cup all-purpose flour, plus more for dusting
- 1 teaspoon baking powder
- ½ teaspoon butter, at room temperature, plus more for brushing
- ¼ teaspoon salt
- ¼ cup water
- ⅛ teaspoon onion powder
- ¼ teaspoon garlic powder
- ⅛ teaspoon seasoning salt
- Cooking spray

Directions:
1. Line the air fryer basket with parchment paper.
2. Mix the flour, baking powder, butter, and salt in a large bowl. Stir to mix well. Gradually whisk in the water until a sanity dough forms.
3. Put the dough on a lightly floured work surface, then roll it out into a ½-inch thick rectangle with a rolling pin.
4. Cut the dough into about twenty 1- or 2-inch squares, then arrange the squares in a single layer in the basket. Spritz with cooking spray.
5. Combine onion powder, garlic powder, and seasoning salt in a small bowl. Stir to mix well, then sprinkle the squares with the powder mixture.
6. Put the air fryer basket on the baking pan and slide into Rack Position 2, select Air Fry, set temperature to 370ºF (188ºC) and set time to 4 minutes.
7. Flip the squares halfway through the cooking time.
8. When cooked, the dough squares should be golden brown.
9. Remove the golden nuggets from the oven and brush with more butter immediately. Serve warm.

567. Baked Cherry Tomatoes With Basil

Servings: 2
Cooking Time: 5 Minutes
Ingredients:
- 2 cups cherry tomatoes
- 1 clove garlic, thinly sliced
- 1 teaspoon olive oil
- ⅛ teaspoon kosher salt
- 1 tablespoon freshly chopped basil, for topping
- Cooking spray

Directions:
1. Spritz the baking pan with cooking spray and set aside.
2. In a large bowl, toss together the cherry tomatoes, sliced garlic, olive oil, and kosher salt. Spread the mixture in an even layer in the prepared pan.
3. Slide the baking pan into Rack Position 1, select Convection Bake, set temperature to 360ºF (182ºC) and set time to 5 minutes.
4. When cooking is complete, the tomatoes should be the soft and wilted.
5. Transfer to a bowl and rest for 5 minutes. Top with the chopped basil and serve warm.

568. Classic Churros

Servings: 12 Churros
Cooking Time: 10 Minutes
Ingredients:
- 4 tablespoons butter
- ¼ teaspoon salt
- ½ cup water
- ½ cup all-purpose flour
- 2 large eggs
- 2 teaspoons ground cinnamon
- ¼ cup granulated white sugar
- Cooking spray

Directions:
1. Put the butter, salt, and water in a saucepan. Bring to a boil until the butter is melted on high heat. Keep stirring.
2. Reduce the heat to medium and fold in the flour to form a dough. Keep cooking and stirring until the dough is dried out and coat the pan with a crust.
3. Turn off the heat and scrape the dough in a large bowl. Allow to cool for 15 minutes.
4. Break and whisk the eggs into the dough with a hand mixer until the dough is sanity and firm enough to shape.
5. Scoop up 1 tablespoon of the dough and roll it into a ½-inch-diameter and 2-inch-long cylinder. Repeat with remaining dough to make 12 cylinders in total.
6. Combine the cinnamon and sugar in a large bowl and dunk the cylinders into the cinnamon mix to coat.
7. Arrange the cylinders on a plate and refrigerate for 20 minutes.

8. Spritz the air fryer basket with cooking spray. Place the cylinders in the basket and spritz with cooking spray.
9. Put the air fryer basket on the baking pan and slide into Rack Position 2, select Air Fry, set temperature to 375ºF (190ºC) and set time to 10 minutes.
10. Flip the cylinders halfway through the cooking time.
11. When cooked, the cylinders should be golden brown and fluffy.
12. Serve immediately.

569. Oven Grits

Servings: About 4 Cups
Cooking Time: 1 Hour 5 Minutes
Ingredients:
- 1 cup grits or polenta (not instant or quick cook)
- 2 cups chicken or vegetable stock
- 2 cups milk
- 2 tablespoons unsalted butter, cut into 4 pieces
- 1 teaspoon kosher salt or ½ teaspoon fine salt

Directions:
1. Add the grits to the baking pan. Stir in the stock, milk, butter, and salt.
2. Select Bake, set the temperature to 325ºF (163ºC), and set the time for 1 hour and 5 minutes. Select Start to begin preheating.
3. Once the unit has preheated, place the pan in the oven.
4. After 15 minutes, remove the pan from the oven and stir the polenta. Return the pan to the oven and continue cooking.
5. After 30 minutes, remove the pan again and stir the polenta again. Return the pan to the oven and continue cooking for 15 to 20 minutes, or until the polenta is soft and creamy and the liquid is absorbed.
6. When done, remove the pan from the oven.
7. Serve immediately.

570. Enchilada Sauce

Servings: 2 Cups
Cooking Time: 0 Minutes
Ingredients:
- 3 large ancho chiles, stems and seeds removed, torn into pieces
- 1½ cups very hot water
- 2 garlic cloves, peeled and lightly smashed
- 2 tablespoons wine vinegar
- 1½ teaspoons sugar
- ½ teaspoon dried oregano
- ½ teaspoon ground cumin
- 2 teaspoons kosher salt or 1 teaspoon fine salt

Directions:
1. Mix together the chile pieces and hot water in a bowl and let stand for 10 to 15 minutes.
2. Pour the chiles and water into a blender jar. Fold in the garlic, vinegar, sugar, oregano, cumin, and salt and blend until smooth.
3. Use immediately.

571. Citrus Avocado Wedge Fries

Servings: 12 Fries
Cooking Time: 8 Minutes
Ingredients:
- 1 cup all-purpose flour
- 3 tablespoons lime juice
- ¾ cup orange juice
- 1¼ cups plain dried bread crumbs
- 1 cup yellow cornmeal
- 1½ tablespoons chile powder
- 2 large Hass avocados, peeled, pitted, and cut into wedges
- Coarse sea salt, to taste
- Cooking spray

Directions:
1. Spritz the air fryer basket with cooking spray.
2. Pour the flour in a bowl. Mix the lime juice with orange juice in a second bowl. Combine the bread crumbs, cornmeal, and chile powder in a third bowl.
3. Dip the avocado wedges in the bowl of flour to coat well, then dredge the wedges into the bowl of juice mixture, and then dunk the wedges in the bread crumbs mixture. Shake the excess off.
4. Arrange the coated avocado wedges in a single layer in the basket. Spritz with cooking spray.
5. Put the air fryer basket on the baking pan and slide into Rack Position 2, select Air Fry, set temperature to 400ºF (205ºC) and set time to 8 minutes.
6. Stir the avocado wedges and sprinkle with salt halfway through the cooking time.
7. When cooking is complete, the avocado wedges should be tender and crispy.
8. Serve immediately.

572. Simple Baked Green Beans

Servings: 2 Cups
Cooking Time: 10 Minutes
Ingredients:
- ½ teaspoon lemon pepper
- 2 teaspoons granulated garlic
- ½ teaspoon salt
- 1 tablespoon olive oil
- 2 cups fresh green beans, trimmed and snapped in half

Directions:
1. Combine the lemon pepper, garlic, salt, and olive oil in a bowl. Stir to mix well.
2. Add the green beans to the bowl of mixture and toss to coat well.
3. Arrange the green beans in the the baking pan.

4. Slide the baking pan into Rack Position 1, select Convection Bake, set temperature to 370ºF (188ºC) and set time to 10 minutes.
5. Stir the green beans halfway through the cooking time.
6. When cooking is complete, the green beans will be tender and crispy. Remove from the oven and serve immediately.

573. Chocolate Buttermilk Cake

Servings: 8
Cooking Time: 20 Minutes
Ingredients:
- 1 cup all-purpose flour
- $2/3$ cup granulated white sugar
- ¼ cup unsweetened cocoa powder
- ¾ teaspoon baking soda
- ¼ teaspoon salt
- $2/3$ cup buttermilk
- 2 tablespoons plus 2 teaspoons vegetable oil
- 1 teaspoon vanilla extract
- Cooking spray

Directions:
1. Spritz the baking pan with cooking spray.
2. Combine the flour, cocoa powder, baking soda, sugar, and salt in a large bowl. Stir to mix well.
3. Mix in the buttermilk, vanilla, and vegetable oil. Keep stirring until it forms a grainy and thick dough.
4. Scrape the chocolate batter from the bowl and transfer to the pan, level the batter in an even layer with a spatula.
5. Slide the baking pan into Rack Position 1, select Convection Bake, set temperature to 325ºF (163ºC) and set time to 20 minutes.
6. After 15 minutes, remove the pan from the oven. Check the doneness. Return the pan to the oven and continue cooking.
7. When done, a toothpick inserted in the center should come out clean.
8. Invert the cake on a cooling rack and allow to cool for 15 minutes before slicing to serve.

574. Air Fried Crispy Brussels Sprouts

Servings: 4
Cooking Time: 20 Minutes
Ingredients:
- ¼ teaspoon salt
- ⅛ teaspoon ground black pepper
- 1 tablespoon extra-virgin olive oil
- 1 pound (454 g) Brussels sprouts, trimmed and halved
- Lemon wedges, for garnish

Directions:
1. Combine the salt, black pepper, and olive oil in a large bowl. Stir to mix well.
2. Add the Brussels sprouts to the bowl of mixture and toss to coat well. Arrange the Brussels sprouts in the air fryer basket.
3. Put the air fryer basket on the baking pan and slide into Rack Position 2, select Air Fry, set temperature to 350ºF (180ºC) and set time to 20 minutes.
4. Stir the Brussels sprouts two times during cooking.
5. When cooked, the Brussels sprouts will be lightly browned and wilted. Transfer the cooked Brussels sprouts to a large plate and squeeze the lemon wedges on top to serve.

575. Dehydrated Bananas With Coconut Sprnikles

Ingredients:
- 5 very ripe bananas, peeled
- 1 cup shredded coconut

Directions:
1. Place coconut in a large shallow dish. Cut Press banana wedges in the coconut and organize in one layer on the dehydrating basket.
2. Hours Put basket in rack place 4 and then press START.
3. Dehydrate for 26 hours or until peanuts are Dry to the touch but still garnish with a sweet, intense banana taste.
4. Let bananas cool completely before storing in an Airtight container for up to 5 months.

576. Sumptuous Vegetable Frittata

Servings: 2
Cooking Time: 20 Minutes
Ingredients:
- 4 eggs
- $1/3$ cup milk
- 2 teaspoons olive oil
- 1 large zucchini, sliced
- 2 asparagus, sliced thinly
- $1/3$ cup sliced mushrooms
- 1 cup baby spinach
- 1 small red onion, sliced
- $1/3$ cup crumbled feta cheese
- $1/3$ cup grated Cheddar cheese
- ¼ cup chopped chives
- Salt and ground black pepper, to taste

Directions:
1. Line the baking pan with parchment paper.
2. Whisk together the eggs, milk, salt, and ground black pepper in a large bowl. Set aside.
3. Heat the olive oil in a nonstick skillet over medium heat until shimmering.
4. Add the zucchini, asparagus, mushrooms, spinach, and onion to the skillet and sauté for 5 minutes or until tender.

5. Pour the sautéed vegetables into the prepared baking pan, then spread the egg mixture over and scatter with cheeses.
6. Slide the baking pan into Rack Position 1, select Convection Bake, set temperature to 380ºF (193ºC) and set time to 15 minutes.
7. Stir the mixture halfway through.
8. When cooking is complete, the egg should be set and the edges should be lightly browned.
9. Remove the frittata from the oven and sprinkle with chives before serving.

577. Buttery Knots With Parsley

Servings: 8 Knots
Cooking Time: 5 Minutes
Ingredients:
- 1 teaspoon dried parsley
- ¼ cup melted butter
- 2 teaspoons garlic powder

Directions:
1. 1 (11-ounce / 312-g) tube refrigerated French bread dough, cut into 8 slices
2. Combine the parsley, butter, and garlic powder in a bowl. Stir to mix well.
3. Place the French bread dough slices on a clean work surface, then roll each slice into a 6-inch long rope. Tie the ropes into knots and arrange them on a plate.
4. Transfer the knots into the baking pan. Brush the knots with butter mixture.
5. Put the air fryer basket on the baking pan and slide into Rack Position 2, select Air Fry, set temperature to 350ºF (180ºC) and set time to 5 minutes.
6. Flip the knots halfway through the cooking time.
7. When done, the knots should be golden brown. Remove from the oven and serve immediately.

578. Creamy Pork Gratin

Servings: 4
Cooking Time: 21 Minutes
Ingredients:
- 2 tablespoons olive oil
- 2 pounds (907 g) pork tenderloin, cut into serving-size pieces
- 1 teaspoon dried marjoram
- ¼ teaspoon chili powder
- 1 teaspoon coarse sea salt
- ½ teaspoon freshly ground black pepper
- 1 cup Ricotta cheese
- 1½ cups chicken broth
- 1 tablespoon mustard
- Cooking spray

Directions:
1. Spritz the baking pan with cooking spray.
2. Heat the olive oil in a nonstick skillet over medium-high heat until shimmering.
3. Add the pork and sauté for 6 minutes or until lightly browned.
4. Transfer the pork to the prepared baking pan and sprinkle with marjoram, chili powder, salt, and ground black pepper.
5. Combine the remaining ingredients in a large bowl. Stir to mix well. Pour the mixture over the pork in the pan.
6. Slide the baking pan into Rack Position 1, select Convection Bake, set temperature to 350ºF (180ºC) and set time to 15 minutes.
7. Stir the mixture halfway through.
8. When cooking is complete, the mixture should be frothy and the cheese should be melted.
9. Serve immediately.

579. Caesar Salad Dressing

Servings: About ⅔ Cup
Cooking Time: 0 Minutes
Ingredients:
- ½ cup extra-virgin olive oil
- 2 tablespoons freshly squeezed lemon juice
- 1 teaspoon anchovy paste
- ¼ teaspoon kosher salt or ⅛ teaspoon fine salt
- ¼ teaspoon minced or pressed garlic
- 1 egg, beaten
- Add all the ingredients to a tall, narrow container.

Directions:
1. Purée the mixture with an immersion blender until smooth.
2. Use immediately.

580. Sweet Cinnamon Chickpeas

Servings: 2
Cooking Time: 10 Minutes
Ingredients:
- 1 tablespoon cinnamon
- 1 tablespoon sugar
- 1 cup chickpeas, soaked in water overnight, rinsed and drained

Directions:
1. Combine the cinnamon and sugar in a bowl. Stir to mix well.
2. Add the chickpeas to the bowl, then toss to coat well.
3. Pour the chickpeas in the air fryer basket.
4. Put the air fryer basket on the baking pan and slide into Rack Position 2, select Air Fry, set temperature to 390ºF (199ºC) and set time to 10 minutes.
5. Stir the chickpeas three times during cooking.

6. When cooked, the chickpeas should be golden brown and crispy. Remove from the oven and serve immediately.

581. Cauliflower And Pumpkin Casserole

Servings: 6
Cooking Time: 50 Minutes
Ingredients:
- 1 cup chicken broth
- 2 cups cauliflower florets
- 1 cup canned pumpkin purée
- ¼ cup heavy cream
- 1 teaspoon vanilla extract
- 2 large eggs, beaten
- ⅓ cup unsalted butter, melted, plus more for greasing the pan
- ¼ cup sugar
- 1 teaspoon fine sea salt
- Chopped fresh parsley leaves, for garnish
- TOPPING:
- ½ cup blanched almond flour
- 1 cup chopped pecans
- ⅓ cup unsalted butter, melted
- ½ cup sugar

Directions:
1. Pour the chicken broth in the baking pan, then add the cauliflower.
2. Slide the baking pan into Rack Position 1, select Convection Bake, set temperature to 350ºF (180ºC) and set time to 20 minutes.
3. When cooking is complete, the cauliflower should be soft.
4. Meanwhile, combine the ingredients for the topping in a large bowl. Stir to mix well.
5. Pat the cauliflower dry with paper towels, then place in a food processor and pulse with pumpkin purée, heavy cream, vanilla extract, eggs, butter, sugar, and salt until smooth.
6. Clean the baking pan and grease with more butter, then pour the purée mixture in the pan. Spread the topping over the mixture.
7. Put the baking pan back to the oven. Select Bake and set time to 30 minutes.
8. When baking is complete, the topping of the casserole should be lightly browned.
9. Remove the casserole from the oven and serve with fresh parsley on top.

582. Potato Chips With Lemony Cream Dip

Servings: 2 To 4
Cooking Time: 15 Minutes
Ingredients:
- 2 large russet potatoes, sliced into ⅛-inch slices, rinsed
- Sea salt and freshly ground black pepper, to taste
- Cooking spray
- Lemony Cream Dip:
- ½ cup sour cream
- ¼ teaspoon lemon juice
- 2 scallions, white part only, minced
- 1 tablespoon olive oil
- ¼ teaspoon salt
- Freshly ground black pepper, to taste

Directions:
1. Soak the potato slices in water for 10 minutes, then pat dry with paper towels.
2. Transfer the potato slices in the air fryer basket. Spritz the slices with cooking spray.
3. Put the air fryer basket on the baking pan and slide into Rack Position 2, select Air Fry, set temperature to 300ºF (150ºC) and set time to 15 minutes.
4. Stir the potato slices three times during cooking. Sprinkle with salt and ground black pepper in the last minute.
5. Meanwhile, combine the ingredients for the dip in a small bowl. Stir to mix well.
6. When cooking is complete, the potato slices will be crispy and golden brown. Remove from the oven and serve the potato chips immediately with the dip.

583. Parmesan Cauliflower Fritters

Servings: 6
Cooking Time: 8 Minutes
Ingredients:
- 2 cups cooked cauliflower
- 1 cup panko bread crumbs
- 1 large egg, beaten
- ½ cup grated Parmesan cheese
- 1 tablespoon chopped fresh chives Spritz the air fryer basket with cooking spray
- Cooking spray.

Directions:
1. Put the cauliflower, panko bread crumbs, egg, Parmesan, and chives in a food processor, then pulse to lightly mash and combine the mixture until chunky and thick.
2. Shape the mixture into 6 flat patties, then arrange them in the basket and spritz with cooking spray.
3. Put the air fryer basket on the baking pan and slide into Rack Position 2, select Air Fry, set temperature to 390ºF (199ºC) and set time to 8 minutes.
4. Flip the patties halfway through the cooking time.
5. When done, the patties should be crispy and golden brown. Remove from the oven and serve immediately.

584. Simple Air Fried Edamame

Servings: 6
Cooking Time: 7 Minutes
Ingredients:
- 1½ pounds (680 g) unshelled edamame
- 2 tablespoons olive oil
- 1 teaspoon sea salt

Directions:
1. Place the edamame in a large bowl, then drizzle with olive oil. Toss to coat well. Transfer the edamame to the air fryer basket.
2. Put the air fryer basket on the baking pan and slide into Rack Position 2, select Air Fry, set temperature to 400ºF (205ºC) and set time to 7 minutes.
3. Stir the edamame at least three times during cooking.
4. When done, the edamame will be tender and warmed through.
5. Transfer the cooked edamame onto a plate and sprinkle with salt. Toss to combine well and set aside for 3 minutes to infuse before serving.

585. Crunchy Green Tomatoes Slices

Servings: 12 Slices
Cooking Time: 8 Minutes
Ingredients:
- ½ cup all-purpose flour
- 1 egg
- ½ cup buttermilk
- 1 cup cornmeal
- 1 cup panko
- 2 green tomatoes, cut into ¼-inch-thick slices, patted dry
- ½ teaspoon salt
- ½ teaspoon ground black pepper
- Cooking spray

Directions:
1. Spritz a baking sheet with cooking spray.
2. Pour the flour in a bowl. Whisk the egg and buttermilk in a second bowl. Combine the cornmeal and panko in a third bowl.
3. Dredge the tomato slices in the bowl of flour first, then into the egg mixture, and then dunk the slices into the cornmeal mixture. Shake the excess off.
4. Transfer the well-coated tomato slices in the baking sheet and sprinkle with salt and ground black pepper. Spritz the tomato slices with cooking spray.
5. Put the air fryer basket on the baking pan and slide into Rack Position 2, select Air Fry, set temperature to 400ºF (205ºC) and set time to 8 minutes.
6. Flip the slices halfway through the cooking time.
7. When cooking is complete, the tomato slices should be crispy and lightly browned. Remove the baking sheet from the oven.
8. Serve immediately.

586. Sumptuous Beef And Bean Chili Casserole

Servings: 4
Cooking Time: 31 Minutes
Ingredients:
- 1 tablespoon olive oil
- ½ cup finely chopped bell pepper
- ½ cup chopped celery
- 1 onion, chopped
- 2 garlic cloves, minced
- 1 pound (454 g) ground beef
- 1 can diced tomatoes
- ½ teaspoon parsley
- ½ tablespoon chili powder
- 1 teaspoon chopped cilantro
- 1½ cups vegetable broth
- 1 (8-ounce / 227-g) can cannellini beans
- Salt and ground black pepper, to taste

Directions:
1. Heat the olive oil in a nonstick skillet over medium heat until shimmering.
2. Add the bell pepper, celery, onion, and garlic to the skillet and sauté for 5 minutes or until the onion is translucent.
3. Add the ground beef and sauté for an additional 6 minutes or until lightly browned.
4. Mix in the tomatoes, parsley, chili powder, cilantro and vegetable broth, then cook for 10 more minutes. Stir constantly.
5. Pour them in the baking pan, then mix in the beans and sprinkle with salt and ground black pepper.
6. Slide the baking pan into Rack Position 1, select Convection Bake, set temperature to 350ºF (180ºC) and set time to 10 minutes.
7. When cooking is complete, the vegetables should be tender and the beef should be well browned.
8. Remove from the oven and serve immediately.

587. Classic Worcestershire Poutine

Servings: 2
Cooking Time: 33 Minutes
Ingredients:
- 2 russet potatoes, scrubbed and cut into ½-inch sticks
- 2 teaspoons vegetable oil
- 2 tablespoons butter
- ¼ onion, minced
- ¼ teaspoon dried thyme
- 1 clove garlic, smashed
- 3 tablespoons all-purpose flour
- 1 teaspoon tomato paste
- 1½ cups beef stock
- 2 teaspoons Worcestershire sauce

- Salt and freshly ground black pepper, to taste
- ²/₃ cup chopped string cheese

Directions:
1. Bring a pot of water to a boil, then put in the potato sticks and blanch for 4 minutes.
2. Drain the potato sticks and rinse under running cold water, then pat dry with paper towels.
3. Transfer the sticks in a large bowl and drizzle with vegetable oil. Toss to coat well. Place the potato sticks in the air fryer basket.
4. Put the air fryer basket on the baking pan and slide into Rack Position 2, select Air Fry, set temperature to 400ºF (205ºC) and set time to 25 minutes.
5. Stir the potato sticks at least three times during cooking.
6. Meanwhile, make the gravy: Heat the butter in a saucepan over medium heat until melted.
7. Add the onion, thyme, and garlic and sauté for 5 minutes or until the onion is translucent.
8. Add the flour and sauté for an additional 2 minutes. Pour in the tomato paste and beef stock and cook for 1 more minute or until lightly thickened.
9. Drizzle the gravy with Worcestershire sauce and sprinkle with salt and ground black pepper. Reduce the heat to low to keep the gravy warm until ready to serve.
10. When done, the sticks should be golden brown. Remove from the oven. Transfer the fried potato sticks onto a plate, then sprinkle with salt and ground black pepper. Scatter with string cheese and pour the gravy over. Serve warm.

588. Butternut Squash With Hazelnuts

Servings: 3 Cups
Cooking Time: 23 Minutes
Ingredients:
- 2 tablespoons whole hazelnuts
- 3 cups butternut squash, peeled, deseeded and cubed
- ¼ teaspoon kosher salt
- ¼ teaspoon freshly ground black pepper
- 2 teaspoons olive oil
- Cooking spray

Directions:
1. Spritz the air fryer basket with cooking spray. Spread the hazelnuts in the pan.
2. Put the air fryer basket on the baking pan and slide into Rack Position 2, select Air Fry, set temperature to 300ºF (150ºC) and set time to 3 minutes.
3. When done, the hazelnuts should be soft. Remove from the oven. Chopped the hazelnuts roughly and transfer to a small bowl. Set aside.
4. Put the butternut squash in a large bowl, then sprinkle with salt and pepper and drizzle with olive oil. Toss to coat well. Transfer the squash to the lightly greased basket.
5. Put the air fryer basket on the baking pan and slide into Rack Position 2, select Air Fry, set temperature to 360ºF (182ºC) and set time to 20 minutes.
6. Flip the squash halfway through the cooking time.
7. When cooking is complete, the squash will be soft. Transfer the squash to a plate and sprinkle with the chopped hazelnuts before serving.

589. Salty Tortilla Chips

Servings: 4
Cooking Time: 10 Minutes
Ingredients:
- 4 six-inch corn tortillas, cut in half and slice into thirds
- 1 tablespoon canola oil
- ¼ teaspoon kosher salt
- Cooking spray

Directions:
1. Spritz the air fryer basket with cooking spray.
2. On a clean work surface, brush the tortilla chips with canola oil, then transfer the chips to the basket.
3. Put the air fryer basket on the baking pan and slide into Rack Position 2, select Air Fry, set temperature to 360ºF (182ºC) and set time to 10 minutes.
4. Flip the chips and sprinkle with salt halfway through the cooking time.
5. When cooked, the chips will be crunchy and lightly browned. Transfer the chips to a plate lined with paper towels. Serve immediately.

590. Herbed Cheddar Frittata

Servings: 4
Cooking Time: 20 Minutes
Ingredients:
- ½ cup shredded Cheddar cheese
- ½ cup half-and-half
- 4 large eggs
- 2 tablespoons chopped scallion greens
- 2 tablespoons chopped fresh parsley
- ½ teaspoon kosher salt
- ½ teaspoon ground black pepper
- Cooking spray

Directions:
1. Spritz the baking pan with cooking spray.
2. Whisk together all the ingredients in a large bowl, then pour the mixture into the prepared baking pan.
3. Slide the baking pan into Rack Position 1, select Convection Bake, set temperature to 300ºF (150ºC) and set time to 20 minutes.
4. Stir the mixture halfway through.

5. When cooking is complete, the eggs should be set.
6. Serve immediately.

591. Fried Dill Pickles With Buttermilk Dressing

Servings: 6 To 8
Cooking Time: 8 Minutes
Ingredients:
- Buttermilk Dressing:
- ¼ cup buttermilk
- ¼ cup chopped scallions
- ¾ cup mayonnaise
- ½ cup sour cream
- ½ teaspoon cayenne pepper
- ½ teaspoon onion powder
- ½ teaspoon garlic powder
- 1 tablespoon chopped chives
- 2 tablespoons chopped fresh dill
- Kosher salt and ground black pepper, to taste
- Fried Dill Pickles:
- ¾ cup all-purpose flour
- 1 (2-pound / 907-g) jar kosher dill pickles, cut into 4 spears, drained
- 2½ cups panko bread crumbs
- 2 eggs, beaten with 2 tablespoons water
- Kosher salt and ground black pepper, to taste
- Cooking spray

Directions:
1. Combine the ingredients for the dressing in a bowl. Stir to mix well.
2. Wrap the bowl in plastic and refrigerate for 30 minutes or until ready to serve.
3. Pour the flour in a bowl and sprinkle with salt and ground black pepper. Stir to mix well. Put the bread crumbs in a separate bowl. Pour the beaten eggs in a third bowl.
4. Dredge the pickle spears in the flour, then into the eggs, and then into the panko to coat well. Shake the excess off.
5. Arrange the pickle spears in a single layer in the air fryer basket and spritz with cooking spray.
6. Put the air fryer basket on the baking pan and slide into Rack Position 2, select Air Fry, set temperature to 400ºF (205ºC) and set time to 8 minutes.
7. Flip the pickle spears halfway through the cooking time.
8. When cooking is complete, remove from the oven.
9. Serve the pickle spears with buttermilk dressing.

592. Golden Salmon And Carrot Croquettes

Servings: 6
Cooking Time: 10 Minutes
Ingredients:
- 2 egg whites
- 1 cup almond flour
- 1 cup panko bread crumbs
- 1 pound (454 g) chopped salmon fillet
- ⅔ cup grated carrots
- 2 tablespoons minced garlic cloves
- ½ cup chopped onion
- 2 tablespoons chopped chives
- Cooking spray

Directions:
1. Spritz the air fryer basket with cooking spray.
2. Whisk the egg whites in a bowl. Put the flour in a second bowl. Pour the bread crumbs in a third bowl. Set aside.
3. Combine the salmon, carrots, garlic, onion, and chives in a large bowl. Stir to mix well.
4. Form the mixture into balls with your hands. Dredge the balls into the flour, then egg, and then bread crumbs to coat well.
5. Arrange the salmon balls on the basket and spritz with cooking spray.
6. Put the air fryer basket on the baking pan and slide into Rack Position 2, select Air Fry, set temperature to 350ºF (180ºC) and set time to 10 minutes.
7. Flip the salmon balls halfway through cooking.
8. When cooking is complete, the salmon balls will be crispy and browned. Remove from the oven and serve immediately.

593. Cinnamon Rolls With Cream Glaze

Servings: 8
Cooking Time: 5 Minutes
Ingredients:
- 1 pound (454 g) frozen bread dough, thawed
- 2 tablespoons melted butter
- 1½ tablespoons cinnamon
- ¾ cup brown sugar
- Cooking spray
- Cream Glaze:
- 4 ounces (113 g) softened cream cheese
- ½ teaspoon vanilla extract
- 2 tablespoons melted butter
- 1¼ cups powdered erythritol

Directions:
1. Place the bread dough on a clean work surface, then roll the dough out into a rectangle with a rolling pin.
2. Brush the top of the dough with melted butter and leave 1-inch edges uncovered.

3. Combine the cinnamon and sugar in a small bowl, then sprinkle the dough with the cinnamon mixture.
4. Roll the dough over tightly, then cut the dough log into 8 portions. Wrap the portions in plastic, better separately, and let sit to rise for 1 or 2 hours.
5. Meanwhile, combine the ingredients for the glaze in a separate small bowl. Stir to mix well.
6. Spritz the air fryer basket with cooking spray. Transfer the risen rolls to the basket.
7. Put the air fryer basket on the baking pan and slide into Rack Position 2, select Air Fry, set temperature to 350ºF (180ºC) and set time to 5 minutes.
8. Flip the rolls halfway through the cooking time.
9. When cooking is complete, the rolls will be golden brown.
10. Serve the rolls with the glaze.

594.Banana Cake

Servings: 8
Cooking Time: 20 Minutes
Ingredients:
- 1 cup plus 1 tablespoon all-purpose flour
- ¼ teaspoon baking soda
- ¾ teaspoon baking powder
- ¼ teaspoon salt
- 9½ tablespoons granulated white sugar
- 5 tablespoons butter, at room temperature
- 2½ small ripe bananas, peeled
- 2 large eggs
- 5 tablespoons buttermilk
- 1 teaspoon vanilla extract
- Cooking spray

Directions:
1. Spritz the baking pan with cooking spray.
2. Combine the flour, baking soda, baking powder, and salt in a large bowl. Stir to mix well.
3. Beat the sugar and butter in a separate bowl with a hand mixer on medium speed for 3 minutes.
4. Beat in the bananas, eggs, buttermilk, and vanilla extract into the sugar and butter mix with a hand mixer.
5. Pour in the flour mixture and whip with hand mixer until sanity and smooth.
6. Scrape the batter into the pan and level the batter with a spatula.
7. Slide the baking pan into Rack Position 1, select Convection Bake, set temperature to 325ºF (163ºC) and set time to 20 minutes.
8. After 15 minutes, remove the pan from the oven. Check the doneness. Return the pan to the oven and continue cooking.
9. When done, a toothpick inserted in the center should come out clean.
10. Invert the cake on a cooling rack and allow to cool for 15 minutes before slicing to serve.

595.Sausage And Colorful Peppers Casserole

Servings: 6
Cooking Time: 25 Minutes
Ingredients:
- 1 pound (454 g) minced breakfast sausage
- 1 yellow pepper, diced
- 1 red pepper, diced
- 1 green pepper, diced
- 1 sweet onion, diced
- 2 cups Cheddar cheese, shredded
- 6 eggs
- Salt and freshly ground black pepper, to taste
- Fresh parsley, for garnish

Directions:
1. Cook the sausage in a nonstick skillet over medium heat for 10 minutes or until well browned. Stir constantly.
2. When the cooking is finished, transfer the cooked sausage to the baking pan and add the peppers and onion. Scatter with Cheddar cheese.
3. Whisk the eggs with salt and ground black pepper in a large bowl, then pour the mixture into the baking pan.
4. Slide the baking pan into Rack Position 1, select Convection Bake, set temperature to 360ºF (182ºC) and set time to 15 minutes.
5. When cooking is complete, the egg should be set and the edges of the casserole should be lightly browned.
6. Remove from the oven and top with fresh parsley before serving.

596.Southwest Corn And Bell Pepper Roast

Servings: 4
Cooking Time: 10 Minutes
Ingredients:
- Corn:
- 1½ cups thawed frozen corn kernels
- 1 cup mixed diced bell peppers
- 1 jalapeño, diced
- 1 cup diced yellow onion
- ½ teaspoon ancho chile powder
- 1 tablespoon fresh lemon juice
- 1 teaspoon ground cumin
- ½ teaspoon kosher salt
- Cooking spray
- For Serving:
- ¼ cup feta cheese

- ¼ cup chopped fresh cilantro
- 1 tablespoon fresh lemon juice

Directions:
1. Spritz the air fryer basket with cooking spray.
2. Combine the ingredients for the corn in a large bowl. Stir to mix well.
3. Pour the mixture into the basket.
4. Put the air fryer basket on the baking pan and slide into Rack Position 2, select Air Fry, set temperature to 375ºF (190ºC) and set time to 10 minutes.
5. Stir the mixture halfway through the cooking time.
6. When done, the corn and bell peppers should be soft.
7. Transfer them onto a large plate, then spread with feta cheese and cilantro. Drizzle with lemon juice and serve.

597. Shrimp Spinach Frittata

Servings: 4
Cooking Time: 14 Minutes
Ingredients:
- 4 whole eggs
- 1 teaspoon dried basil
- ½ cup shrimp, cooked and chopped
- ½ cup baby spinach
- ½ cup rice, cooked
- ½ cup Monterey Jack cheese, grated
- Salt, to taste
- Cooking spray

Directions:
1. Spritz the baking pan with cooking spray.
2. Whisk the eggs with basil and salt in a large bowl until bubbly, then mix in the shrimp, spinach, rice, and cheese.
3. Pour the mixture into the baking pan.
4. Slide the baking pan into Rack Position 1, select Convection Bake, set temperature to 360ºF (182ºC) and set time to 14 minutes.
5. Stir the mixture halfway through.
6. When cooking is complete, the eggs should be set and the frittata should be golden brown.
7. Slice to serve.

598. Simple Butter Cake

Servings: 8
Cooking Time: 20 Minutes
Ingredients:
- 1 cup all-purpose flour
- 1¼ teaspoons baking powder
- ¼ teaspoon salt
- ½ cup plus 1½ tablespoons granulated white sugar
- 9½ tablespoons butter, at room temperature
- 2 large eggs
- 1 large egg yolk
- 2½ tablespoons milk
- 1 teaspoon vanilla extract
- Cooking spray

Directions:
1. Spritz the baking pan with cooking spray.
2. Combine the flour, baking powder, and salt in a large bowl. Stir to mix well.
3. Whip the sugar and butter in a separate bowl with a hand mixer on medium speed for 3 minutes.
4. Whip the eggs, egg yolk, milk, and vanilla extract into the sugar and butter mix with a hand mixer.
5. Pour in the flour mixture and whip with hand mixer until sanity and smooth.
6. Scrape the batter into the baking pan and level the batter with a spatula.
7. Slide the baking pan into Rack Position 1, select Convection Bake, set temperature to 325ºF (163ºC) and set time to 20 minutes.
8. After 15 minutes, remove the pan from the oven. Check the doneness. Return the pan to the oven and continue cooking.
9. When done, a toothpick inserted in the center should come out clean.
10. Invert the cake on a cooling rack and allow to cool for 15 minutes before slicing to serve.

599. Air Fried Blistered Tomatoes

Servings: 4 To 6
Cooking Time: 10 Minutes
Ingredients:
- 2 pounds (907 g) cherry tomatoes
- 2 tablespoons olive oil
- 2 teaspoons balsamic vinegar
- ½ teaspoon salt
- ½ teaspoon ground black pepper

Directions:
1. Toss the cherry tomatoes with olive oil in a large bowl to coat well. Pour the tomatoes in the baking pan.
2. Put the air fryer basket on the baking pan and slide into Rack Position 2, select Air Fry, set temperature to 400ºF (205ºC) and set time to 10 minutes.
3. Stir the tomatoes halfway through the cooking time.
4. When cooking is complete, the tomatoes will be blistered and lightly wilted.
5. Transfer the blistered tomatoes to a large bowl and toss with balsamic vinegar, salt, and black pepper before serving.

600. Lemony And Garlicky Asparagus

Servings: 10 Spears
Cooking Time: 10 Minutes

Ingredients:
- 10 spears asparagus (about ½ pound / 227 g in total), snap the ends off
- 1 tablespoon lemon juice
- 2 teaspoons minced garlic
- ½ teaspoon salt
- ¼ teaspoon ground black pepper
- Cooking spray

Directions:
1. Line the air fryer basket with parchment paper.
2. Put the asparagus spears in a large bowl. Drizzle with lemon juice and sprinkle with minced garlic, salt, and ground black pepper. Toss to coat well.
3. Transfer the asparagus to the basket and spritz with cooking spray.
4. Put the air fryer basket on the baking pan and slide into Rack Position 2, select Air Fry, set temperature to 400ºF (205ºC) and set time to 10 minutes.
5. Flip the asparagus halfway through cooking.
6. When cooked, the asparagus should be wilted and soft. Remove from the oven and serve immediately.

CPSIA information can be obtained
at www.ICGtesting.com
Printed in the USA
LVHW101546300321
682970LV00006B/350